Essentials of
Clinical
Diagnosis

Ninth Edition

Sunil K Sen

MBBS (cal, FRCP (Edin), FICP, FIAMS, FIMSA, FICC, FACC

Hony. Professor of Cardiology, Medical College, Calcutta (1977-1987)
Fellow Emeritus, American College of Cardiology
Emeritus Adviser, Royal College of Physicians of Edinburgh, UK
Overseas Adviser, Royal College of Physicians of Edinburgh
UK (1986-98)
Dr BC Roy National Award—1989
President, Association of Physicians of India, WB (1988-90)
President, Cardiological Society of India (1979-81)
International Man of the Year (1993-94) IBC Cambridge. England
Rajiv Gandhi Memorial Award (1996)

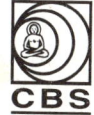

CBS

CBS Publishers & Distributors Pvt Ltd

New Delhi • Bengaluru • Chennai • Kochi • Kolkata • Mumbai
Hyderabad • Nagpur • Patna • Pune • Vijayawada

Disclaimer
Science and technology are constantly changing fields. New research and experience broaden the scope of information and knowledge. The author has tried his best in giving information available to him while preparing the material for this book. Although, all efforts have been made to ensure optimum accuracy of the material, yet it is quite possible some errors might have been left uncorrected. The publisher, printer and the author will not be held responsible for any inadvertent errors, omission or inaccuracies.

Essentials of
Clinical Diagnosis
Ninth Edition

ISBN: 978-93-85915-22-2

Copyright © Mrs Manju Sen

CBS Reprint: 2016 2019
Ninth Edition: 2011

All rights reserved. No part of this book may be reproduced or transmitted in any form or by any means, electronic or mechanical, including photocopying, recording, or any information storage and retrieval system without permission, in writing, from the author and the publisher.

Published by Satish Kumar Jain and produced by Varun Jain for

CBS Publishers & Distributors Pvt Ltd
4819/XI Prahlad Street, 24 Ansari Road, Daryaganj, New Delhi 110 002, India.
Ph: 23289259, 23266861, 23266867   Website: www.cbspd.com
Fax: 011-23243014   e-mail: delhi@cbspd.com; cbspubs@airtelmail.in.
Corporate Office: 204 FIE, Industrial Area, Patparganj, Delhi 110 092
Ph: 4934 4934   Fax: 4934 4935   e-mail: publishing@cbspd.com;
publicity@cbspd.com

Branches

- **Bengaluru:** Seema House 2975, 17th Cross, K.R. Road, Banasankari 2nd Stage, Bengaluru 560 070, Karnataka
  Ph: +91-80-26771678/79   Fax: +91-80-26771680   e-mail: bangalore@cbspd.com
- **Chennai:** 7, Subbaraya Street, Shenoy Nagar, Chennai 600 030, Tamil Nadu
  Ph: +91-44-26680620, 26681266   Fax: +91-44-42032115   e-mail: chennai@cbspd.com
- **Kochi:** Ashana House, No. 39/1904, AM Thomas Road, Valanjambalam, Ernakulam 682 018, Kochi, Kerala
  Ph: +91-484-4059061-65   Fax: +91-484-4059065   e-mail: kochi@cbspd.com
- **Kolkata:** 6/B, Ground Floor, Rameswar Shaw Road, Kolkata-700 014, West Bengal
  Ph: +91-33-22891126, 22891127, 22891128   e-mail: kolkata@cbspd.com
- **Mumbai:** 83-C, Dr E Moses Road, Worli, Mumbai-400018, Maharashtra
  Ph: +91-22-24902340/41   Fax: +91-22-24902342   e-mail: mumbai@cbspd.com

Representatives

- **Hyderabad** 0-9885175004
- **Patna** 0-9334159340
- **Vijayawada** 0-9000660880
- **Nagpur** 0-9021734563
- **Pune** 0-9623451994

Printed at Swastik Packaging, Patparganj, Delhi 92

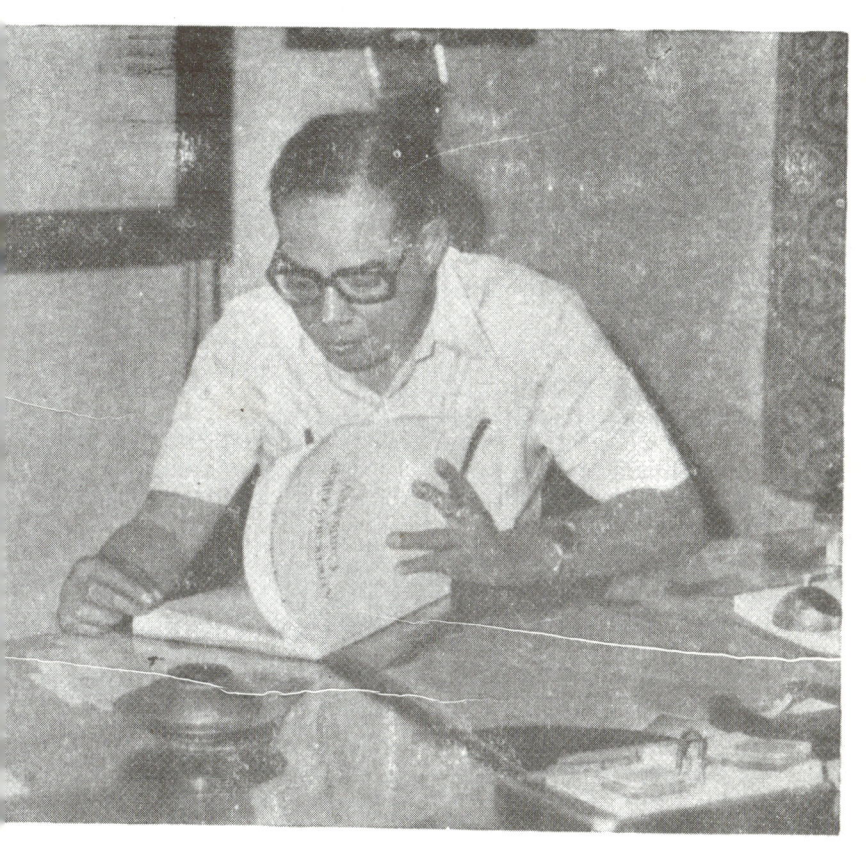

Dr. SUNIL K. SEN

B I O - D A T A

Name   : SEN SUNIL KUMAR
Address   : 2, Woodburn Park , Calcutta -700 020
               West Bengal, India.
Date of birth   : 1st January, 1932

Qualification   :

(1) Graduated in Medicine from Medical College,West Bengal under the University of Calcutta in 1954.

(2) Obtained Membership of Royal College of Physicians. Edinburgh with Advanced studies in cardiology inJanuary, 1959.

Special Academic Honours :

(1) Elected fellow of Royal College of Physicians Edinburge in 1968.

(2) Elected Fellow of College of Chest Physicians (U.S.A) in 1970.

(3) Elected Fellow of American College of cardiology in 1973.

(4) Elected Fellow of international College of Engiology in 1975

(5) Elected Founder Fellow of the IMA Academy of Medical Specialities. New Delhi in 1982.

(6) Elected Member, The New York Academy of Sciences 1985.

(7) Appointed as the Representative of the Royal College of Physicians of Edinburgh, U.K. January, 1987-1994

(8) Elected fellow international Medical Sciences Academy, New Delhi 1994.

(9) Elected Vice - President, Cardiological Society of India in 1976.

(10) Elected President Cardiological society of India (1979-1981).

(11) Elected Executive committee Member of Association of Physicians of India (West Bengal Branch)1982.

(12) Elected as Adviser on Coronary Heart Disease to the Editorial Board of the Indian Heart Journal in 1982.

(13) Elected Vice - President of Association of Physicians of India (West Bengal Branch) 1984.

(14) Elected as a Founder Fellow of the Association of Physicians of India . November, 1987.

(15) Elected President Association of Physicians of India (West Bengal Branch) 1988-89.

Special Honour at Medical College, Calcutta W.B :

Elected President, Ex. Student Association of Medical College, Calcutta-1977.

Member of the Associations :
(1) Life Member , Association of Physicians of India as well as its West Bengal chapter.
(2) Life of Member Cardiological Society of India and its West Bengal Chapter.
(3) Member for the last 35 Years of Indian Medical Association.

Special Honour at University of Calcutta West Bengal, India :
(1) Elected member of the post-graduate Council of Medicine, University of Culcutta from1973-1978.
(2) Member of the Faculty of Medicine , University of Calcutta , West Bengal , India from 1973-1978.
(3) Appointed as an Examiner of Under - graduate Examinations in Medicine, 1969,1970,1974,1978.
(4) Appointed as an Examiner of Post - graduate Diploma in Cardiology from 1960 to 1980.
(5) Appointed as an Examiner of Doctorate of Medicine in 1971 and post Doctoral Degree in Cardiology Examinations from 1982 to 1984.

Highest Teaching post Held at Medical college, Calcutta, West Bengal, India:
Professor of Medicine and Cardiology, Department of Medicine, Medical college, Calcutta from 1977 to1987.

Teaching Experience:
(1) Under Graduate Medical teaching 1965 to 1987 in different teaching posts like Lecturer. Assistant Professor R e a d e r, Associate Professor and Professor.
(2) Post Graduate Medical Teaching, 1960 to 1987.

Field of specialisation:
(1) Internal Medicine.
(2) Cardiology.

National Award:
DR. B.C. ROY NATIONAL AWARD AS AN EMINENT TEACHER 1989, OF INDIA,

Publications in Foreign Journal:
(1) "A Giant arterio Venous Aneurysm of the Abdominal Aorta and inferior vena Cava, a rare case" in International Journal of " **ANGIOLOGY**" U.S.A.- June, 1975

PREFACE

The aim of bringing out this Re- prient 9th edition is to cater to the ever increasing demand of the book amongest medicos, both students as well as practitioners. This treatise of clinical diagnois, provides much needed basic clinical knowledge for undergraduates as well as a sound background for senior students.

Basic clinical methods have not undergone drastic changes though medical technology have undergone tremendous changes in the recent timies in technological and investigational aspect. Due attention have been paid in this edition to orientation of basic clinical medicines in terms of modern devices and advances. This book will be useful to all those who aspire to gain such knowledges of modern technological advances.

But for the sincere efforts of Dr. Rupasri Bhattacharya MD(Cal), Dr. Saktirup Sen MD (Cal), Mrs. Rajashri Chowdhuri M.Sc., this Reprint 9th edition would not have seen the light of the day. To these junior colleagues of mine I remain extremely thankful and express my sincere gratitude.

It is sincerely hoped that this edition will meet the demands of new entrants of medical faculty in their guest to find reliable and sound treatise for understanding the science of clinical diagnosis.

Thanks are due to all whose names have not been specifically mentioned and publisher for their instinted co-operation without which it would have been impossible to bringout this Reprint 9th of this edition. I shall appreciate constructive suggestion from readers for future guidance.

2, Woodburn park, Kolkata- 700 020   **Sunil k. Sen**

Dated: **3.7.2011**

Acknowledgements of Past Editions

The author expresses his utmost gratitude and heartfelt thanks to the following colleagues who helped most generously in preparing the previous editions of the book.

Drs. Satya Prasad Chakraborty F.R.C.P.(U.K),Dilip Majumdar MD(Cal) F.R.C.P(U.K.),Samarendranath Roy MD(Cal), Chitra Ranjan Banerjee MD(Cal), S.Khanra MD(Cal), P.P. Mitra MD(Cal), Sankar Pal MD (Cal), Ashim Kumar Basu F.R.C.P.(U.K.) Bhabani Goswami MD(Cal), Sudarshan Chakraborty MD (Cal), Dipankar Dutta MD(Cal), Arun Chatterjee MD (Cal) DMRD, Debabrata Banerjee MD (Cal) Amalendu Sarker, Ashok Mukherjee, Joytirmoy Dutta F.R.C.G.P.(UK), Rajat Subhra Sanyal,Shymal Das, Goutam Maity, Nirmal Palle **Dwark Nath Bhadra MD (Cal)** and Others.

C O N T E N T S

Part --- 1

Chapter

REFERENCES

British Medical Journal, The New England Journal of Medicine, The lancet and Journal of the American Medical Association in addition to **Principles of Neurology** by Adams & Victor, **Brain's clinical Neurology** and Textbook of **Neurology, Neurological** Examination in Clinical Practice by Bickerstaff, Heart Disease by Braunwald, Correlative **Neuroanatomy** and Functional Neurology by Chusid,**Clinical Haematology** in Medical Practice by Degruchy, Hematology by **jw** williams, Blood Pure and Eloquent by MM Wintrobe,Dermatology in General Practice by Fitzpatrick, Essential Paediatrics by OP Ghai, Common symptoms of Disease In Children by RS **Illingworth, Diseases of the Chest** by Hinshaw & Murray, The Heart by Hurst Clinical Heart Disease by Oram, **Bedside Cardio logy by jules Constant Physical Examination of the Heart** and Circulation by Perloff, Harrison's Principles of **Internal Medicine Oxford Textbook of Medicine.**
Diseases of the Liver and **Biliary Tract by** Sheila sherlock, Nelson Textbook of **Paediatrics and General pathology by Walter & Israel.**

PART-I

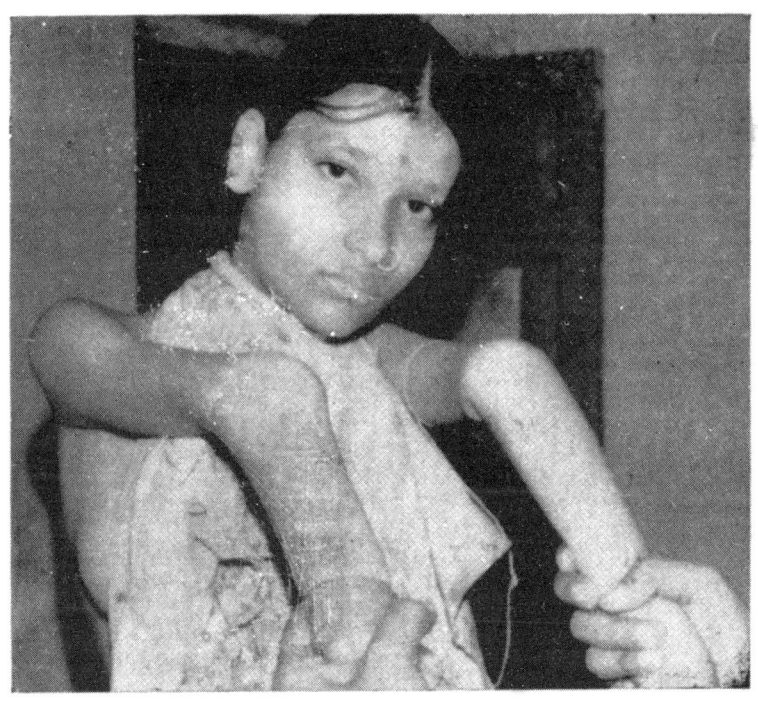

Fig. A : Ehlers Danlos Syndrome ; note the
hyperextensible joints.

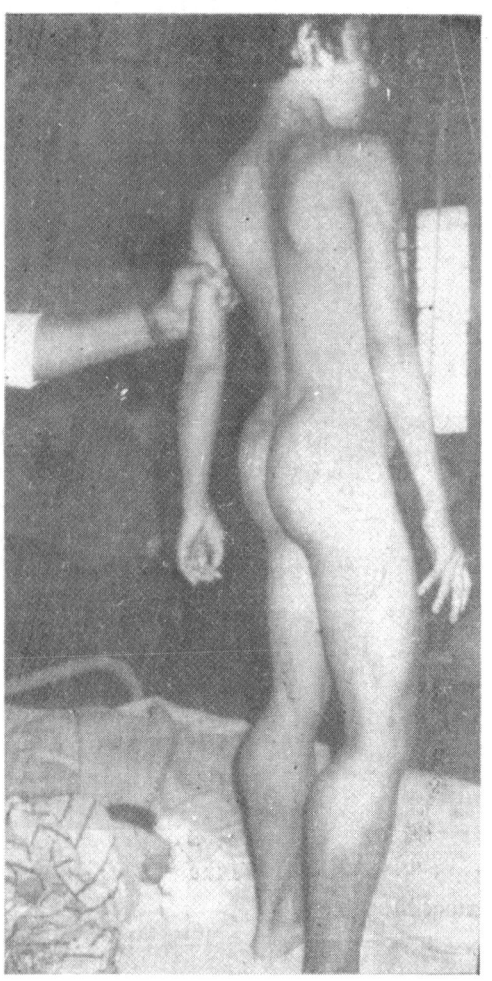

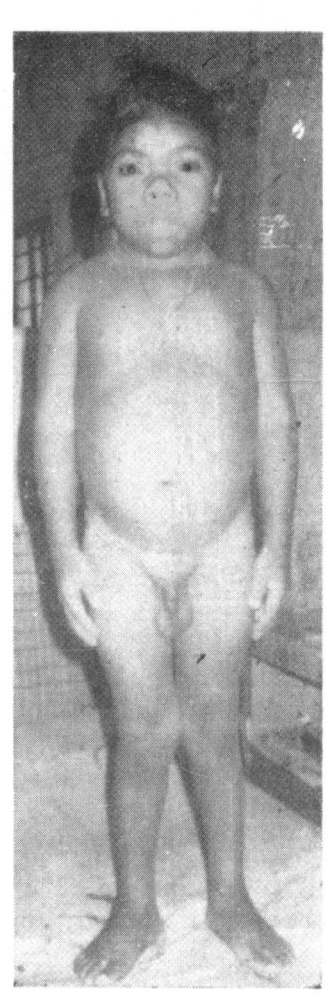

Fig. B : Duchenne's Pseudohypertrophic
muscular dystrophy.

Fig.C: A cretin.

| CHAPTER 1 | GENERAL EXAMINATION |

> *Young man, go to the bedside of the patient, there only can you learn medicine—Thomas Sydenham*

PRINCIPLES OF HISTORY TAKING

The patient's complaints as regards his illness is the most important part in history taking. A detailed history from the patient gives clue to the correct diagnosis of the disease. Sympathetic attitude and keen observations are essential to properly elicit the history and get to the real malady of the patient. It is preferable to note down the history of the illness in the same way as expressed by the patient as far as practicable. Repetition of same complaint or irrelevant facts should be ignored intelligently. Leading questions are to be avoided during enquiry except where the patient is confused or is unable to express himself intelligently because of, say, mental dullness. It is imperative to exercise the restraint everytime a history is taken as leading questions suggest to the patient the symptoms the examiner expects to find or brings about an unconscious distortion of the patient's history. Making bedside notes is very essential.

The following points in the history should be noted in a routine way :

A. Name – This is asked as a rule for identification of the particular individual for future references.

B. Age – It is a very important clinical data in history -taking as some diseases are prevalent in particular age

3

groups. For example–arteriosclerosis, ischaemic heart disease, menopausal syndrome, malignancy etc. are maladies of older age group whereas acute rheumatic fever, congenital heart diseases, acute nephritic syndromes, congenital haemolytic anaemias, infectious diseases like measles, diphtheria are found in infancy and childhood. Chronic leukaemias, gall-bladder diseases, peptic ulcers are the diseases common in middle life.

C. Sex– Diseases like mitral regurgitation, cirrhosis of liver, chronic duodenal ulcer are more common in males whereas atrial septal defect, chronic cholecystitis, hypo and hyperthyroidism, anaemia of nutritional origin, are most commonly seen in females. Haemophilia and Duchenne muscular dystrophy are found almost exclusively in males.

D. Occupation– Enquiry about the patient's occupation may give some hints to the diagnosis of many diseases. Examples :

(i) A person long employed in a printing press having blue line in the gum and suffering from abdominal colic, paraesthesias in the extremities and revealing punctate basophilia in the peripheral blood smear has certainly been suffering from chronic lead poisoning.

(ii) In an individual working in a coal mine and suffering from breathlessness, cough with expectoration for a long time and clinically showing features of pulmonary emphysema,—the most possible diagnosis is coal miner's pneumoconiosis.

(iii) A sewer of paddy-field worker who suddenly develops high temperature with rigor, muscle pain, nausea and vomiting with jaundice, evidences of anaemia and haemorrhagic episodes with leucocytosis, positive guineapig inoculation test (with blood in the first week or with urine in the second and third weeks) and revealing leptospira in smears from liver, kidney and blood culture–is a patient of Weil's disease.

(iv) Chances of coronary arterial diseases are more in businessmen, persons of sedentary habit, and those with type A personality.

(v) Men working in plastic and rubber industries are prone to develop bronchial asthma and cancers of genitourinary tract, particularly those who handle chemicals like benzidine.

(vi) Workers in mines (gold, copper, coal) pottery and sand blasting may develop silicosis, a type of pneumoconiosis. Pulmonary tuberculosis is very often a complication of silicosis.

(vii) Workers in printing industry who handle gum acacia often develop bronchial asthma.

(viii) Asbestosis is a type of pneumoconiosis that is common in persons working in textile industries and in persons engaged in construction work. Pleural plaques, bronchogenic carcinoma and pleural mesothelioma are often associated with asbestosis.

Persons suffering from these occupational chronic debilitating illnesses may legally claim for compensation and physicians are likely to be called into diagnose the condition and assess the severity.

E. Marital Status–The matrial status of the patient must be noted– diseases like haemophilia A, nephrogenic diabetes insipidus, Duchenne muscular dystrophy, glucose 6–phosphate dehydrogenase deficiency are X-linked recessive and hence are usually carried asymptomatically by females while male offsprings are unfortunate victims. Marriage in extremes of age results in babies with congenital cardiac defects, abortion etc. and this is exemplified by the common occurrence of Down's syndrome (Trisomy 21) in children of elderly mothers and increasing frequency of Marfan's syndrome with increasing paternal age.

Psychiatric disturbances are sometimes precipitated by marital disharmony.

Marriage between close relatives or consanguineous marriages result in more frequent expression of genetic defects in the offsprings.

F. Address–Diseases like malaria, kala-azar, blackwater fever and filaria are common in West Bengal and parts of Orissa, whereas pernicious anaemia and subacute combined degeneration are rarely encountered in the tropics, but quite commonly seen in temperate countries.

Intestinal and extraintestinal (e.g. hepatic) amoebiasis. giardiasis, ascariasiss, hookworm infection are very common in West Bengal, and other regions of Eastern India particularly along the Gangetic plains.

G. Chief complaints–It is essential to note down three or four most important symptoms of the patient in chronological order along with their durations.

H. History of present illness– The patient should be allowed to narrate the history of the present complaints from the beginning of its development in sequences, without any leading questions being put in as far as practicable.

Unnecessary elaboration and repetition of symptoms should be tactfully avoided. Intelligent and educated patients sometimes narrate their complaints in medical terms e.g. acidity, rheumatism etc. In such cases, they should be asked to describe what discomfort they actually feel.

Details of previous treatments should be enquired about particularly the name and duration of drugs taken and any adverse reactions out of them (e.g. hypersensitivity to penicillin), previous surgical procedures, irradiation or psychotherapy. These information may have influenced the presenting symptoms or disease. For example, a female patient presenting with symptoms suggestive of diabetes mellitus may have history of long continued intake of corticosteroids for her rheumatoid arthritis.

The patient should also be asked to produce the previous records, if possible. In case of children and very old or mentally sick patients, close relatives should be asked about the previous treatment.

I. Past illness–The history or relevant diseases from which the patient has suffered in the past should be elaborated; e.g.

(i) Rheumatic fever; (ii) Malaria and kalaazar; (iii) Infectious diseases e.g. diphtheria, scarlet fever, small pox; (iv) Infective hepatitis; (v) Syphilis and gonorrhoea etc.

There might be some correlation of the above mentioned diseases with the present clinical signs–e.g. hepatomegaly, hepatosplenomegaly, features of portal hypertension due to cirrhosis, rheumatic valvular heart disease, cardiomyopathy, tabes dorsalis, syphilitic aortic incompetence, gonococcal arthritis etc.

J. Family history and Personal history–(i) Enquiry about the health of parents and causes of death if they are not alive should be made because diseases like diabetes mellitus, hypertension, coronary arterial disease etc. run in family and they are usually multifactorial.

(ii) As regards brothers and sisters, it is of same value because hypertension, congenital heart diseases, diabetes mellitus, ischaemic heart diseases, congenital haemolytic anaemias may be frequent amongst the brothers and sisters of the same family, In such cases a family tree should be constructed.

(iii) Food habit is very important because malnutrition, iron deficiency anaemia, avitaminosis etc. are very common in the tropics.

(iv) Chronic alcoholism may lead to diseases like cirrhosis of liver, coronary arterial disease, peripheral neuritis whereas excessive smoking may lead to chronic bronchitis with emphysema, Buerger's diseases, bronchogenic carcinoma etc.

(v) Regular habits of physical exercise may prevent obesity, coronary arterial disease etc.

K. Psychological history– Psychological disturbances should be elicited very carefully while taking the history as psychoneurosis and psychosomatic disorders like peptic ulcer, hyperthyroidism, bronchial asthma, ulcerative colitis, irritable bowel etc. are encountered daily in the practice of medicine.

Type of work, social and sexual relationships should be asked when neurotic and psychosomatic disturbances are clinically suspected. Common psychoneurotic symptoms like anxiety, depression, obsessive thoughts should be elicited. History of delusions or false beliefs and hallucinations or false sensation or perceptions should be carefully enquired about if severe mental disorders like schizophrenia is suspected.

L. Menstrual History–In females, menarche or age of onset of menstruation, duration of menstruation and quantity of blood loss in each menstrual cycle or any abnormalities thereof should be noted.

Number of birth and complication during pregnancy or/ and birth (too early birth, sectio etc.) should be asked.

History of amenorrhoea, if any, should be asked for. Onset of menopause or stoppage of menstruation and symptoms attributed to premenopausal syndrome should be enquired about in elderly females.

Excessive blood loss due to gynaecological causes like fibroid uterus or cancer cervix may be a clue to the search for a cause of anaemia.

Perimenopausal bleeding, endometrial carcinoma, dysfunctional uterine haemorrhage are sometimes associated with excessive bleeding.

History of taking oral contraceptives with its duration should be noted. Obesity, hypertension, deep vein thrombosis, jaundice and sometimes breast carcinoma may occur as complications of these drugs.

M. Social Background—The living condition should be noted :

Patient is living on street, in a hut, house, flat.

Patient has to climb e.g. three stages to get at home.

There is freshwater available, or not; electricity or not. Note, if necessary situation how patient is coming with other people e.g. relatives, friends etc.

Is there any other social pressure or environmental disorder which might cause unwell feeling or even disease (eg home near a big and busy street, lot of noise, no proper sleep possible etc.

There could be much more of interest, which you find out after a second or third talk with the patient. The social and environmental sorrounding is one of the basic items. This conditions decides at last whether we were able to cure the patient or only "repair" a symptom.

PHYSICAL EXAMINATION

GENERAL SURVEY (Decubitus, build, nutrition, facies, anaemia, cyanosis, jaundice, pigmentation, oedema, clubbing, temperature, pulse, respiration, blood pressure).

1. DECUBITUS

Definition– The posture of the patient in bed. The different types are—

(i) Decubitus of choice— The patient does not feel uncomfortable in any particular position.

(ii) Propped up, which may be grossly generalised as follows :
45"–mild dyspnoea
60^0—moderate dyspnoea
90^0—Severe dyspnoea (also known as orthopnoea). However, even a mildly dyspnoeic patient may be most comfortable at 60^0 or even at 90^0 elevation. This is because dyspnoea is a subjective phenomenon and patients vary from one to another in tolerance or endurance.

Causes of propped up decubitus :

(a) *Cardic–*Left ventricular failure due to mitral incompetence. aortic valvular disease. hypertension, myocardial infarction, cardiomyopathy, patent ductus arterisous, coarctation of aorta etc. Left atrial failure due to mitral stenosis, myxoma of left atrium, ball valve thrombus in the left atrium, mitral atresia etc. Massive pulmonary embolism (acute corpulmonale). Chronic corpulmonale.

(b) *Respiratory–*Bornchial asthma, pleural, effusion, pneumothorax and hydropneumothorax, bronchogenic carcinoma, chronic bronchitis with or without emphysema, pulmonary arteriovenous fistula, acute pulmonary oedema due to over transfusion, carbon monoxide poisoning etc.

(c) *Gastrointestinal—*Huge ascities—mechanically pushing the diaphragm upwards causes a de crease in vital capacity and leads to reduced air entry into the lungs.

(d) *Neurological*–Any lesion below the level of pons that causes paralysis of respiratory muscles (including Guillain-Barre syndrome), recurrent laryngeal nerve palsy causing stridor and maysthenias and myopathies causing respiratory muscle weakness or paralysis.

(iii) *Trepopnoea*—Patient feels comfortable lying on the affected side and becomes dyspnoeic if he lies on the opposite side e.g. pleural effusion, hydropneumothorax, pneumothorax etc.

(iv) Curled up decubitus is seen in acute renal colic, acute biliary colic meningitis etc.

(v) Opisthotones—seen in tetanus, strychnine poisoning spinal meningitis, maple syrup urine disease (leucinosis) or may occur as a hysterical manifestation.

(vi) Listless attitude— is seen in unconsciousness, peritonitis, parkinsonism, hysteria.

COMMON CAUSES OF UNCONSCIOUSNESS

Neurological λ Cerebral haemorrhage λ Cerebral embolism λ Subarachnoid haemorrhage λ Cerebral thrombosis λ Postepileptic coma and status epilepticus λ Encephalitis and encephalomyelitis λ Meningitis.

Endocrine λ Diabetic coma (hyperglycaemic diabetic ketoacidosis or hyperosmolar nonketotic) λ Addisonian crisis λ Hypothyroidism (Myxoedema coma) λ Pituitary coma (Pituitary apoplexy)

Cardiovascular λ Adams-Stokes syndrome λ Syncopal attack due to severe aortic stenosis, pulmonary stenosis, aortic, stenosis Fallot's tetralogy etc. λ Hypertensive encephalopathy.

Respiratory λ Carbon dioxide narcosis, respiratory failure.

Gastrointestinal   λ   Hepatic coma (encephalopathy associated with hepatic failure)

Renal	λ Terminal stage of uraemia.
Poisoning	λ Barbiturate, morphin etc.
Traumatic	λ Head injury.
Psychogenic	λ Hysteria.

2. BUILD

Definition — Build is the skeletal structure in relation to age and sex of the individual as compared to a normal person. Build is short in those in whom it is below the 3rd centile of a normal population of same age and sex and tall when the height is above the 97th centile for normal population.

Types—(1) Short—the common causes are—

(a) Normal genetic variation.

(b) Chromosomal abnormalities e.g. Down's syndrome, Turner's syndrome, Noonan's syndrome.

(c) Childhood diseases e.g. marasmus, kwashiorkor, rickets, tuberculosis, fibrocystic disease, gluten, enteropathy, hookworm infestation, congenital cyanotic or acyanotic heart diseases, thalassaemia major, chronic renal disease, congenital syphilis glycogen storage diseases etc.

(d) Skeletal abnormalities, e.g. Achondroplasia, gargoylism, Ellis van Creveld syndrome, rickets, poliomyelitis, Still's disease.

(e) Endocrine disorders, e.g. craniopharyngiomas or other pituitary tumours, idiopathic hypopituitarism. Frohlic's syndrome, Laurence-Moon Biedl syndrome, hypothroidism, sexual precocity, Cushing's syndrome, congenital adrenal hyperplasia.

(f) Intrauterine maldevelopment e.g. foetal alcohol syndrome, progeria etc.

(g) Drug induced e.g. glucocorticoids, androgens, anabolic steroids, oestrogens, antithyroid drugs, vitamin D etc.

(2) Tall— This is mostly inherited from tall parents and pathological causes are not common. The different causes are—

(a) Constitutional

(b) Overnutrition causing tallness before fusion of epiphyses

(c) Chromosomal abnormalities e.g. Klinefelters syndrome (47 XXY). Supermale (XYY) and superfemale (XXX)

(d) Miscellaneous causes include Marfan's syndrome, homocystinuria, cerebral gigantism, lipodystrophy and Beckwith Wiedemann syndrome.

3. NUTRITION

Definition— It means nourishment of the body which is assessed by

(i) Subcutaneous fat,

(ii) Bulk of muscle

(iii) Features of vitamin deficiency, if any.

However, in a recent study logistic regression analysis has shown that mid-upper arm circumference is as effective as other nutritional indices and combinations of different indices have not been shown to be better especially in predicting death in malnourished children (BMJ. 1986, 293, 373).

Types (1) Subnutrition—Body weight 10% less than that of a standard person in relation to age and sex. It is due to quantitative dietary deficiency.

(2) Starvation–Body weight 25% less than that of a standard person in relation to age and sex.

(3) Malnutrition Deficiencies of vitamins, minerals and essential amino acids are characteristic. It is due to qualitative dietary deficiency. But overnutrition is also a form of malnutrition.

(4) Cachexia–A cachectic shows anaemia, evidences of vitamin deficiency and features of starvation.

(5) Emaciation—Loss of subcutaneous fat and diminution of muscle bulk.

CAUSES OF PATHOLOGICAL SUBNUTRITION :

(i) Pulmonary tuberculosis (due to anorexia as well as defective utilisation of nutrients).

(ii) Diabetes mellitus (loss of calorie due to glycosuria and malabsorption may be associated due to various gastrointestinal disorders).

(iii) Thyrotoxicosis
(iv) High fever   ⎫ due to increased metabolic rate
(v) Malignancy   ⎭

(6) Obesity–It means an excess of adipose tissue that imparts a health risk. The degree of excess adiposity is difficult to quantity; but the Framingham study has shown that a 20% excess over ideal weight imparts a definite health risk.

Causes of obesity : These may be either (a) primary or idiopathic where the precise mechanism remains unknown, or (b) secondary, which may be due to (i) hypothyroidism, (ii) Cushing's syndrome, (iii) hypothalamic disorders, (iv) pinealomas, (v) pseudohypoparathyroidism, (vi) Pancreatic insulinomas, (vii) testicular hypogonadism, (viii) polycystic ovarian disease, (ix) induced by drugs e.g. insulin, oral hypoglycaemic agents, glucocorticoids oestrogents etc. (x) abnormal distributions of fat e.g. lipodystrophies, (xi) or may be associated with syndromes or unknown aetiology e.g. Laurence- Moon-Biedl syndrome, Prader-Willi syndrome, Alstrom syndrome etc.

(7)   Nutritional oedema–This includes
  (i) Wet beriberi.
  (ii) Famine oedema with hypoproteinaemia
  (iii) Famine oedema without hypoproteinaemia (isohydraemic famine oedema)
  (iv) Epidemic dropsy.

(8) Protein Energy Malnutrition (i) *Kwashiorkor* : It is a clinical condition characterised by retardation of growth, wasting of muscles, grey or lustreless hair, pigmentation, desquamation and ulceration of skin, oedema and signs of vitamin deficiency occurring in infants and children due to dificiency of protein with adequate calorie intake. Commonly, it occurs due to prolonged breast feeding.

  (ii) *Nutritional marasmus* : Here also infants usually under one year of age suffer from retardation of growth, loss of weight, wasting of muscles and subcutaneous fats but the precipitating factor is the severe restriction of all foods, reproteins, calorie, vitamins etc. One-fifth to one-third of the body weight is lost and the face is pinched and has a curiously senile expression with sunken eyes. The thorax is particularly wasted with prominent ribes. Early weaning and rapid succession of pregnancies are common causes in our country.
  (iii) *Marasmic Kwashiorkor* : In this variety, the children have some clinical features of both the above disorders.

4. FACIES

Definition—Expression in the face of patient.
Types —

(i) Anxious— It indicates awareness or apprehension of the patient about the disease. It may be found in nervous individuals.

(ii) Dull and vacant look of mentally retarded children Mongoloid facies is characterised by slanting eyes, epicanthic fold, small nose with a small oral cavity. This is characteristically seen in Down's syndrome (trisomy 21).

(iii) Masked facies—Parkinsonian syndrome. This facies is characterised by wide palpebral fissures, infrequent blinking, and spontaneous ocular movements are lacking. This is also seen in bilateral facial paralysis, facial myopathies, myasthenia, gravis, progressive systemic sclerosis etc. The face remains devoid of any expression.

(iv) Hepatic facies—This is characterised by shrunken eyes, hollowed temporal fossa, pinched up nose, parched lips, muddy complexion, icteric tinge.

(v) Tabetic facies—Features are persistent wrinkling of the forehead in an attempt of compensate for the drooping of eyelids due to pseudoptosis caused by paralysis of Muller's muscle.

(vi) Thyrotoxic facies—Staring look and exophthalmos are the characteristic features.

(vii) Coarse facial appearance, wrinkling of eyebrows and thick tongue are the characteristic features of cretinism. Apathy of hypothyroidism should draw the attention of the clinician.

(viii) 'Moon' facies the bloated appearence of the face and rounding of the features are caused by—
Cushing's syndrome and disease,
Steroid therapy for a prolonged period,

Acute (proliferative) glomerulonephritis, Minimal lesion and membranous glomerulonephritis, Myxoedema etc.

Superior mediastinal syndrome and pulmonary stenosis.

(In glomerulonephritis the lower eyelids become puffy because of less subcutaneous fat and low tissue tension).

(ix) Facies of bilateral facial palsy—a face devoid of any expression with loss of nasolabial and other promiment furrows (vide supra).

The commonest cause is Guillain-Barre Syndrome of acute infective polyneuritis (when bulbar nuclei are affected. Other rare causes are sarcoidosis, leukaemias and lymphomas, Melkersson's syndrome. In infants forceps delivery in an important cause.

(x) Flushed facies—(a) Malar flush–High colour of the cheek as seen in mitral stenosis particularly with severe pulmonary hypertension in fair skinned individuals. Another cause is myxoedema.

Severe flushing of the cheeks hectic flush is encountered in pulmonary tuberculosis. Facial flushing is characteristic of patients with Cushing's syndrome, polycythaemia, emphysema (pink puffers) and carcinoid syndrome. Postprandial facial flushing occurs in rosacea. In congestive cardiac failure the cheeks may be red and high coloured and a bluish tint may be evident.

(b) Generalised flush—May be caused by–(i) High fever (ii) Severe hypertension (iii) Thyrotoxicosis (iv) Chronic alcoholism (v) Carcinoid syndrome (vi) Pheochromocytoma (vii) Drugs like atropine, nicotinic acid (niacin) and percutaneous absorption of monosulfiram, (viii) Systemic mastocytosis (ix) Toxic erythemas (x) Measles rubella, scarlet fever (xi) Lupus erythematosus etc. Localised flushing is seen in erythromelalgia and also in systemic lupus erythematosus (SLE).

(xi)   Pallor—It is seen in shock where blood flow through the capillaries diminished, in syncopal attack, left heart failure, peripheral vascular diseases like Raynaud's phenomenon and arterial spasm on exposure to cold. Generalised pallor is found in severe anaemia.

(i) Pallor with anaemia—found in all types of severe anaemia, infective endocarditis, acute rheumatic fever etc.

(2)   Pallor without anaemia—The cardiovascular causes are—Tight mitral stenosis, Severe aortic stenosis, Acute myocardial infarction, Acute left ventricular failure, Acute peripheral circulatory failure and other causes are—

(i) Nephrotic syndrome, (ii) Causalgia, (iii) Acute alcoholic coma, (iv) During paroxysm of vertigo in Meniere's disease and (v) Acute nephritic syndrome especially when there is anaemia.

(xii)   Risus sardonicus—The eyebrows are raised and the angles of the mouth drawn out due to tonic spasm of the muscles of the face in tetanus.

(xiii)   Photophobia–in meningitis and also seen in meningisms.

(xiv)   Elfin facies —Found in supravalvular aortic stenosis (William's syndrome) that may be associated with hypercalcemia.

5. ANAEMIA

Definition — Qualitative or quantitative reduction of circulating RBC and/or of the percentage of haemoglobin concentration in relation to standard age and sex. Normal blood count—

RBC — Male   } — 5 to 6 million /cmm
       Female }   — 4.5 to 5.5 million/cmm
WBC— Male   }   4,000 – 11,000 cmm
       Female }

Haemoglobin—

Male–14.6 to 15.5 gm per 100 ml (100.11%)

Female–13.3 to 14.6 gm per 100 ml (90.100%)

[100% = 14.6 gm per 100 ml]

Reticulocyte — o to 1%

Platelet — 1.5 to 4 lacs/cmm.

Anaemia is said to be severe when heamoglobin is less than 40% moderate when 40.50% mild when 50.60%

Sites to be looked for—

(i) Lower palpebral conjunctiva,

(ii) Tip and dorsum of tongue,

(iii) Soft palate,

(iv) Nail beds—

(v) General skin, palm and sole.

Colour of the mucous membrane of the conjunctiva and the tongue is more reliable than the general skin. Estimation of percentage of haemoglobin and examination of stained films indicate the severity and aetiology of anaemia.

Symptoms referable to anaemia :

General—Fatigue and lassitude.

Neurological—Giddiness vertigo, dimness of vision, headache, insomnia, tingling and numbness of extremities.

Cardiovascular—Palpitation, dyspnoea, anginal attack.

Gastrointestinal—Indigestion diarrhoea, anorexia,

Signs due to anaemia :

General–Pallor, oedema.

Cardiovascular—Water-hammer pulse, pistol shot sound, capillary pulsation forceful apex, haemic murmur over the pulmonary area in left second of third space or in the apical region, ejection click and nonrumbling soft diastolic murmur in mitral area. This is due to relative stenosis of mitral or tricuspid valve secondary to greatly increased blood flow. This murmur is encountered in sickle cell anaemia where the anaemia is very severe and chronic.

(Noncardiac cuses of water-hammer pulse are thyrotoxicosis, high fever, Paget's disease, arteriovenous fistula, wet beriberi, chronic annoxic, corpulmonale, hepatic coma etc.)

Respiratory—Crepitations in lung bases.

Neurological features of polyneuritis or subacute combined degeneration of spinal cord and papilloedema.

Renal—Albuminuria.

Gastrointestinal—Enlarged liver and spleen due to proliferation of reticuloendothelial cells.

Types of anaemia—

I. Iron deficiency (Hypochromic microcytic) (a) Haemorrhagic acute post haemorrhagic anaemia following trauma or intestinal bleeding and chronic post haemorrhagic anaemia in bleeding from haemorrhoids, from peptic ulcer, due to hookworm infestation or chronic menorrhagia;

(b) Nutritional deficiency :

(c) After gastrectomy ;

(d) Malabsorption synurome.

II. Megaloblastic—This is due to vitamin B12 and/or folate deficiencies leading to arrest to maturation of the cells. The causes are Nutritional; Pregnancy; Liver diseases; Malabsorption syndrome; Drugs e.g. (a) Folate antagonists e.g. methotrexate and pyrimethamine, (b) Anticonvulsants eg Phenytoin, (c) Cytosine arabinoside by interfering with DNA synthesis. The causes that are rare in our country are (a) Pernicious anaemia (b) In Leukaemias and haemolytic anaemias—due to excess utilisation of folate; (c) Diphyllobothrium latum infestation.

III. Dimorphic anaemia—Presence of the picture of both iron deficiency and megaloblastic anaemia in peripheral blood. This type is quite common in our country. The causes are − (i) Hookworm infection with nutritional deficiency state. (ii) Pregnancy.

    IV. Anaemia of scurvy.

    V. Anaemia of hypothyroidism.

    VI. Haemolytic anaemias—

(1) Hereditary disorders of RBC :

(a) Congenital spherocytosis;

(b) Haemoglobinopathies like sickle cell anaemia, thalassaemia, haemoglobin C disease and haemoglobin E disease;

(c) Glucose-6-phosphate dehydrogenase (66PD) and other enzyme deficiencies in RBC.

(2) *Due to antibody formation against erythrocytes :*

(i) Haemolytic disease of newborn;

(ii) Autoimmune (acquired) haemolytic anaemia;

(iii) Symptomatic haemolytic anaemia;

(iv) Paroxysmal haemoglobinuria;

(v) Rh incompatibility :

(vi) Mismatched blood transfusion.

(3) *Due to infective or toxic factors :*

(i) Organisms like haemolytic streptococci, staphylococci, Clostridium welchii etc.

(ii) Malaria : Blackwater fever.

(iii) Arsenic, lead and other heavy metals and drugs like sulphonamides, potassium chlorate, methyldopa and chemicals like napthalene etc.

(vi) Anaemia due to bone-marrow depression—causing pancytopaenia or aplastic or hypoplastic anaemia.

(a) Idiopathic

(b) Secondary to :

(I) Drugs like chloramphenicol, trinitrotoluene, gold, anticonvulsants (troxidone), arsenic, following use of cytotoxic drugs—due to idiosyncratic reaction.

(II) Idiosyncrasy to certain chemicals and insecti cides–benzol and its derivatives like trinitrophenol.

(III) Repeated exposure to X-rays and radioactive substances.

VII. Myelosclerosis, myelofibrosis, myelophthisic anaemia, multiple myeloma lead to simultaneous pres -ence of myelocytes and normoblasts in the peripheral blood and is referred to as *leucoerythroblastic* blood picture and is due to bone-marrow infiltration.

VIII. Anaemia of uncertain origin :

(a) Uraemia (partially due to deficiency of erythro - poietin in chronic renal failure);

(b) Malignancy, chronic infections, hepatic cirrhosis, rhuematoid-arthrities etc. lead to *anaemias of chronic disorders.*

IX. Sideroblastic anaemia —— It is a type of dyshaemopoietic anaemia where peripheral blood picture is hypochromic microcytic or dimorphic in type but the bone-marrow contains ringed sideroblasts. Sideroblasts are nucleated red blood cells having excess iron containing granules in the cytoplasm. Here utilisation of iron is impaired due to defect in erythropoiesis. These are either hereditary (sex-linked partially recessive) or acquired. The latter may be (i) primary (idiopathic) or (ii) secondary. The secondary anaemias may be due to— (a) Drugs like anti-tuberculous, paracetamol, phenacetin; (b) nutritional disorder e.g. chronic alcoholism, nutritional megaloblastic anaemia, malabsorption; (c) increased haemopoietic cell proliferation e.g. myeloproliferative disorders, leukaemias haemolytic anaemias. Nearly one-third of the sideroblastic anaemias respond to large (e.g. 100 mg) daily doses of pyridoxine.

In all cases of severe anaemia apart from routine examination of blood, bone-marrow study should be carried out, Coomb's test may have to be done in some forms of haemolytic anaemia. In hereditary spherocytosis, the test is negative; it is positive in immune haemolytic anaemias.

6. CYANOSIS

Definition — Bluish discolouration of the skin and mucous membrane due to excessive amount of reduced haemoglobin in the blood (more than 5 gms/100 cc.) Clinical cyanosis is present when oxygen saturation is below 85%. Types :

1. *Peripheral cyanosis*—This occurs in the presence of normal arterial oxygen saturation and is due to pronounced oxygen unsaturation of the venocapillary and capillary blood.

Sites—Tip of nose, fingers and toes, ear lobule, palm and sole.

Mechanism—

    (a) Vasconstriction (peripheral),

    (b) Low cardiac output,

    (c) Sluggish circulation in extremities.

       Causes—

(i) Acute left ventricular failure or acute left atrial failure with peripheral stasis.

(ii) Shock from severe burns or severe haemor-rhage.

(iii) Exposure to cold.

(iv) Cryoglobulinaemia–Cryogobulin is an abnormal plasma protein (globulin) which forms get at low temperature; may be found in lym-phoma, nephrosis, multiple myeloma, collagen diseases, kala azar etc.

(v) Raynaud's phenomenon–characterised by bluish colouration of the digits due to excessive vasoconstrictor response to cold to mechanical stimuli.

(vi) Venous obstruction due to any cause and local vasomotor disturbances may give rise to local cyanosis.

II. *Central cyanosis*—Due to excessive oxygen unsaturation of the arterial blood.

Sites—Tongue, inner surface of lip and also sites for peripheral cyanosis.

Causes—

(a) Pulmonary–Corpulmonale, pleural effusion, pneumothorax, respiratory failure, pneumonia, absorption collapse etc.

(b) Cardiac–Congenital cyanotic heart diseases with right to left shunt–e.g. Fallot's tetralogy, Eisenmenger complex and syndrome. The syndrome is characterised by pulmonary hyper tension with reversal of shunt, the term Eisenmenger's complex is used when the reversed shunt is at the ventricular level. Cyanosis tardive or late cyanosis may be found in A S D with reversal of shunt due to increased pulmonary and right ventricular resistance because of heart failure of pulmonary compli cations.

(c) Vascular—Pulmonary arteriovenous fistula.

III. *Enterogenous*—This group includes—

(i) Sulphaemoglobinaemia–55–68 band in spectroscopy.

(ii) Methaemoglobinaemia—Cyanosis is due to formation of methaemoglobin where ferrous iron of the haem of haemoglobin is converted into ferric ($Fe^{++} \rightarrow Fe^{++}$) form in excessive amounts.

Causes :

(a) Inherited defects like haemoglobin M or deficiency of cytochrome b5 reductase.

(b) Poisoning with chemicals e.g. aniline, nitrobenzene etc.

(c) Drugs e.g. phenacetin, dapsone, sulphonamides etc.

(iii) Cherry red colouration of skin is produced in carbon monoxide poisoning.

Clinical effects of cyanosis—

(1) Hypertrophy of and bleeding from gum,

(2) Recurrent arthritis, gout and tophi formation,

(3) Plumonary osteoarthropathy.

(4) Secondary polycythaemia—e.g. in corpulmonale or cyanotic congenital—heart diseases,

(5) Embolic manifestation–e.g. pulmonary embolism.

IV. *Differential cyanosis—*

(a) Hands blue but feet red—in coarctation of aorta with transposition of great vessels.

(b) Hands red but feet blue–in patent ductus arteriosus

with reversal of shunt due to pulmonary hypertension.

7. JAUNDICE

Definition—Yellowish discolouration of the skin and mucous membrane due to excessive bilirubin in the blood. [Normal range is 0.2 to 0.8 mg/100 ml serum]

Latent jaundice [1 mg–1.9 mg/100 mm serum] can be detected only by serum analysis.

Sites— (i) Upper bulbar conjunctiva,
     (ii) Soft palate,
     (iii) Undersurface of tongue,
     (iv) Skin,
     (v) Palm and sole.

Internal tissues are also stained when the jaundice is severe.

Types—(a) Obstrcutive, (b) Haemolytic, (c) Toxic or Hepatocellular or combination of any of these.

Obstructive Jaundice : This is due to a block in the pathway between the site of conjugation of bilirubin in the liver cells and entry of bilirubin in the intestine.

Clinical effects—
     (i) Greenish-yellow bulbar conjunctiva.
     (ii) Petechial haemorrhage (due to vit K deficiency which being a fat soluole vitamin is not absorbed from the intestine and hence the bleeding disorder).
     (iii) Sinus bradycardia—increase in the vagal inhibitory tone due to circulating bile salt.
     (iv) Marks of scratching due to pruritu–possibly a reflex; bile acids acting as irritants on the nerve endings.

(v) Enlarged liver.

(vi) Gall bladder may or may not be palpable depending upon the cause. (According to Courvoisier's law, gall bladder is usually not palpable in jaundice due to a stone in the common bile duct whereas in carcinoma of the head of pancreas gall bladder becomes distended).

(vii) Splenomegaly due to associated biliary cirrhosis (rarely).

(viii) Mustard oil coloured urine.

(ix) Clay coloured stool.

(x) Xanthelasma, xanthoma tuberosum etc. in about 20% of cases.

Liver function tests which are mainly dependent upon the patency of the bile ducts are impaired. In obstructive jaundice. serum alkaline phosphatase level varies between 30 and 100 KA units. [Normal serum value in adult is 3 to 13 King-Armstrong (KA) Units per 100 ml or 40–100 i u l.]

Causes of obstructive jaundice :

(A) Intrahepatic—

(a) Viral infection—infective hepatitis;

(b) Drugs like (i) Chlorpromazine, (ii) Para aminosalicylic acid, (iii) Sulpha drugs—Sulphadiazine, (iv) Chlorpropamide, (v) Methyl testosterone and other anabolic steroids, (vi) MAO inhibitors, (vii) oral contraceptives, (viii) Alcohol, (ix) INH etc.

(c) Active chronic hepatitis :

(d) Cirrhosis of liver

(e) In pregnancy—due to cholestasis;

(f) Lymphoma e.g. Hodgkin's disease;

(g) Secondary carcinoma of liver;

(h) Sometimes in severe bacterial infection;

(i) Pericholangitis in chronic ulcerative colitis.

(B) Extrahepatic—

    (i) Impacted gall stone;

    (ii) Enlarged glands at porta hepatis;

    (iii) Carcinoma of head of the pancreas;

    (iv) Carcinoma of ampulla of Vater or bile duct;

    (v) Carcinoma of gall bladder;

    (vi) Rarely a duodenal ulcer involving the commonbile duct;

    (vii) Stricture of common bile duct, viz after surgery;

(viii) Sclerosing cholangitis complicating ulcerative colitis.

Haemolytic Jaundice : This is due to excessive destruction of red blood cells– resulting in increased bilirubin load on the liver.

Clinical features :

    (i) Lemon-yellow bulbar conjunctiva.

    (ii) Anaemia, the degree of which varies with the severity of haemolytic process and power of bone-marrow to regenerate.

    (iii) Splenomegaly—due to excessive activity of the reticuloendothelial system.

    (iv) High-coloured stool containing large amount of stercobilinogen and stercobilin.

    (v) Freshly voided urine is of normal colour since no bilirubin is present but oxidation of excess urobilinogen to urobilin quickly turns the urine dark.

    (vi) Examination of blood reveals reticulocytosis.

    (vii) Liver function tests dependent upon meta bolic activities of the parenchymal cells are normal.

Causes :
(i) Congenital
  (a) Hereditary spherocytosis;
  (b) Haemoglobinopathies (sickle cell anaemia, thalassaemia etc.);
  (c) Glucose-6-phosphate dehydrogenase (G6PD) and pyruvate kinase deficiencies.
(ii) Acquired
  (a) Mismatched blood transfusion;
  (b) Rh-incompatibility;
  (c) Following poisonous snake bite;
  (d) Drugs e.g. primaquin, phenacetine, sulphonamides causing haemolysis due to G6PD deficiency in RBC;
  (e) Infection by parasites–malaria and kala azar;
  (f) Acquired immune haemolytic anaemia.
  (g) Marchiafava Micheli syndrome or paroxysmal nocturnal haemoglobinuria (PNH)–due to unusual sensitivity of RBC to complement;
  (h) Paroxysmal cold haemoglobinuria (PCH) secondary to syphilis (congenital syphilis);
  (i) March haemoglobinuria—due to external trauma to small vessels.

Toxic or Hepatocellular Jaundice : This is due to damage of liver cells by toxic or infective agents.
Causes :
(A) Infective :
  (i) Viral––Hepatitis A, B, C, D, E, Cytomegalovirus, Epstein Barr and Yellow fever virus.
  (ii) Spirochaetal—Leptospira icterohaemorrhagia (Weil's disease).
  (iii) Protozoal—Toxoplasma gondii.

(iv) Rickettsia—Coxiella burnetti (Q fever agent).

(B) Toxic—(1) Drugs :

    (i) Chlorpromazine and other phenothiazine derivatives;

    (ii) MAO inhibitors;

    (iii) Imipramine, amitryptiline;

    (iv) Erythromycin, tetracycline (in high doses particularly in pregnancy and in impaired renal function), rifampicin.

    (v) Isoniazid and para aminosalicylic acid;

    (vi) Methyldopa

    (vii) Phenylbutazone, indomethacin and gross overdosage of paracetamol.

    (viii) Halothane, the anaesthetic agent (idiosyncratic reaction).

(2) Poisons and Toxins :

    (i) Carbon tetrachloride,

    (ii) Yellow phosphorus,

    (iii) Copper Sulphate,

    (iv) Alcohol.

    (v) A fungal toxin used as poison (amanita phalloides).

(C) Other conditions– In pregnancy (besides cholestasis) jaundice may be due to acute fatty liver, toxaemias or hyperemesis, both the latter being rare causes.

Some other important causes of jundice :

(a) Primary defect in bilirubin transport of conjugation in the liver cells particularly in premature infants is known as physiological jaundice of the newborn. The defect in conjugation is due to immaturity of the enzyme mechanism.

(b) Gilbert's syndrome–the fault is in the uptake

of bilirubin by liver cells and a partial defici
ency of glucuronyl transferase enzyme. This
is an inherited autosomal dominant disorder.
(c) Dubin-Johnson syndrome is an autosomally
inherited benign defect in the transport of
bilirubin glucuronide from the liver cells into
the bile canaliculi. Rotor syndrome is some
what similar.
(d) Crigler-Najjar syndrome—An autosomal recessive condition, consists of the two types :

Type 1—Total absence of the enzyme glucuronyl
transferase. It is the severe form. Unconjugated
hyperbilirubinaemia may lead to kernicterus in
newborn and ultimately to death.

Type II—Partial deficiency of the enzyme
glucuronyl transferase is present. The patient
may survive to adult life.

Jaundice in cardiovascular disorders
(a) Congestive cardiac failure—hepatic conges
tion and hepatocellular hypoxia is congestive
cardiac failure are associated with disturbance
in the function of the liver. This may give rise
to icteric tinge.
(b) Recurrent and/or multiple pulmonary
infarctions.
(c) May be associated with repeated myocardial
infarction.
(d) Latrogenic.

8. PIGMENTATION

Usual sites that are to be examined are —
(i) Face,
(ii) inside the cheek,

(iii) Creases of palms,

(iv) Skin particularly pressure points and areas exposed to light.

Causes of pigmentation—

(A) Physiological

(i) Pregnancy–e.g. chloasma, linea nigra, sec -ondary areola etc.

(ii) Racial.

(iii) Bluish black pigmentation of the mongols.

(B) Pathologial

Congenital–(a) Von Recklinghausen's disease– typical *cafe-au-lait* pigmentation.

[N. B.–other causes of cafe-au-lait pigmenta- tion are–(i) tuberous sclerosis or epiloia (ii) Polyostotys tic fibrous dysplasia – Albright's syn-drome; (iii) Watson syndrome–pulmonic stenosis with cafe-au-lait patches, (iv) nor- mally in 10% of all people, (v) infective endocarditis etc.

(b) Xeroderma, pigmentosum.

(c) Peutz-Jeghers syndrome.

(d) Multiple polyposis of colon.

(e) Acanthosis nigricans juvenile variety.

(f) Blooms syndrome characterised by typical facies, retardation of growth and photosensi- tive telangiectatic erythema on face.

(g) Nevus.

Acquired– (a) Physical agents :

(i) Exposure to radiation;

(ii) Exposure to sun-rays and heat;

(iii) Erythema ab igne–caused by local heating in domestic conditions.

(b) Skin diseases :

(i) Lichen planus, (ii) Exfoliative dermatitis,

(iii) Pityriasis versicolor, (iv) Dermatitis herpetiformis, (v) Patchy pigmentation may alternate with white patches in leucoderma, (vi) Lichen simplex chronicus, (vii) Psoriasis, (viii) Discoid lupus erythematosus, (ix) Acanthosis nigricans–associated with diabetes mellitus, gross obesity or internal malignancies e.g. carcinoma stomach.

(c) Poisoning :
  (i) Chronic arsenical poisoning
  (ii) Argyria–diffuse slaty grey colouration due to deposition of silver in the skin.

(d) Endocrine :
  (i) Addison's disease–increased pigmentation in skin and mucous membrane varying from light to dark brown in colour.
  (ii) Pituitary tumours—particularly ACTH and· MSH producing tumours; Nelson's syndrome.
  (iii) Thyrotoxicosis;
  (iv) Diabetes mellitus;
  (v) Prolonged steroid therapy.

(e) Parasitic–chronic malaria, kala-azar.

(f) Nutritional deficiency :
  (i) Malabsorption syndrome, chronic cachexia, chronic liver disease kwashiorkor, etc :
  (ii) Pellagra :

(g) Metabolic :
  (i) Haemochromatosis (bronze diabetes)–generalised, bronze colouration ;
  (ii) Prophyria (congenital, variegate and cutanea tarda);
  (iii) Willson's disease (Hepatolenticular degeneration).

(h) Drugs : Busulphan, fixed drug eruption as may occur with sulphur drugs; steroids etc.

Causes of hypopigmentation :

Congenital–

    (a) Albinism–Congenital absence of pigment in the skin either localised (piebaldism) or gen eralised;

    (b) Vitiligo;

    (c) Fanconi's syndrome;

    (d) Phenylketonuria.

Acquired–

    (a) Infections :

      (i) Hypopigmented anaesthetic patches in tuberculoid leprosy (associated nerve thickening confirms the diagnosis);

      (ii) Pityriasis alba;

      (iii) Tinea versicolor—a fungal infection;

      (iv) Eczematous dermatitis;

      (v) Psoriasis.

(b) Endocrine factors :

      (i) Hypopituitarism; (ii) Hypogonadism.

(c) Others :

      (i) Alopecia areata; (ii) Chloroquine.

Varieties of skin eruptions :

    (a) Macule– Abnormal colour of the skin in a localised area without elevation of depression, e.g. haemorrhages into the skin, rose spots of typhoid fever, secondary syphilis.

    (b) Papule–A raised area from the surface, size about 5 mm. e.g. acne lichen.

    (c) Vesicle–Raised from the surface and contains milky or serous fluid (size about 5 mm) eg chicken pox, small pox.

(d) Pustule–Raised from the surface, size about 5 mm. contains pus e.g. chicken pox, small pox.
(e) Bigger than papule involving epidermis and dermis e.g. leprosy.

Diets :

(f) Wheal–Raised from the surface of the skin with a pale centre and red periphery. Mainly type II.
(g) Blebs–Area of the epidermis raised from the surface, size more than 5mm; contains milky or serous fluid e.g. herpes, impetigo pemphigus vulgaris.

Haemorphagic spots (Purpura) :

(1) Petechiae : The spot is less than 1 mm in diameter and does not disappear on pressure by a glass slide.
(2) Suggillations : These are larger macules, more than 2 cm, in diameter and does not disappear on pressure.
(3) Ecchymoses : These are extensive purpuric macules.
(4) Haematoma : These are large haemorrhages in the skin causing elevation of the skin.

Causes of haemorrhagic spots (purpura) in the skin :
(A) Capillary endothelial defect :
　(a) Vascular purpura (Sympatomatic)–
　　(i) Anaphylactoid purpura e.g. Henoch–Scchoenlein, purpura simplex.
　　(ii) Infections : infective endocarditis, septicaemia, meningococcal meningitis, typhoid fever etc.
　　(iii) Chemical agents and drugs (e.g. phenylbutazone, aspirin, indomethacin. Phenobarbitone, penicillin, sulphonamide, snake venom.)

   (iv) Metabolic : uraemia, hepatic failure.

   (v) Other symptomatic vascular purpura (e.g. Cushing's diseases, scurvy, dysproteinaemias like cryoglobulinaemia multiple myeloma, etc)

(b) Miscellaneous :

   (i) Systemic disorders like collagen diseases e.g. polyarteritis nodosa, allergy;

   (ii) Mechanical ;

   (iii) Orthostatic.

(c) Congenital :

   (i) Hereditary haemorrhagic telangiectasia (Osler-Rendu Weber disease);

   (ii) von Willebrand's disease;

   (iii) Hereditary capillary fragility;

   (iv) Ehlers Danlos syndrome.

(B) Due to deficiency of blood platelets :

   (1) Primary, idiopathic thrombocytopenic purpura

   (2) Secondary :

(I) Common causes :

   (i) Drug and chemicals–Cytosin arabinoside, busulphan, methotrexate, vincristine–all cause purpura by depressing the bone-marrow.

   (ii) Aplastic anaemia.

   (iii) Leukaemias, Lymphomas, myelofibrosis. disseminated carcinomas – cause thrombocytopenia by infiltrating the bone-morrow.

   (iv) Hypersplenism–platelets are sequestered in the spleen.

   (v) Systemic lupus erythematosus–autoimmunity

   (vi) Liver diseases;

   (vii) Infective eodocarditis;

(viii) Deficiency of vit B_1–defective maturation;

(ix) After massive blood transfusion.

(x) Disseminated intravascular coagulation–excessive consumption of clotting factors.

(II) Rare causes :

(i) Wiskott-Aldrich syndrome–hereditary defect in maturation of platelet;

(ii) Trombotic thrombocytopenic purpura;

(iii) After prosthetic valve replacement;

(iv) Food allergy etc.

9. OEDEMA

Definition–A local or generalised condition in which the body tissues and/or the serous sacs contain an excessive amount of tissue fluid. In a restricted sense it means an increase in the extravascular component of the extracellular body fluid.

Sites–

( ) Dependent oedema or pitting oedema is classically found in congestive cardiac failure in ambulent patients; (a) at the ankle (b) on the dorsum of the foot, (c) and gradually ascends upward along the leg, thigh and trunk with increasing severity of the failure.

In patients confined to bed. examine the skin over the sacrum (small of the back). Other places like eyelids, abdomen (parietal oedema) should also be looked for. Oedema of the face, particularly puffiness of the lower eyelids is found in acute nephritic and nephrotic syndromes.

(II) Solid oedema of myxoedema of chronic lymphostatic disorders e.g. filariasis does not pit on pressure.

Method of demonstration :

Firm pressure for 5 seconds over the medial malleolus, medial surface of lower end of tibia and sacral region will produce a relatively persistent dimple.

Types of oedema : (A) Symmetrical and (B) Asymmetri cal. Symmetrical oedema may be either generalised or localised.

Causes of generalised symmetrical oedema :

(a) Congestive cardiac failure–Possible mecha- nisms are—

(i) Impairment of renal blood flow leading to a fall in the glomerular filtration rate resulting in excessive reabsorption of water and salt by the renal tubules.

[Normal renal blood flow–1.3 litres/minute. Glomerular filtration rate–180 litres/day of which 1.5 litres are excreted as urine.]

(ii) Increased central venous pressure→increased capillary pressure→transudation of fluid into interstitial space.

(iii) Secondary hyperaldosteronism and sodium retention. (ADH is found in the urine of patient with congestive cardiac failure)→increased retention of water in distal tubules.

(iv) Lymphatic factors like lymphangiectasis, incompetent valve, poor drainage also play important roles.

(v) Chronic passive congestion of liver (so reduc- tion of albumin synthesis in the liver), poor appetite and loss of protein into the oedema fluid and in urine cause hypoalbuminaemia leading to interstitial fluid accumulation.

(b) Renal :

(i) Nephrotic syndrome–Due to excessive loss of protein in the urine leading to diminished colloidal oncotic pressure (ii) Acute nephritis–inflammatory swelling of the glomeruli causes fall of glomerular filtration rate leading to relative increase in tubular reabsorption with consequent reduction in urine volume and expansion of intravascular fluid volume.

(c) Hypoproteinaemia : Oncotic pressure is mostly maintained by serum albumin, fall in concentration of which predisposes to oedema etc. The causes are–(i) Inadequate protein intake–e.g. (kwashiorkor, famine, pyloric obstruction with vomiting). (ii) Failure of digestion or absorption e.g. malabsorption syndrome, chronic pancreatitis, resection of considerable length of small intestine etc. (iii) Reduced synthesis in liver diseases like cirrhosis or chronic active hepatitis. (iv) Excessive loss of protein in the gastrointestinal tract (e.g. gluten enteropathy, ulcerative colitis, Crohn's disease, chronic gastrointestinal infection) (v) Excessive loss of protein in urine e.g. nephrotic syndrome.

Generalised symmetrical oedema may rarely be due to– (d) angioneurotic oedema, (e) idiosyncratic reaction of aspirin, potassium iodide, (f) excessive arsenic ingestion, (g) beriberi etc.

Localised symmetrical oedema may be caused by– (i) Obstruction of the superior vena cava or its main branches by mediastinal neoplasms, chronic mediastinal fibrosis, thoracic aneurysms, thrombosis etc. (ii) Erysipelas, cellulitis,

Ludwig's angina, (iii) Angioneurotic oedema, (iv) Dermatoses of various aetiologies, (v) inferior vena cava obstruction of various aetiologies, (vi) Milroy's disease (vii) Pretibial myxoedema, (viii) Epidemic dropsy etc.

Asymmetrical oedema is mainly due to (a) Local causes e.g.–(i) arteriovenous aneurysms, (ii) Milroy's disease, (iii) superficial or deep tissue infections, (iv) venous obstruction, (v) lymphatic obstruction e.g. by filariasis, metastatic carcinoma etc., (vi) Stings, bites and other causes of local inflammation; and rarely due to (b) General causes e.g. toxins, drugs angioneurotic oedema etc.

10. TEMPERATURE

Normal 98°F to 99°F, (normal body temperature shows a diurnal variation of 1.5°F with an increase towards evening, reaching the peak between 6 pm and 10 pm).

Subnormal–Below 98°F. (36. 7°C)

Pyrexia–Above 99°F. (37.2°C). An increase in the diurnal variation of more than 1.5°F is the rule, but the pattern of diurnal variation is commonly maintained.

Hyperpyrexia–Above 106°F (41.1°C)

Hypothermia–Below 95°F (35°C).

Causes of hyperpyrexia :

(1) Septicaemia (2) Lobar pneumonia (3) Heat stroke (4) Malaria (5) Pontine haemorrhage (6) Encephalitis (7) Pyelitis (8) Thyroid storm (9) Malignant hyperthermia (e.g. caused by halothange or succinylcholine) (10) Neuroleptic Malignant syndrome or NMS (caused by potent neuroleptics in therapeutic doses).

Causes of hypothermia :

(1) Myxoedema coma.

(2) Peripheral circulatory failure, congestive cardiac failure.

(3) Enteric fever, when there is haemorrhage or perforation.

(4) Accidental prolonged exposure to cold.

(5) Hypoglycaemia.

(6) Acute respiratory failure.

(7) Renal failure.

(8) Extreme wasting as in malignancy or starvation.

(9) Coma due to alcohol, barbiturates, chlorpromazine, tricyclic antidepressants, morphine etc.

Types of fever :

Continuous–The daily fluctuation is less than 1·5°F and temperature does not touch the baseline. This is commonly encountered in pneumococcal pneumonia, in second week of enteric fever, lobar pneumonia, rheumatic fever, miliary tuberculosis, meningitis etc.

Remittent—The diurnal fluctuation exceeds 2°F and does not touch the base line. This is commonly found in pulmonary tuberculosis, amoebic liver abscess, urinary tract infection etc.

Intermittent—Fever continues for several hours (usually 104°–105° F), and returns to normal sometime during the day, as occurs in vivax malaria, Types–(a) quotidian, (b) tertian, and (c) quartan.

(a) Quotidian–The paroxysm of intermittent fever occurs daily, as in septicaemia, double infection with p. vivax etc.

(b) Tertian–The paroxysm occurs on alternate

days as in benign tertian malaria due to p. vivax or malignant tertian due to p. falciparum.

(c) Quartan–The interval between the two consecutive paroxysmal attacks is two days as in quartan malaria due to p. malariae.

A combination of the above three types of fever may be found in a case of typhoid, i.e., remittent in the first week, continued in the second week and fluctuation, of 3° or 4°F in the third week.

Hectic–Temperature is characterised by a great swing e.g. a rise by 5°F during the night returning to normal in the morning accompained by sweating. This type is commonly found in septicaemia, empyema, advanced tuberculosis etc.

Shivering, commonly referred to as rigor (due to constriction of the skin vessels) occurs in infection by parasites (e.g. malaria); E coli infection, occasionally following transfusions or infusions due to some pyrogen reaction, and may be produced and perpetuated by intermittent administration of aspirin or other effective antipyretics.

The rise of temperature in acute E coli pyelitis and in pneumonia is very abrupt whereas in typhoid fever and in miliary tuberculosis the process in a gradual one. In typhoid fever, the temperature rises in a series to steps classically known as 'staircase phenomenon.'

The fall of temperature may occur by *crisis* or by *lysis.* The temperature falling quickly 6 to 12 hours is known as a crisis and is found in lobar pneumonia. Alternately the fever subsides gradually over several days by lysis infections untreated by antibiotics (as occurred in typhoid fever before the introduction of chloramphenicol) and in bronchopneumonia.

The course of fever may be regular (as in lobar pneumonia and malaria) or irregular (as in tuberculosis or bronchopneumonia).

Regular alternation of recurrent bouts of pyrexia with a period of apyrexia is known as Pel-Ebstein temperature and is sometimes seen in lymphomas (e.g. Hodgkins' disease) and an irregular alternation may sometimes be noticed in infective endocarditis.

Relapsing fever–This comprises a group of acute infectious diseases clinically characterised by cyclic periods of fever and apyrexia. Malaria is a good example, but the term is classically used for the fever caused by spirochaetes of the genus Borrelia recurrentis.

Pyrexia of unknow origin : (PUO or FUO)

I. Definition : When a fever of more than 101°F, persists for 2-3 weeks with the cause remaining obscure despite intensive study for 1 week, the fever is called pyrexia of unknown origin.

II. Causes : Some of the common causes are Hodgkin's and non-Hodgkin's lymphoma, carcinoma of lung, liver and other sites with or without metastasis, connective tissue disorders like systemic lupus erythematosus, polyarteritis nodosa, infections like tuberculosis brucellosis, subacute infective endocarditis subphrenic abscess, pyeloneph itis and hypersensitivity to a drug.

III. Investigations : PUO requires systematic and thorough clinical examination and intensive laboratory investigation to detect the cause.

Preliminary investigation (Step I) —

    (i) History (including drung history) and thorough clinical examination etc.

    (ii) Routine haemogram including differential leu cocyte count and ESR to exclude abnor malmononuclear cells suggestive of glan dular fever, leucopenia for enteric fever, viral fever and brucellosis, high ESR for collagen disease and paraprotinaemia, tuberculosis etc.

(iii) Midstream urine for routine examination microscopy, culture and sensitivity test for 6 consecutive days.

(iv) Liver function tests

(v) Plain X-ray of chest, (both P-A and lateral views)—to exclude tuberculosis, sarcoidosis and other chest infections.

(vi) For female patient—a high vaginal swab for culture and sensitivity test.

(vii) Venous blood culture, 3, taken at intervals of 1 hour, when temperature is > 101, 3°F(38.5°C) or more usually suffice, but for those who have received antimicrobials within the last 2 weeks and in whom endocarditis remains a possibility a total of 6 cultures should be taken over a 2 day period. And in emergent conditions 2 cultures are to be taken simultaneously from different anatomical sites. The femoral vein should preferably by avoided.

(viii) Plain X-ray of abdomen – so exclude subphrenic abscess enlargement of organs like kidney, liver, spleen, appendicular abscess etc.

(ix) Mantoux test.

(x) Throat swab for culture and sensitivity.

(xi) Routine examination of stool—for Entamoeba histolytica etc.

Step II :

(i) Stool culture and sensitivity for enteric fever and other salmonella infection.

(ii) Widal test–for enteric fever.

(iii) Intravenous pyelogram–when pathology in kidney is suspected or where size of the kidney is enlarged (perinephric abscess etc.)

(iv) Paul-Bunnell-test–for infectious mono-nucleosis, cytomegalovirus complement fixation test and test for toxoplasmosis–if atypical lymphocytosis or mononucleosis found in peripheral blood.

(v) Test lupus erythematosus or LE cell, antinulcear factor, rheumatoid factor or latex fixation tests if ESR is above 50 mm in first hour and clinically collagen disease is sus-pected.

(vi) Antistreptolysin (ASO) titre–if throat swab shows β-haemolytic streptococci and rheu-matic fever is suspected.

(vii) Study of plasma proteins particularly immunoglobulins–when ESR is > 50 mm and multiple myeloma or paraproteinaemia is suspected.

(Viii) Liver scan–for primary or secondary liver cancer or amoebic liver abscess. If primary cancer is suspected it can be confirmed by alpha fetoprotein (AFP) level of blood.

(ix) Coomb's test for autoimmune haemolytic anaemia.

(x) Wassermann Reaction–for secondary syphilis.

(xi) Amoeba complement fixation test.

xii) Complement fixation test for Q–fever.

Step III :

    (i)   Arterial blood culture have shown to have no additional advantage over venous blood cultures. Bone-marrow cultures may help (when blood culture is negative) in patients with disseminated salmonellosis. tuberculosis, deep mycoses etc.

    (ii)   Cholecystogram.

    (iii)   Plain X-ray of skull and paranasal sinuses.

    (iv)   Liver biopsy–for primary liver cancer cryptic form of miliary TB.

    (v)   Screening of diaphragm when plain X-ray of abdomen suggests a subphrenic abscess.

    (vi)   Bone marrow–stained film to exclude multi ple myeloma and marrow culture for AFB and Brucella.

    (vii)   Kveim test–when plain X-ray chest and nega tive Mantoux test suggest sarcoidosis.

    (viii)   Biopsy of lymph gland–for tuberculosis; lymphoma etc.

Step IV :

The following tests are to be done only for rare disorders and for unusual presentation of common diseases :

    (i)   Dental X-ray – for dental abscess which may be painless and is overlooked.

    (ii)   Bipedal Lymphangiogram–for lymphoma.

    (iii)   Fibrin degradation product in plasma and urine–for disseminated intravascular coagulation.

    (iv)   Weil-Felix-reaction–for Rickettsial diseases.

Step V :

    (i)   Laparotomy–This is done when the above

procedures fail and when factitious fever is excluded. Lymphoma, granuloma retroperitoneal abscess or arteritis may be con firmed and staged if required after biopsy.

MALARIA

Malaria is the most common infectious disease in the world (300–500 mio newly infected people per year India 2.3 Mil in 1991). There are three different types of malaria, all transmitted by female anophelese mosquitos (see fever period pages before) :

Benign type (1/3) : λ Malaria quartana (Plasmodium malaria)

λ Malaria tertiana (Pl. vivax and ovale)

Malignant type (2/3) λ malaria tropica (Pl. falciparum)

Double infections are possible, too.

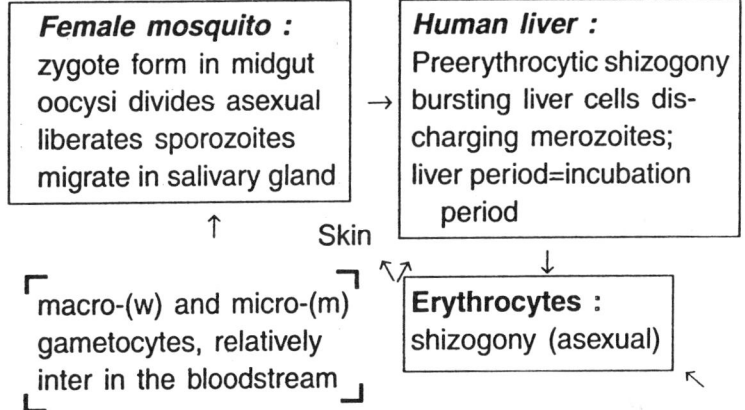

| Female mosquito : zygote form in midgut oocysi divides asexual liberates sporozoites migrate in salivary gland | $\rightarrow$ | Human liver : Preerythrocytic shizogony bursting liver cells discharging merozoites; liver period=incubation period |

↑ Skin

| macro-(w) and micro-(m) gametocytes, relatively inter in the bloodstream | Erythrocytes : shizogony (asexual) |

[release of 6-24 merozoites]

Clinical features : Malaria is an acute febrile illness with a periodic picture. The dangerous, life threatening malaria is caused by pl. falciparum, with the shortest incubation period of about 7 days. Relapses may occur in malaria tertiana as a result of reactivated liver hypnozoites. The general development is shown below :

Cold stage : Feeling of cold and apprehension, chills, malaise, headache, fatigue, shakes of the whole body (15 min-1h). chest, back abdominal and joint pain nausea vomiting clinically anaemia possible, mild jaundice with soft hepato/splenomegaly, skin cold, cyanotic and dry. pulse, low volume tachycardia.

Hot stage (2-6th) flush fever>40°C(<104°F). tachypnoea, nausea, vomiting weakness, confusion, delirious skin dry burning and flushed; pulse : high volume tachycardia.

Sweating stage (2–4th) : immense sweating temperature weak and sleepy, but more or less O.K.

Malaria	Fever perioidicity
–quartana	quartan (72h)
–tertiana	tertian (48h)
–tropica	irregular : sub-bi-tertian, (24/36/48h), quotidian

Thrombocytopenia is a marker of the severity of malaria.

Complications due to a disorders of the microcirculation is severe cases of malaria tropica (seldom in others) :

- λ Cerebral malaria → consiousness, generalized convulsion up to persisting coma (open-eyed), opisthotonos
- λ Cerebellar syndrome (common. in India) → taxia, Intention tremor, hypotonia, dysarthria and nystogymus
- λ Pulmonary oedema → possible at any stage, dyspnoea. crepitations ARDS (adult respiratory distress syndrome)

λ **Cardiovascular shock** → collapse, skin extremely cold temp.

λ **Renal dysfunction** → combined with jaundice, pro longed coma, hypoglycaemia and hypovolaemia.

Chronic malaria : large spleen and anaemia.

Malaria in infants appear with anaemia and paleness within a day or two children being breast fed and less likely to get malaria.

Diagnosis : History and examination

Blood examination :

Thick film : taken from the side of the fingerball. You should be able to read through the patch. if posssible use Field's stain.

Thin film : smaller drop than needed in thick film. Stain with Giemsa. In doubtful cases repeat blood examination every four hours. One negative slide does not mean no infection. Every   'or should be able to carry out this two blood examinations.

Fluorescent stain : (a) quantified Buffy coat technique (QBC),

(b) RNA-specific fluorochrome-benzothiocarboxypurine (BPC).

Serological tests (a) indirect fluorescent antibody test (IFAT).

Positive 6-10 days after beginning of sease (wildly used).

(b) indirect haemoagglutination test (IHA); only simple equipment necessary, but less sensitive.

(c) enzyme-linked immunosorbent assay (ELISA) small quantity of antigen required.

(d) radioimmunoassay (RIA); for research items.

Other tests : (a) Pl. falciparum-histidin-rich protein. 2 (PFIHRP-2) paper-strip test prepared with monoclonal antibodies to detect malaria tropica, but less sensitive than microscopic examination.

(b) polymerase chain reaction (PCR) and transcript amplification system (TAS) to detect DNA and RNA.

Start immediatly after diagnosis if the species in not known or you face a mixed infection treat as falciparum malaria.

Generally keep in mind :

1. Select falciparum drug treatment according to your local resistant pattern!

2. There are chloroquine-resistant species in some regions, so be aware of if success stays away!

3. Do not treat with chloroquine when used as prophylaxis!

4. Reexamine patient after some weeks for signs of recrudescence !

Drug groups	Effectivity	Side effect
Arylaminoalcohols	blood schizontocides	
λ Quinine/Qinidine (i.v.,p.o.)	severe m. tropical and in pregnancy	hypoglycaemia, allergy
λ Mefloquine (p.o.)	prophylaxis	bradycardia, acute brain syndrome not in pregnancy!
λ Halofantrine (p.o.)	multiresistant malaria tropica (MRPE)	prolongation of ECG QT interval !not in pregnancy!
4. aminoquinolines: λ Chloroquine (i.v.,p.o.)	blood schizontocides benign malaria uncomplicated m. tropica (not everywhere)	i.v. hypotension. longterm : blurring of vision, pruritus
λ Pyronaridine	MRPF	dizziness, headache GI-disorders

Drug groups	Effectivity	Side effect
8. aminoquinolines:	hypnozoites, gameto-cytocides	
λ Primaquine	redical cure of P. vi vaxlovale, eliminates sexual cycle in p. falciparum	haemolysis in G6PD deficiency methaemoglobin-aemia
λ WR-238.605	ten times more effective	new drug with less experience
Biguanides :	blood schizonticides	
λ Pyrimethamine	in combination with sulfonamides for acute treatment and prophylaxis of falciparum malaria	not in pregnancy and 6 weeks child Steven-Johnson syndrome
Sulfonamides :	blood schizonticides	
λ Sulfadoxine	in combination with	Urticaria, hepatitis,
λ Cotrimoxazole	pyrimethamine and proguanil	agranulocytosis; ! not in pregnancy!
Peroxides :	blood schizontocides	
λ Artemisinin	severe complicated falciparum; cerebral malaria	experimental stage new drugs; erytrotoxic bone-mar-
λ Artemether	severe falciparum	.row, cardiotoxic
λ Artesunate	uncomplicated falciparum; better combined with mafloquine	Feticide
Naphthoquinones :	all growing stages	
λ Atavaquone	experimental drugs in	
λ BW566C80	research stage	

1997 the WHO announced that malaria becomes a major problem in the future. The scientific re-search dominated by the rich countries (USA and Europe) have no further interest in developing new effective drugs or vaccination against malaria. There are some ideas about future treatment, but not yet in research state. The most difficult matter in malaria is the fast development of resistance especially plasmodium falciparum, which causes malaria tropica.

Treatment Table

Falciparum malaria

11. PULSE

(i) Definition–Pulse is the lateral expansion of the

Drug	Dosage
Quinine salt (not bisulphate type)	600 mg/8h po for 7 days in severe ill patients : 20mg/kg over 4th iv (max. 1.4g).
Next	followed by 10 mg/kg iv over 4h after 8-12h interval (max. 0.7g) this repeated untill pat can swallow to complete 7 days treatment 3 tablets as a single dose
Pyrimethamine plus Sulfadoxine or in Fansidar-resistant areas Tetracycline	250 mg/6th for 7 days
Mefloquine	20 mg/kg (base) divided in two doses with 6-8h interval po
Halofantrine	3 × 500 mg 6h in between and repeated after one week (on empty stomach)

Benign malaria

Drug	Dosage
Chloroquine base 150 mg = phosphate (po) 250 mg =sulphate (iv) 200 mg in P vivax and ovale cradieation therapy is to be added after above course with	initially 600 mg (base) followed by 300 mg single dose 6-8h later next two days 300 mg single dose total amount of 3 days should be 25 mg/kg chloroquine base.
Primaquine	15 mg/d for 14-21 days

arterial wall imparted by the column of arterial blood due to contraction of the left vantricle.

(ii) Rate–Beats per minute, normal 60 to 100 per minute, average 72 beats per minute in adult and 130 per minute at birth.

Bradycardia–Rate less than 60 per minute.

Causes : (1) Physiological–in trained athletes, during sleep etc.

(2) Pathological

Vasovagal attacks.

Myxoedema.

Obstructive jaundice.

Raised intracranial tension.

Drug e.g. digitalis propranolol.

Different types of heart block; the rate is 20 to 40 beats per minute in complete heart block.

Sick sinus syndrome.

Other causes include hypothermia, acute nephritis, phaeochromocytoma, aortic stenosis, carotid sinus synciope etc.

Tachycardia–Rate more than 100 per minute, found normally in infants and in anxiety state.

Relative bradycardia–When with per degree rise of temperature [F] the pulse rate increase is less than 10 beats per minute, the condition is called relative bradycardia. For example, when temperature rises to 100°F pulse rate should be about 82 per minute normally, but less than this if there is relative bradycardia. Relative bradycardia is found in first week of enteric fever meningitis etc.

Relative tachycardia– Here pulse rate rises by more

than 10 beats per minute per degree rise of temperature and is seen in rheumatic carditis, tuberculosis etc.

Sinus tachycardia–Pulse rate varying between 100-160 per minute, It indicates that the cardiac impulse arises from the sino atrial node.

Physiological causes of sinus tachycardia : Exercise, emotion, belladonna group of drugs amyl nitrite or other vasodilators etc. are known to produce sinus tachycardia.

Pathological causes : Shock acute haemorrhage, fever, thyrotoxicosis, severe anaemia, congestive cardiac failure, cardiac neurosis, toxaemia, phaeochromocytoma, severe myocardial disease etc.

Paroxysmal tachycardia–more than 160 beats per min, usually between 180 and 200 per minute. The ventricles almost always respond to each atrial beat, rarely there may be 2 : 1 atrioventricular block.

Causes of paroxysmal atrial tachycardia (PAT) : Rheumatic carditis, mitral stenosis, ischaemic heart disease, hypertensive heart disease, thyrotoxicosis, atrial septal defect. Wolf-Parkinson-White (WPW) syndrome (characterised by paroxysmal atrial tachycardia short P-R interval, wide QRS complex, a slur on the initial phase of the QRS complex–the delta wave), cardiomyopathy functional e.g. anxiety state etc.

Exertion, emotion, coffee, alcohol etc. are the aggravating factors. PAT with block is sometimes encountered in digitalis intoxication with hypokalaemia.

(iii) *Rhythm*–Spacing of successive pulse waves in time. The rhythm may be regular or irregular, the latter may be completely irregular (irregularly irregular) or the rhythm is occasionally interrupted by slight irregularity or a recurring pattern of irregularity (regularly irregular). Thus the pulse in atrial fibrillation, multiple extrasystoles, partial heart block with dropped beats, atrial flutter with varying degrees of A-V block are *irregularly irregular* whereas in premature beats, sinus arrhythmia and atrial flutter with 2 : 1 block it is *regularly irregular*

Sinus rhythms : Impulse originates in the SA node. Types–(a) sinus bradycardia, (b) sinus tachycardia, (c) sinus arrhythmia in which the heart rate increase with inspiration and slows down in expiration. It is increased by deep breathing and abolished by exercise. This variety is normally encountered in children and young people and usually absent in elderly individuals large ASD, heart failure sick sinus syndrome etc.

Ectopic rhythms : Here the impulse arises from a site other than the S-A node e.g. in the atria, A-V node or ventricles. The rhythm may be regular or irregular.

Premature (Ectopic) beat or Extrasystole–It arises from some abnormal focus in the heart, occurs prematurely, is small and followed by a compensatory pause. It may be caused by overindulgence in coffee, tobacco and alcohol; dyspepsia, anxiety or organic heart disease like rheumatic carditis, ischaemic heart disease, hypertension or cardiomyopathy etc. When a premature beat follows each normal beat, the pulse is said to be coupled and designated as *pulsus begeminus.*

Atrial fibrillation, atrial flutter and atrial tachycardia may be regarded as similar ectopic rhythms which differ only in the rate of the ectopic atrial focus. A rate of 140 to 220 per minute result in atrial tachycardia; a rate of 250 to 350 per minute is atrial flutter and rates above 350 per minute is atrial fibrillation.

Paroxysmal tachycardia may be supraventricular (atrial, atrial tachycardia with A-V block nodal) or ventricular. Ventricular tachycardia (VT) is commonly encountered in ischaemic heart disease, digitalis toxicity, electrolyte and or acid base imbalance etc.

Atrial flutter–Rapid regular generation of impulse occurs at a rate of 250-350 per minute in the atria, all of which cannot traverse the A-V node and so usually there is 2 : 1 physiological heart block. The block may increase to 3 : 1 or 4 : 1 when carotid pressure is applied, (due to increased vagal tone) and so the ventricular rate diminishes transiently but the sinus rhythm is not restored. Vagal stimulation in a case of paroxysmal supraventricular tachycardia (PSVT) will either terminate the paroxysm or have not effect. Rheu-matic heart disease, ischaemic heart disease and thyrotoxicosis are the common causes of atrial flutter.

Atrial fibrillation–Rapid fibrillation waves (f waves in ECG take the place of normal atrial contractions and ventricles respond at random. The atrial rate is between 350 and 600 per minute. The A-V node cannot conduct so many impulses and varying degrees of heart block always exist in an untreated patient as a result of concealed conduction. The ventricular rate is usually 100–150 per minute. It is recognised clinically by complete irregularity of the pulse both in rate and volume and the varying intensities of the irregular heart sounds. pheumatic, ischaemic, hypertensive and thyrotoxic heart diseases are the common causes of atrial fibrillation.

Heart block–It is either S-A of A-V block. In S-A block a complete cardiac cycle is missed so that a gap appears in the pulse and is due to increased vagal tone or intrinsic SA nodal disease. Conduction between the atria and the ventricles is impaired in A-V block, which may be of three types :

(a) First degree block : detected most commonly by the ECG which reveals P-R interval more than 0.2 second.

(b) Second degree of partial heart block : Some impulses from the atrial do not reach the ventrical. It may be of three types :–

(1) Mobitz Type I or Wenckebach type : Gradual prolongation of P-R interval followed by a dropped beat–the cycle is repeated; better prognosis.

(2) Mobitz Type II (periodic block)–The P-R or P-P intervals remain unaltered and any one P-wave is not followed by QRS complex e.g. 6 : 5 A-V block.

(3) Second degree constant block e.g. 2 : 1, 3 : 1 or 4 : 1 A-V blocks.

(c) Third degree or complete heart block : In this type no impulse from atria reaches the ventricles and hence the atria and ventricles contract independent of each other and the ventricular rate is usually between 20 to 40 per minute. Ischaemic heart disease, calcific aortic stenosis rheumatic cardiovascular diseases, syphilitic heart disease, congenital cardiac lesions, digitalis, infectious diseases like diphtheria etc. are the common causes of heart block.

Ventricular fibrillation (VF) : This arrhythmia is characterised by rapid, irregular, uncoordinated and ineffective contractions of the ventricles. It may occur in acute myocardial infarction as a complication of general anaesthesia by chloroform of cyclopropane, after toxic doses of digitalis or quinidine etc. Clinical presentation may be as Stocks-Adams syndrome with syncope and convulsion.

(iv) *Volume* : It is defined as amplitude of pulse wave. It signifies left ventricular output per beat.

Causes of high volume pulse : Hyperkinetic circulatory

states eg, fever severe anaemia, thyrotoxicosis, aortic incompetence and corpulmonale, atheros clerosis of aorta, complete heart block or gross bradycardia from any cause etc.

Causes of low volume pulse : aortic stenosis, tight mitral stenosis, pulmonary stenosis, severe pulmonary hypertension, obstructive cardiomyopathy, pericardial effusion, shock due to any cause etc.

(v) *Tension* : Pressure required to obliterate the pulse is known as systolic tension. Optimum pressure exerted by the proximal finger to have the maximum thrust felt by the middle finger is said to be diastolic tension. Sphygmomanometry being such a simple, easy, and accurate procedure, estimation of tension had become obsolete.

(vi) *Condition of arterial wall* : It should be noted for evidence of arterial thickening or undue mobility. Using 3 fingers, exsanguinate the artery and then roll over the bony surface. Sufficient pressure is applied on the brachial artery to abolish pulsation in the radial artery which should then be rolled over the bony surface. Normally the arterial wall is not palpable. It may be palpable in old age due to arteriosclerosis (tortusity and cord like thickening).

(vii) *Equality* : Comparison of volume of pulse of two upper and lower extremities. *Causes of inequality between the radial pulses are—*

(i) Anatomical variations.

(ii) Thoracic inlet syndrome.

(iii) Pre-subclavian coarctation.

(iv) Pressure over axillary artery.

(v) Volkmann's ischaemic contracture.

(vi) Aortic arch syndrome.

(vii) Supravalvular aortic stenosis etc.

N.B.– Radial artery and femoral artery should be palpated simultaneously to detect coarctation of aorta. Delayed pulsation of femoral artery compared to that of radial artery, i.e. radio femoral delay suggests coarctation of aorta. Difference of timing of radial and dorsalis pedis pulse is 0.02 to 0.03 second. Inequality of brachial pulse may be due to thrombosis, embolism or atherosclerosis of aorta.

Bounding pulse : A large pulse wave signifying a high pulse pressure, associated with increased blood flow, seen in hyperkinetic circulartory states.

12 RESPIRATION

The rate, rhythm and type of breathing are determined by placing the hand over the epigastrium and noting the features of respiration without the patient's knowledge.

(a) *Rate :* 18-20 per minute in adults.

Increased rate (tachypnoea)

- (i) Fever
- (ii) Exertion
- (iii) Excitement and emotion
- (iv) Pulmonary diseases e.g. pneumonia pulmonary embolism etc.
- (v) Hypoxaemia from cardiac or pulmonary causes as in interference with reflex control of respira tion by structural changes in lung e.g. fibrosing alveolitis.
- (vi) Shallow and frequent breathing in pleurisy and peritonitis.

(b) Rhythm : Varies considerably even among nor mal individuals

Biot's breathing : This is a type of periodic breathing where periods of apnoea are interrupted by a phase of hyperpnoea consisting of four or five breaths only all of which are of the same amplitude and the beginning and the end of the phases are abrupt but no waxing and waning of respiration is seen. This is commonly found in children suffering from meningitis, but may occur in primary brainstem lesions and in increased intracranial tensions.

Inspiration may be unduly prolonged in laryngeala or tracheal diseases, whereas expiration may be prolonged in bronchial or pulmonary disease.

Cheyne-Stoke breathing : This is the commonest variety of periodic breathing (independently described by John Cheyne in 1818 and William Stokes in 1846) in which the respiration becomes gradually deeper until a peak is reached and this is followed by a complete pause of breathing or apnoea. The pause lasts for 10 to 30 seconds while the hyperpnoeic phase of 30 or more breaths lasts for 1 to 3 minutes. The patient may remain asymptomatic; it is usually prominent at night.

Causes of Cheyne-Stokes respiration :

- (i) Left ventricular failure : Commonest cause, par ticularly in those with degenerative arterial diaeases.
- (ii) Renal failure.
- (iii) Morphine poisoning.
- (iv) Bronchopneumonia or other respiratory infec- tions in the elderly.
- (v) Occasionally during recovery from Stokes- Adams attacks.
- (vi) Increased intracranial tension, cerebral haemor- rhage, thrombosis cerebral tumours and severe head injuries.
- (vii) In sleep in apparently healthy elderly subjects.
- (viii) In normal subjects at high altitudes and after hyper ventilation.

(c) *Types* :		
(i) Thoracic. e.g. In women*	(ii) Abdominal e.g.	(iii) Abdominc-thoracic e.g. In men
Anxiety states	young children	
Hysteria,	Pneumothorax,	Pleurisy (restriction
Diphragmatic	chest movement due	of severe pain).
palsy. Acute	to losing spondylitis.	Anky-Intercostal
peritonitis.		paralysis.
Huge ascites.		

13. BLOOD PRESSURE

Blood pressure is measured by the sphygmomanometer. The width of the cuff is 12 cm for an adult, 3 inches for young children. 1 inch for infants and the length should be no less than 25 cm. To avoid a falsely high blood pressure in the leg a wider (8 inch) cuff should be used as this compresses the thigh more effectively than the narrower one which is used for the arm.

Casual recording of the blood pressure may not give the true figure due to exercise, fear of emotion and thus it varies from time to time. So the blood pressure should be recorded with the patient at rest in a comfortable position.

To measure blood pressure in the arm the patient should lie flat, on his back, whereas for that of the leg the patient should lie prone (as the systolic pressure will be much higher if the patient sits or stands up). Before commencing the recording of blood pressure, the patient should remain at rest in supine (or prone) positions for 5 minutes.

In recording the blood pressure, particular care should be taken to wrap the cuff firmly and evenly around the base of the arm about 2.5 cm above the elbow joint, with the middle of the rubber bag over the brachial artery. The arm

---

* in last trimen on of pregnency

should not be hyperextended as it may introduce error in recording the diastolic pressure. The cuff should then be inflated till the radial pulse disappears and then deflated slowly. The point at which radial pulse first reappears indicates the systolic pressure. As the cuff is further deflated, pulsation of radial artery gradully assumes a water hammer character and then all on a sudden resumes its normal character, the reading corresponding to the sudden change represent the diastolic pressure.

In auscultatory method the diaphragm of the stetho-scope should be placed over the brachial artery close to or under the edge of the sphygmomanometer cuff. Care should be taken that the diaphragm is not pressed heavily over the artery as it may give wrong diastolic pressure. The cuff is then inflated quickly to 20 mm above the systolic pressure recorded by palpation and slowly deflated.

The highest level at which successive clear, tapping sounds (Korotkoff's phase I) are heard is the systolic pressure. As the pressure is further lowered in the cuff, the point at which louder and sharper sounds suddenly become muffled (Korotkoff's phase IV) or inaudible (Korotkoff's phase V) indicate the diastolic pressure. Normally sounds disappear few mm below the change over/but in aortic incompetence sounds may be audible even at zero pressure. Experimentally it has been shown that direct record-ing of intraarterial diastolic pressure more closely corre-lates with mufling than when the sounds completely disap-pear.

To measure the blood pressure in the thigh the sphygmomanometer cuff should be adjusted around the lower part of the bare thigh with the patient in prone position. The diaphragm of the stethoscope is to be placed over popliteal artery.

N. B. – If anaeroid gauges are used, they must be calibrated every 6 months against a mercury manometer.

Auscultatory (silent) gap–

Sometimes as phase of silence may separate the first appearance of Korotkoff's sounds from their second appearance at a lower pressure and this the auscultatory gap. The phenomenon tends to occur in–(i) venous distension, (ii) reduced arterial flow velocity into the arms as in severe aortic stenosis. In such cases the diastolic pressure will be overestimated if recorded at the point of first muffling of sounds and the systolic one will be underestimated if recorded at the point of second appearance of sounds. The auscultatory gap is of obvious clinical importance in systemic hypertension.

In an arrhythmia, the higher pressure of the beat following an ectopic beat should be ignored.

In atrial fibrillation the systolic pressure should be taken at the point where the majority of beats come through and the diastolic pressure where the majority of beats become muffled.

When there is a differnece of pulse volumes between the two arms as in presubclavian coarctation, aortic arch syndrome. supraclavicular aortic, stenosis, pressure over the brachial artery by enlarged lymph gland etc. blood pressure in both the arms should be recorded. Slight disparity (less than 5 mm Hg) between reading from each arm is common in atherosclerotic and hypertensive patients and is not of much clinical significance.

Blood pressure should also be recorded in both arms and legs when there is feeble or delayed pulsation in femoral, popliteal, posterior tibial or dorsalis pedis arteries as may occur in saddle shaped embolism at the bifurcation of the abdominal aorta and more significantly in coarctation of aorta.

Normal Blood pressure :

In infancy the systolic pressure is 75 to 90 mm Hg; in childhood 90 to 110 mm Hg : and in puberty 100 to 120 mm Hg. The diastolic pressure varies from 50 to 70 mm Hg. till puberty. Blood pressure varies widely in healthy adult subjects. Systolic pressure varies from 100 to 145 mm Hg and diastolic from 60 to 90 mm Hg. The upper limit of the normal blood pressure for adults below 45 years is 130/80 mm Hg, for adults above 45 years 140/90 mm Hg; the systolic pressure in legs is up to 20 mm Hg above that in the arms in a normal individual in the horizontal position, but the diastolic ones are almost identical.

Pulse pressure is the difference between systolic and diastolic pressures. Normally it is 30 to 60 mm Hg.

In children below 15 years, systolic pressure over 130 mm Hg and diastolic pressure over 80 mm Hg is considered hypertension.

In adult individuals, if the blood pressures are in excess* (160/100 MHg) of the above mentioned values after several controls, hypertension should be diagnosed.

Divergent blood pressures (eg 160/20 mm Hg) are found in arteriosclerosis, aortic incompetence, pheochromocytoma etc.

Systolic hypertension is encountered in atherosclerosis, aortic incompetence, complete heart block with severe bradycardia etc. Diastolic hypertension is encountered in essential hypertension, renal diaseases, eclampsia, Coushing's syndrome, pheochromocytoma etc.

N.B.– Very recently a simple method has been devised that records only the systolic blood pressure. The instruments is known as finger sphygmomanometer and can be used on any of the four fingers. Compared to the conven-

---

*(>160/100 mm Hg)

tional device, it is claimed to be a more reliable indicator for making diagnostic and therapeutic decisions and in one recent study it had a specificify of 98.5% during routine screening compared to the conventional mercury column device that had a specificity of 97.6% (BMJ, 1986, 293; 775). To sum up a few recent recommendations of the British Hypertension Society (BMJ, 1986, 293 611) are outlined here with some modifications.

(i) An anaeroid type loses accuracy over time and so it should be checked at different pressure levels by connecting with a Y piece to the tubing of a standardised mercury manometer.

(ii) Bladder lengths should be 80 cm of arm circumference; 35 cm for a normal and lean arm, 42 cm for a muscular and obese arm, < 12 cm for children below 5 years.

(iii) Sitting and supine pressures make little difference in BP and arm must be at heart level and supported during measurement otherwise the BP reading will be falsely high.

(iv) The mercury manometer must be vertical, at eye level and not more than 3 feet from the observer.

(v) A digit preference bias is best avoided by recording to the nearest 2mm Hg.

(vi) The auscultatory (silent) gap occurs when Korotkoff sounds disappear between the systolic and diastolic pressure and may lead to underestimation of the systolic pressure unless first recorded by palpation and if a silent gap is present, it must be clearly recorded.

(vii) The BP of children below 5 years cannot be measured easily by the usual BP instrument and in them the BP measured on different occasions varies considerably. Thus only when clinically indicated measurement of BP in them should be undertaken and moderate deviations from normal should be ignored.

REGIONAL EXAMINATION

HEAD AND NECK

(a) Inspection and palpation. Look for any abnormalities in or for position, size, shape, any asymmetry, deformity, irregularity and depression or elevation. in Kippel-Feil syndrome, the neck is short mobility restricted, a characteristic posture of the neck is seen and there may be mirror movements of the limbs. Slight bending may be noticed in a defect of vision (an attempt by the patient of compensate as occurs in head tilting to the opposite side with *superior oblique paralysis* of one side) or in abscesses or localised infections of the neck avoid discomfort. Hypertrophic changes in bones as with an underlying *meningioma* without any defect in the scalp may occasionally be found. Bossing of skull bones and a square shape may be found in *rickets*. The frontal eminences are very much exaggerated, the bridge of the nose is depressed and the forehead is vertical in *congenital syphilis*. The skull assumes a globular form in *hydrocephalus*. The sutures are opened up and imperfectly ossified areas are seen in *craniotabes*. The skull is bigger particularly in the transverse diameter in Paget's disease. Skull appears large in contrast to short stature in *achondroplasia*. Skull appears small compared to prominent supraorbital ridges and lower jaw in *acromegaly*. Long headed skull is known as *dolicocephaly* where as a bulletheaded skull is called *brachycephaly*. In *oxycephaly* or "steeple head" the skull is conical or tower shaped because the coronal and saggital sutures undergo premature synostosis and is seen in *gargoylism*,

Apert's syndrome etc. Oxycephaly is also known as *acrocephaly* and shows overgrowth of the vertex, exophthalmos, optic atrophy and a divergent squint.

Localised swelling of the skull may be present due to sebaceous cyst, tumours like osteoma, fibroma, sceondary deposit, acute leukaemias, dermoid cyst, encephalocele etc. *Leontiasis ossea* is a progressive irregular enlargement of the cranial and facial bones resulting in asymmetry and the superior maxilla is especially prominent. In Parry-Romberg disease there is facial hamiatrophy.

(b) Occasionally a bruit may be audible on auscultation over the temporal parietal and forntal regions, and may be due to—

(i) Carotido-cavernous fistula (thrills and bruits over the eyes).

(ii) Intracranial aneurysms.

(iii) Intracranial angiomas e.g. Struge-Weber syndrome (haemangiomas of leptomeninges with mucocutaneous haemangiomas along the distribution of trigeminal nerve and facial naevus one on side).

(iv) Angiomas of scalp.

(v) Brain tumours.

(vi) Paget's disease.

(c) Neck rigidity (must be seen as a routine).

(d) Any evidence of exophthalmos should be looked for.

(e) Involuntary movements of the head in diseases e.g.— (i) Park-insonism—constant tremor. (ii) Habit spasms—sudeen jerky movement with facial grimace. (iii) de Musset's sign—jerky head movements with each heart beat seen in severe aortic regurgitation (iv) Chorea–sudden, jerky movements.

(f)   *Neck Veins :* The patient should be propped up by a back rest to any angle that best and *maximally* demonstrates the jugular venous pulsation (the angle is that between the trunk and the level of the bed at the hip joint). The top to the oscillating venous blood column should be identified and the different waves determined. Normally the pulsations of the neck veins should not be above the root of the neck at an angle of 45% If it is significantly above that level most possibly the patient is in congestive cardiac failure. If the vein is engorged but not pulsatile *superior mediastinal syndrome* is suspected where there is obstruction to venous return in the SVC.

The internal jugular vein is ideally examined in preference to the external jugular and venous pulsations both sides of neck should be seen as a routine, but that of the right side is a better indicator of the activities of the right heart.

Hepato Jugular reflex : Increased jugular venous pulsations can be demonstrated incongestive cardiac failure by applying pressure on the liver or the anterior abdominal wall. This increases the intraabdominal venous pressure leading to increased venous return to the right heart which cannot be compensated in heart failure and even early congestive cardiac failure can be diagnosed. It is better termed as abdominojugular reflux.

Carotid artery : Normally the carotid artery pulsation is seen anterior to the sternomastoid muscle. The pulsation is exaggerated in nervous individuals, in normal persons during excitement, aortic incompetence, thyrotoxicosis, fever severe anaemia pregnancy, patent ductus arteriosus, coarctation of the aorta and kinking of the carotid artery (kinked carotid) due to elevation of the aortic arch as a result of hypertension or atherosclerosis, particularly in females, on the right side. Carotid kinking may be confused with the pulsating aneurysm at the base of the right common carotid artery.

The pulsation is *diminished* in carotid artery stenosis, aortic arch syndrome, severe aortic stenosis, mitral stenosis and pulmonary stenosis.

The exaggerated carotid pulsation in aortic incompetence is known as Corrigan's sign. Inspection of carotid pulsation may reveal atrial or ventricular premature beats as also atrial fibrillation. Enlargement of the carotid artery with each pulsation is seen in aneurysm of the carotid artery as well as on the right side in kinked carotid. Silent carotid pulsation is a common feature in severe aortic stenosis and severe pulmonary stenosis.

(g) *Thyroid Gland* : The gland should ideally by palpated from behind after well exposure of the neck which is slightly flexed. Patient must be in the sitting posture. The patient is asked to swallow and note whether the gland moves up and down. The gland should also be examined from the front by Kocher's method with the patient supine and the neck adequately extended by placing a pillow in the nape of the neck. The isthmus and the two lobes are to be palpated. Thrills or bruits over the gland may be found on routine examination.

(h) *Lymph Glands* : Cervical lymph glands are examined from behind with the neck slightly flexed. Glands should be palpated in a definite order starting from the occipital lymph glands and gradually proceeding to postauricular, anterior auricular, tonsillar, submandibular and submental lymph glands, glands of the anterior and posterior triangles of the neck both on the upper and lower parts and lastly the supraclavicular lymph glands.

After the examination of the cervical lymph glands, the axillary, the epitrochlear and the inguinal lymph glands are palpated as a routine. The group or groups of glands affected, their consistency, tenderness and whether these are discrete or matted are to be noted very carefully to arrive at a clinical diagnosis.

Cervical lymph glands may be enlarged in—

1. *Infections e.g.—*
   - (a) Infections from the surrounding area, e.g. aural infection, throat infection, scalp infection. Usually caused by pyogenic streptococci and staphylococci.
   - (b) Tuberculosis (Cervical adenitis or scrofula).
   - (c) Infectious mononucleosis.
   - (d) Syphilis.
   - (e) Rubella.
   - (f) Viral (e.g. cytomegalovirus infection and pharyngoconjunctival fever caused by adenovirus).
   - (g) Toxoplasmosis.
   - (h) Histoplasmosis.
   - (i) Brucellosis.

II. *Neoplastic condition e.g.—*
   - (1) Hodgkin's and non-Hodgkin lymphomas.
   - (2) Chronic lymphatic leukaemia.
   - (3) Acute leukaemias.
   - (4) Metastases from solid tumour e.g. carcinoma of head, neck, thyroid, lung, stomach, breast etc.

III. *Miscellaneous conditions e.g.—*
   - (1) Sarcoidosis.
   - (2) Connective tissue diseases like systemic lupus erythematosus (SLE) rheumatoid arthritis, dermatomyositis etc.

CAUSES OF GENERALISED LYMPHADENOPATHY

(Involving more than two separate node groups)
  I. Hodgkin's and non-Hodgkin lymphomas,
 II. Acute and chronic lymphatic leukaemias,
III. Miliary tuberculosis,
 IV. Infectious mononucleosis,
  V. Sarcoidosis,
 VI. Toxoplasmosis and histoplasmosis,
VII. Secondary syphilis,
VIII. Brucellosis,
 IX. Histiocytosis,
  X. Infectious hepatitis,
 XI. Immunoblastic lymphadenopathy,
XII. Persistent generalised lymphadenopathy. (PGL)
     and
XIII. Acquired Immune Deficiency Syndrome (AIDS).

When there is generalised lymphoglandular enlargement, routine clinical examination of liver and spleen
should be done and any tenderness in the sternum or iliac
crest or other bones (due to marrow hyperplasia) is to be
found out. In leukaemia, sarcoidosis and tuberculosis chest
X-rays should be taken. When leukaemia and lymphomas
are suspected, examination of peripheral blood for the
detection of abnormal cells and examination of bone-
marrow by sternal puncture of iliac crest biopsy are
essential for confirmation of the diagnosis. Next procedure
is to remove a lymph gland (gland biopsy) for histological
examination. The gland which is most superficial and
isolated should be selected. This procedure may be helpful
in differentiating tuberculosis from lymphoma at a certain
stage of the disease. Lung tomography (to demonstrate
mediastinal and hilarlymphadenopathy), lymphangiography
(to exclude involvement of abdominal lymph glands) and

bone scan (to note whether any skeletal structure is involved or not), are done in a suspected case of lymphoma. Even laparotomy and splenectomy are needed for confirmaion of the diagnosis and staging of lymphomas.

CLUBBING : This is physical sign characterised by bulbous changes and diffuse enlargement of the terminal phalanges of the fingers and toes and is due to an increase in the volume of the soft tissues as well as increased curvature of the nails in both longitudinal and transverse plains. The angle between the nail and nail bed (the Lovibond's angle), gets obliterated and hence clubbing is also known as *Lovibond's sign.* The phenomenon of clubbing is also termed *Hippocratic fingers.* Hypertrophic osteoarthropathy is usually considered as a further extension of the clubbing process and in this the changes are in the larger bones and joints of distal parts of limbs.

Pathology–Proliferation of subungual connective tissue.

Degree : (a) First degree–There is only increased fluctuation of the nail bed.

(b) Second degree–There is an increased anteroposterior and transverse diameter in addition to fluctuation.

(c) Third degree–Combination of the changes described above and increased pulp tissue.

(d) Fourth degree–Combination of the above changes and subperiosteal thickening in bones of wrist and ankle.

In hypertrophic osteoarthropathy there is thickening of the periosteum of radius, ulna, tibia and fibula in addition to the clubbing of fingers, Hypertrophic osteoarthropathy is also known as secondary hypertrophic osteoarthritis. It is frequently associated with disorders of the lungs particularly bronchial carcinoma. It also occurs in association with pleural tumours but is quite rare in secondary tumours of lung. It may also be either familial or idiopathic. When sufficiently progressed, ribs, clavicles and scapulae may be involved. Any disorder causing clubbing may cause hypertrophic pulmonary osteoarthropathy. The most reliable sign for mild clubbing is the obliteration of the Lovibond's angle.

Mechanism : It is known that clubbing mostly occurs first in the thumb and index fingers, subsequently spreading to the other digits but the exact mechanism is not definitely known. Some theories have been postulated. These include—(i) Toxic e.g. infective endocarditis. (ii) Anoxia e.g. congenital cyanotic group of heart diseases (e.g. Fallot's tetralogy (iii) Reflex phenomena–Improvement of clubbing in bronchogenic carcinoma after vagotomy supports reflex theory. (iv) Metabolic–clubbing in thyrotoxicosis and in acromegaly may probably be due to abnormal metabolic process. (v) Alteration of the pressure gradient between the radial artery and digital artery may play some role in the formation of clubbing.

Lobectomy in Pancoast's tumour and decortication in empyema may produce some improvement of clubbing. All these also may improve hypertrophic pulmonary osteoarthropathy.

Causes of Clubbing : These may be remembered by the following mnemonic :

C	L	U	BB	I	N	G
Cardiac diseases like congenital cyanotic heart diseases, infective endocarditis, cardiac tumours.	Lung disease (a) Bronchiectasis (b) Lung abscess (c) Empyema. (d) Fibrocaseous also type of tuberculosis (e) Bronchogenic carcinoma.	Ulcerative colitis	Biliary and other types of cirrhosis	Intestinal (Steatorrhoea) Regional enteritis intestinal tuberculosis, abdominal Hodgkin's chronic bacillary and amoebic dysentery	Normal in some people	Genetic factors

Miscellaneous Causes

(1) Occupational (2) Thyrotoxicosis (3) Acromegaly (4) Carpal tunnel syndrome (5) Sarcoidosis (6) Asbestosis

Unilateral clubbing may be found in presubclavian coarctation, bronchogenic carcinoma and in aneurysm of right subclavian artery.

Painful clubbing may be in bronchogenic carcinoma.

In the presence of hypertrophic osteoarthopathy the most important condition to be excluded is an intrathoracic neoplasm and it has been said that osteoarthropathy militates against a diagnosis of tuberculosis.

UPPERLIMBS : EXAMINATION OF ARMS AND HANDS :

(A) Length of both arms and arm span is compared with the trunk;–this may help in the diagnosis of Marfan's syndrome.

(B) Following points are noted in examination of hand:

(i) Clubbing–Vide supra.

(ii) Digital throbbing–It signifies vasodilatation, it can be demonstrated by holding the fingers of the patient's right hand with the fingers of the examiner's right hand in the position of flexion.

(iii) Capillary pulsation–This is classically demonstrated on the inner surface of the lower lip which is everted and a glass slides is pressed firmly on the mucous membrane to produce an area of blanching. The blanched area becomes pink with each systole in aortic incompetence. This can be demonstrated in the nails also.

Nails may show significant *pitting* in psoriasis.

(iv) Splinter haemorrhages under the nails may be

present in infective endocarditis, scurvy, rheumatic heart disease, occasionally in normal subjects trichinosis, rheumatoid arthritis SLE etc.

(v) Osler's node–It has a pale centre with surrounding
erythema due to arteriolar embolism. The lesion
is characteristic of infective endocarditis and is
found in fingers or toes, in the palms or in the sole.

(vi) Hand may be warm and signifies thyrotoxicosis,
wet beri-beri, chronic respiratory failure and Paget's
disease of bone. Cold hand may be due to
exposure to cold, neurosis, low cardiac output
states and Raynaud's phenomenon.

(vii) Flat (even concave), fragile or spoon shaped nail
(koilonychia) may be found in iron deficiency
anaemia, thyrotoxicosis or it may be congenital;
white nails (leuconychia) may be found in chronic
liver diseases (like portal cirrhosis) including cardiac cirrhosis.

(viii) Palmar erythema may be found in physiological
conditions like pregnancy and in pathological
conditions like fever, thyrotoxicosis, rheumatoid
arthritis, anoxic corpulmonale, hepatic failure,
chronic alcoholism etc.

(ix) Any wasting of muscle is to be noted. This is
commonly found in motor neurone diseases, thoracic inlet syndrome, carpal tunnel syndrome, lead
neuritis and leprosy etc.
Any atrophy of the skin is to be noted which is
commonly found in old age, reumatoid arthritis
and in osteoarthritis.

(x) Presence of only one crease in palm (simian

crease) is found in mongolism 21.

(xi) Tremor : This may be physiological due to anxiety, fear and in old age. Pathological causes of tremor are as follows : familial toxic (chronic alcoholism or tobacco), thyrotoxicosis, uraemic twitchings flapping tremor of portocaval (hepatic) encephalopathy, static tremor of parkinsonism, dynamic tremor of cerebellar disorder, tremor due to belladonna poisoning.

(xii) Involuntary movements like chorea, athetosis, hemiballismus must be noted. Similarly other abnormal movements like tics, myoclonus and fasciculation may be present in different neurological disorders.

(xiii) Joints may show either evidence of osteoarthritis, rheumatoid arthritis, psoriatic arthropathy, features of gout and pulmonary osteoarthropathy.

(xiv) Congenital deformities : (a) Arachnodactyly–characterised by elongated spider fingers and toes (found in Marfan's syndrome), (b) Syndactyly and polydactyly : These may be hereditary or familial and may be found in association with ventricular septal defect, Fallot's tetralogy, Laurence -Moon-Biedl syndrome, Apert's syndrome, Chondroectodermal dysplasia (Ellis-van Creveld syndrome) etc.

(xv) Heberden's nodes : These are hard bony nodules found at the base of the distal phalanges or at the distal ends of middle phalanges. These are found in osteoarthrosis of finger joints and in women as a hereditary condition.

(C)   Different groups of lymph nodes of axilla (apical, medial and lateral groups, central anterior and posterior groups) should be examined by palpation.

(D)   Nutrition of the muscles of the upper limb is assessed. It may be altered in disorders of nervous system and myopathies.

THORAX :

The type of chest, obvious deformity if any, rate and depth of respiration are noted. Prominent veins in the chest wall and different pulsation accessory nipple and sinuses, if any, are to be looked for. Routine inspection of the posterior aspect of the chest must be done for the detection of any spinal deformity like kyphosis, scoliosis or gibbus.

ABDOMEN :

Movement of the abdominal wall, distension either localised or generalised any scar mark or operation mark, dilated vein, shape and position of the umbilicus, any visible peristalsis and the hernial orifices are to be noted in the regional survey of the abdomen.

Visible peristalsis may be seen in pyloric stenosis. small or large gut obstructions. Prominent veins may be due to portal vein or inferior vena cava obstruction. Generalised distension of the abdomen may be due to intestinal obstruction or paralytic ileus or acute dilatation of stomach. Umbilicus may be everted in huge ascites.

LOWER LIMBS :

Legs are examined for clubbing, oedema, varicose veins, varicose ulcer, vascular disturbances like diminished pulsation of dorsalis pedis artery, phlebitis or a gangrene of the toe. Bony deformities such as bowing of the legs may be noticed in Paget's disease of bone and in rickets; *locked knee* and *sabre tibia* may be found in syphilis. There may be evidence of post polio contracture.

Pes cavus : In which there is a fixed deformity of the foot with a high arc is associated with Friedreich's ataxia, muscular dystrophy, peroneal muscular atrophy, poliomyelitis, spastic hemiplegia etc. or may be idiopathic.

Measurement from the highest point of iliac crest to the medial melleolus should be done—as a routine and compared to that of the opposite side.

———

CARDIOVASCULAR SYSTEM

CHAPTER 2

Borders :

The base of the heart is represented by a line joining the right 3rd sternocostal articulation and a point at the level of the left 2nd intercostal space just internal to the parasternal line.

The *right border* extends from the right 3rd sternocostal articulation above up to the right 7th sternocostal articulation below. This is a slightly curved line with convexity to the right side. The *left border* is traced by a line joining the point at the level of the left 2nd intercostal space above just internal to the parasternal line and the apex beat below. This border is concave to the left in the upper 1/3 while the lower 2/3 is slightly convex.

The apex beat is normally situated in the left 5th intercostal space $\frac{1}{2}$" inside the midclavicular line. In children it is in the left 4th space on the midclavicular line.

Position of valves

(1) Mitral valve is obliquely placed behind the inner end of the left 4th costal cartilage and the adjoining part of the sternum.

(2) Tricuspid valve is situated obliquely behind the right 5th costal cartilage.

(3) Pulmonary valve is placed horizontally at the upper border of the left 3rd costal cartilage.

(4) Aortic valve corresponds to a line drawn obliquely

across the left half of the sternum at the level of the lower border of the left 3rd costal cartilage.

Auscultatory areas

The heart sounds and murmurs are best heard in these areas.

(1)   Mitral area– It corresponds with the apical area situated in the left 5th space 1″ inside the midclavicular line. It varies with the size of the heart i.e., it is not fixed.

(2)   Tricuspid area–It is situated in the left 4th intercostal space near the sternal edge and also in the lower part of the sternum.

(3)   Pulmonary area–The pulmonary murmurs are best heard in the 2nd left intercostal space close to the parasternal line.

(4)   Aortic area–The aortic murmurs are best audible over the right 2nd costal cartilage.

Sometimes an aortic murmur is heard only in the left 3rd space close to the sternum (*Erb's point*).

EXAMINATION OF THE CARDIOVASCULAR SYSTEM

GENERAL EXAMINATION

(a) *Feel the temperature of the extremities.* Warm hands are observed in hyperkinetic circulatory states such as pregnancy, thyrotoxicosis, chronic anoxic cor pulmonale, beriberi, Paget's disease of bones aortic regurgitation etc.–

Hands may be cold due to exposure to cold, anxiety neurosis, low cardiac output (as occurs in mitral stenosis, aortic stenosis, left ventricular failure, peripheral circulatory failure and severe pulmonary hypertension).

(b) *Look for dilated veins over the dorsum of hand.* These are found in chronic cor pulmonale, beriberi, Paget's disease, pericardial effusion, old age etc.

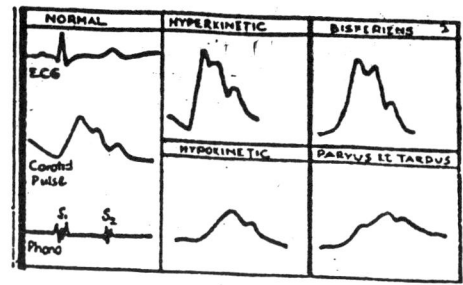

Fig. 3A : Normal Carotid and 4 abnormal Carotid Pulses.

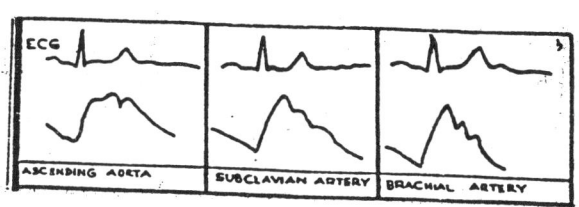

Fig. 3B : Changes in the Contour of the arterial pressuae pulse during a
Pullback of a micro manometer catheter from the central.
aorta to the brachial artery.

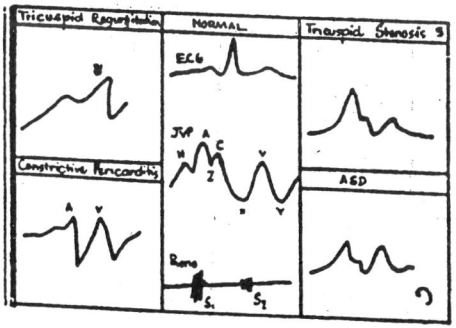

Fig. 3C : The normal and 4 abnormal
types of Jugular venous
pulse (JVP).

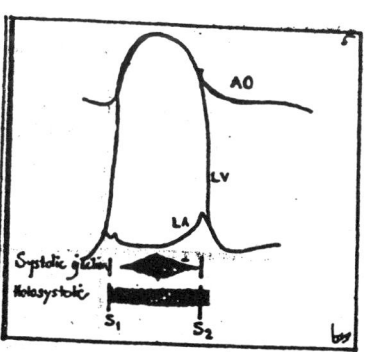

Fig. 3D: Characteristics of a
systolic ejection and a pansystolic regurgitant murmur.
AO- Aortic pressure tracing.
LA and LV: Left atrial and
left ventricular pressure
tracing, s_1 and s_2 : First and
second Heart Sounds.

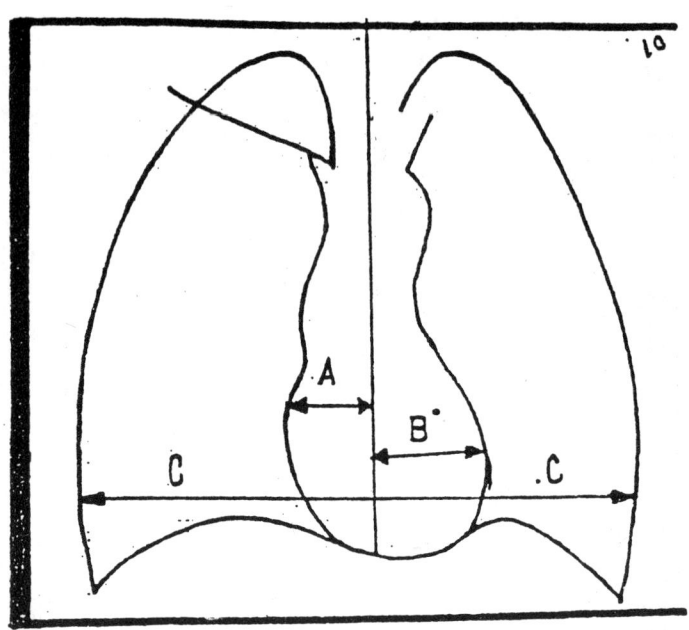

Fig. 3E: Diagrammatic representation of the measurements of the cardiothoracic ratio. A+ B= Maximum transverse diameter of the heart. C=Maximum transverse diameter of the chest.
C T Ratio = A+B/C (Normal Value: about 0.5)

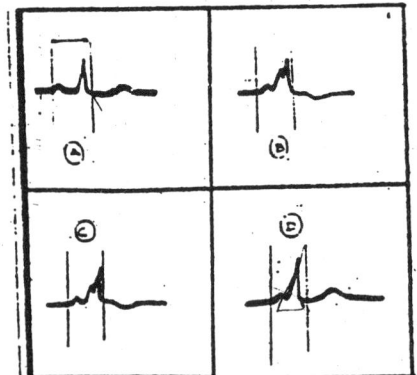

Fig. 3F: Variations in the ECG pattern of preexcitation. A- Normal sinus Beat. B- usual preexcitation beat. Normal PJ but short PR interval. C- short PJ interval. D- short PR and PJ interval with normal QRST complex. Note the Delta waves in B and C.

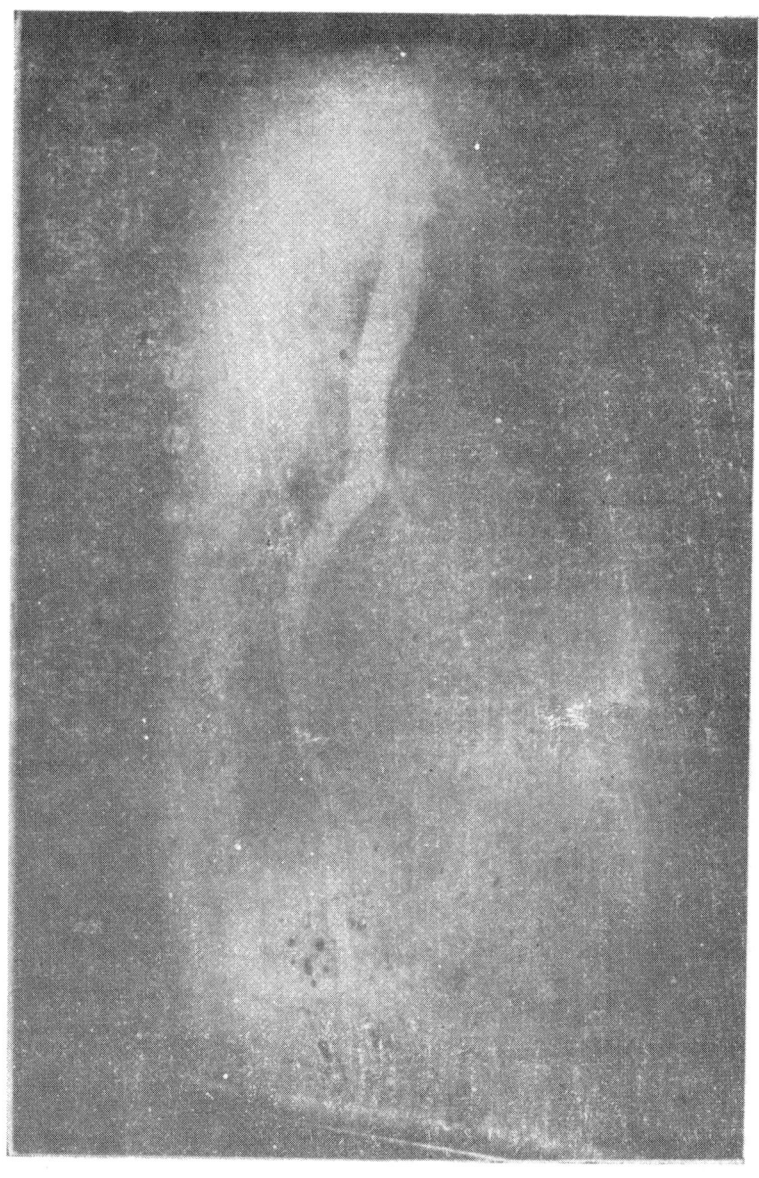

Fig. 3G : Left lateral view with Barium Oesophagus showing
sickle shaped pattern of the oesophagus due to left
atrial hypertrophy.

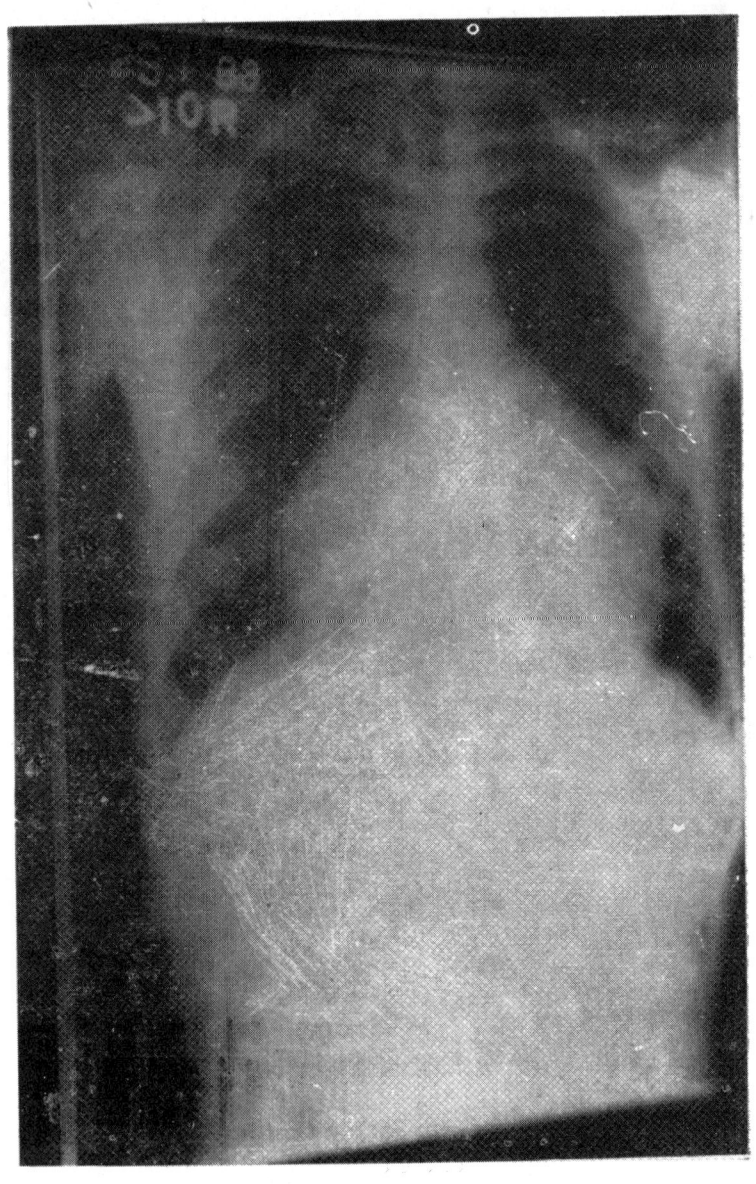

Fig. 3H : Globular appearance of the heart due to
pericardial effusion.

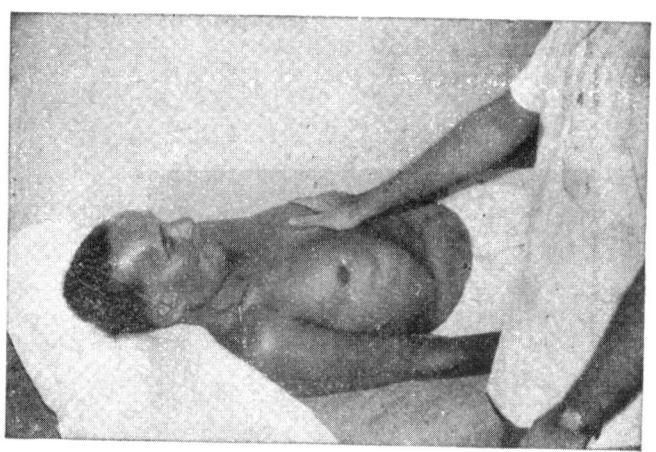

Fig. 3I : Demonstrating Palpation of
the apical Impulse

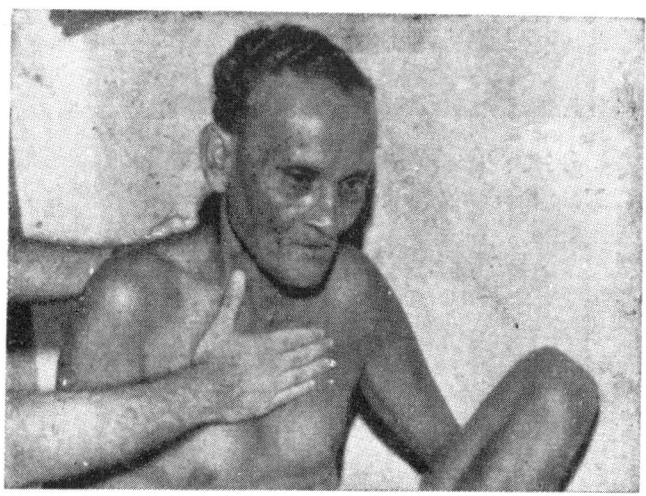

Fig. 3J : Demonstrating Palpation of the base of heart.
Note that the patient is in a Sitting posture.

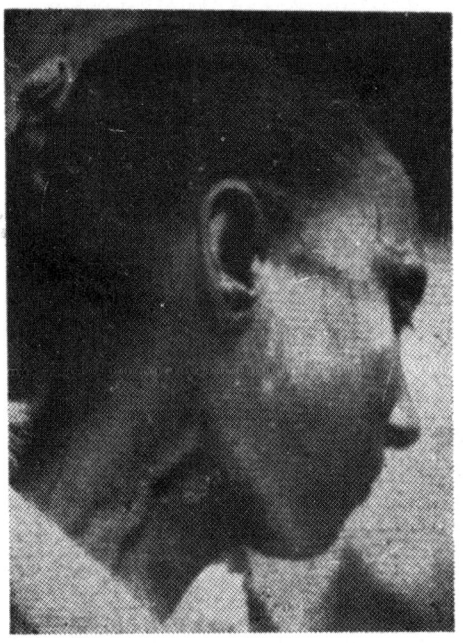

Fig. 3K : Case of congestive heart failure.
Note the engorgement of the neck veins.

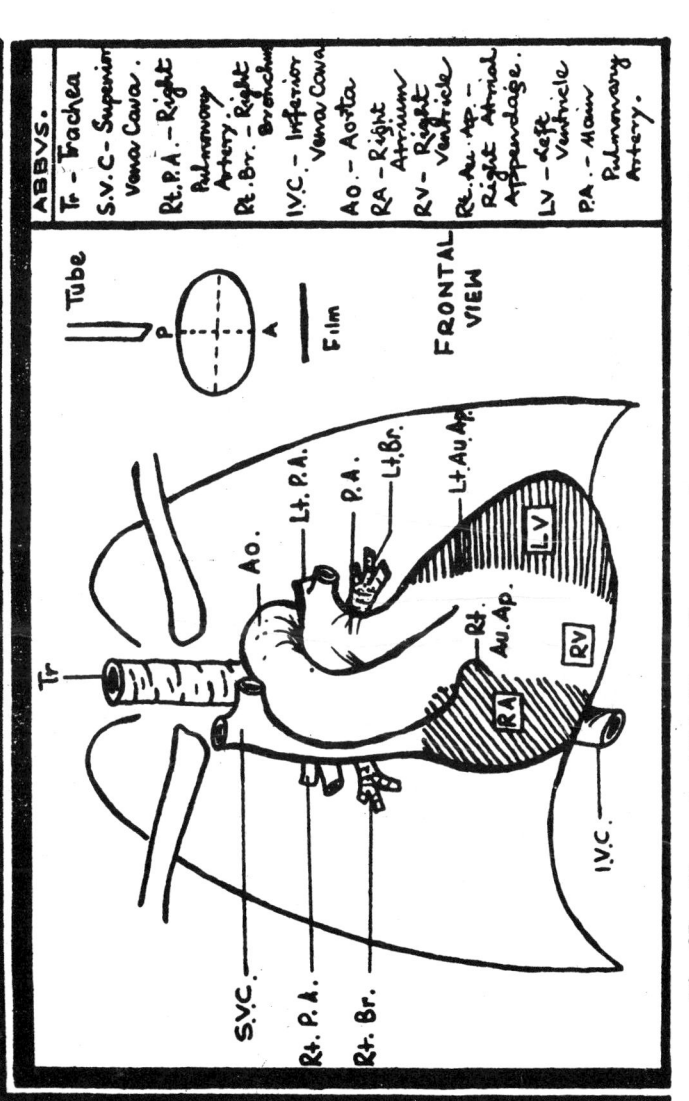

ABBVS.

Tr. – Trachea

S.V.C. – Superior Vena Cava.

Rt.P.A. – Right Pulmonary Artery.

Rt. Br. – Right Bronchus.

IVC. – Inferior Vena Cava.

Ao. – Aorta.

RA – Right Atrium.

RV – Right Ventricle.

Rt. Au. Ap. – Right Atrial Appendage.

LV – Left Ventricle.

PA. – Main Pulmonary Artery.

Tube

P

A

Film

FRONTAL VIEW

Tr.

Ao.

Lt. P.A.

P.A.

Lt. Br.

Lt. Au. Ap.

LV

Rt. Au. Ap.

RV

RA

S.V.C.

Rt. P.A.

Rt. Br.

I.V.C.

Fig. 3L : X-ray chest PA View-diagrammatic representation of the different Cardiovascular structures

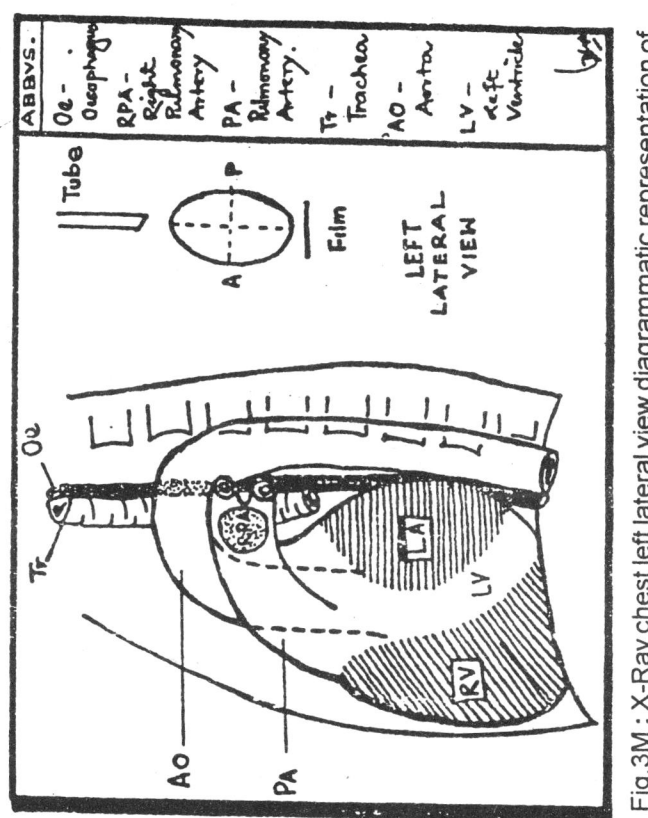

ABBVS.
Oe – Oesophagus
RPA – Right Pulmonary Artery
PA – Pulmonary Artery.
Tr – Trachea
AO – Aorta
LV – Left Ventricle

Tube

A B

Film

LEFT
LATERAL
VIEW

Oe

Tr

AO

PA

LA

LV

RV

Fig.3M : X-Ray chest left lateral view diagrammatic representation of the different cardiovascular structures.

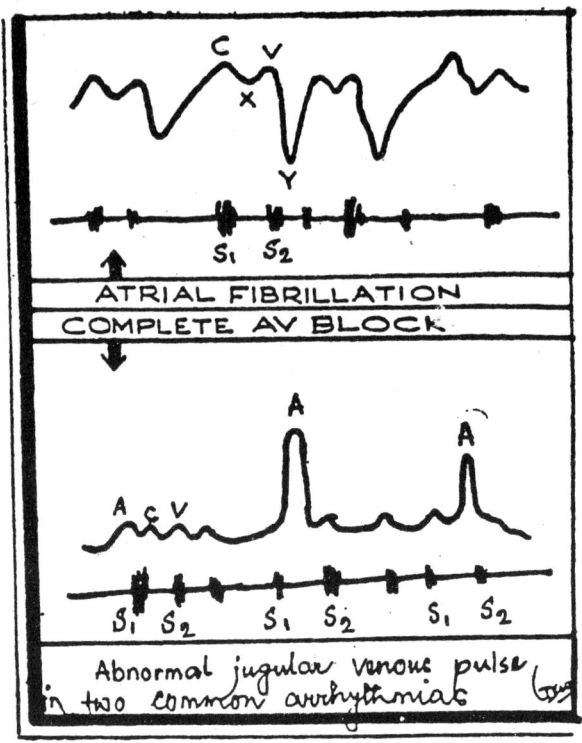

Fig. 3N : Two abnormal JVP's.

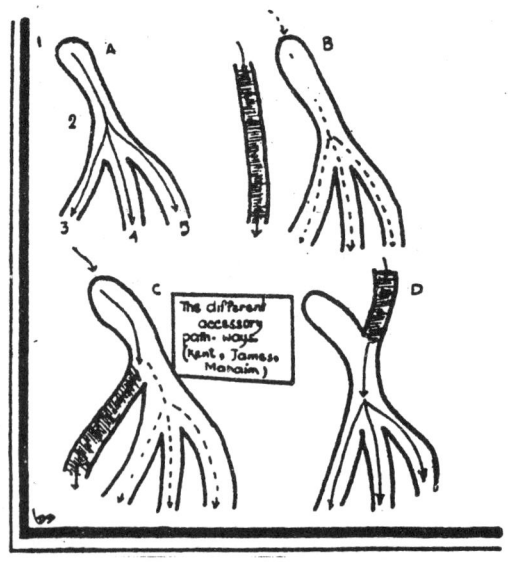

Fig. 3O : B-Kent; C- james; D- Mahaim.

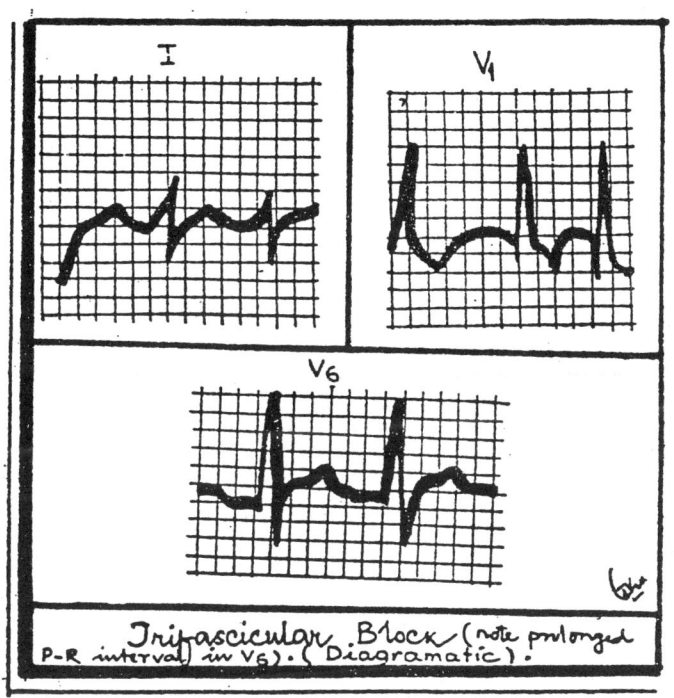

Fig. 3P : ECG of Trifascicular Block.

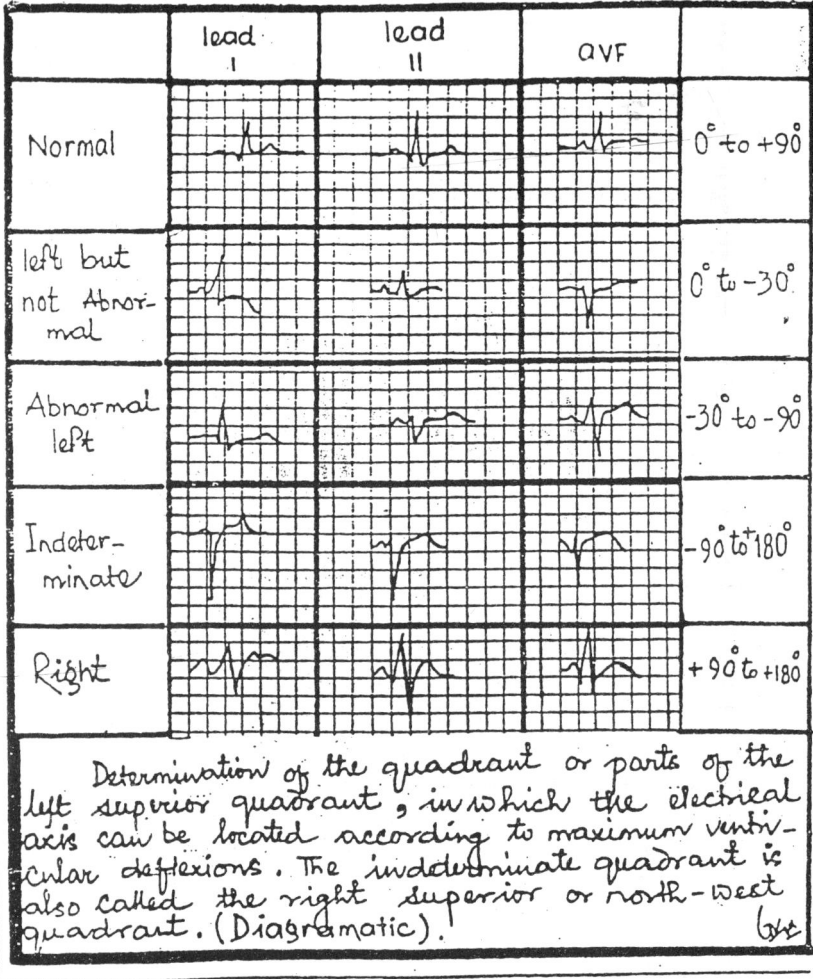

	lead I	lead II	aVF	
Normal				$0°$ to $+90°$
left but not Abnormal				$0°$ to $-30°$
Abnormal left				$-30°$ to $-90°$
Indeterminate				$-90°$ to $^+180°$
Right				$+90°$ to $+180°$

Determination of the quadrant or parts of the left superior quadrant, in which the electrical axis can be located according to maximum ventricular deflexions. The inddeterminate quadrant is also called the right superior or north-west quadrant. (Diagramatic).

Fig. 3Q : ECG showing different types of axis deviations.

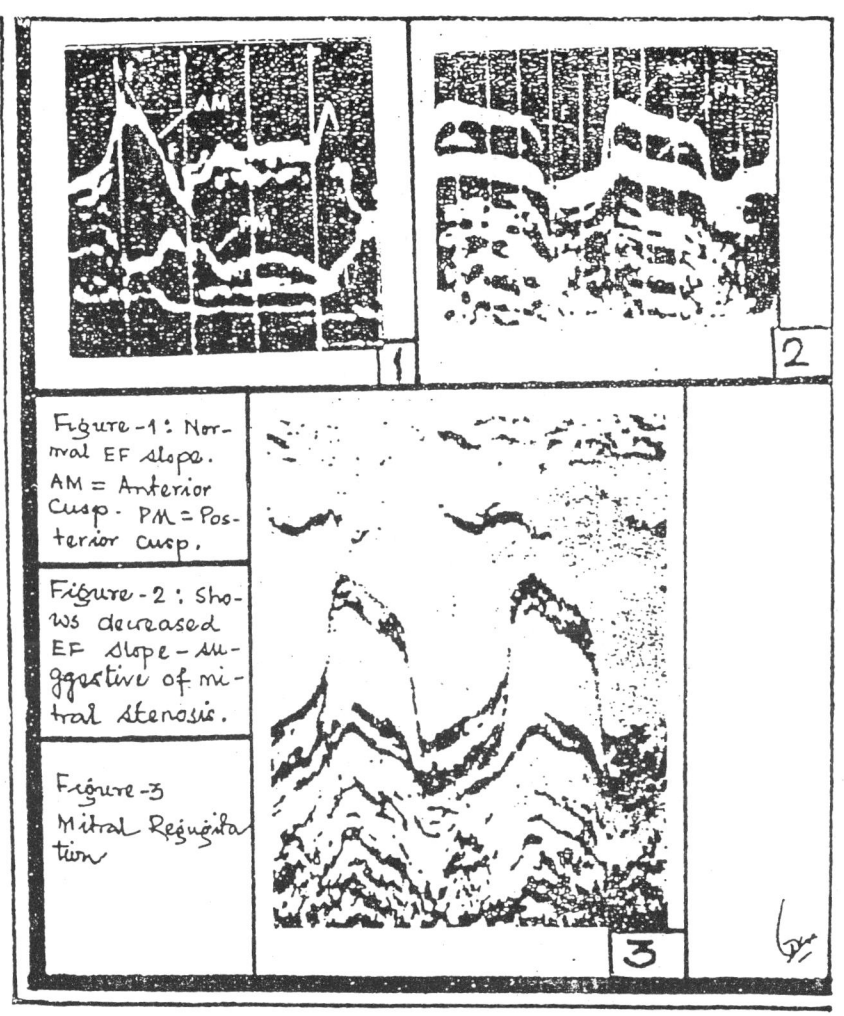

Figure-1: Normal EF slope. AM = Anterior Cusp. PM = Posterior Cusp.

Figure-2: Shows decreased EF slope - suggestive of mitral stenosis.

Figure-3 Mitral Regurgitation

Fig. 3R : Echocardiogram of the mitral valve.

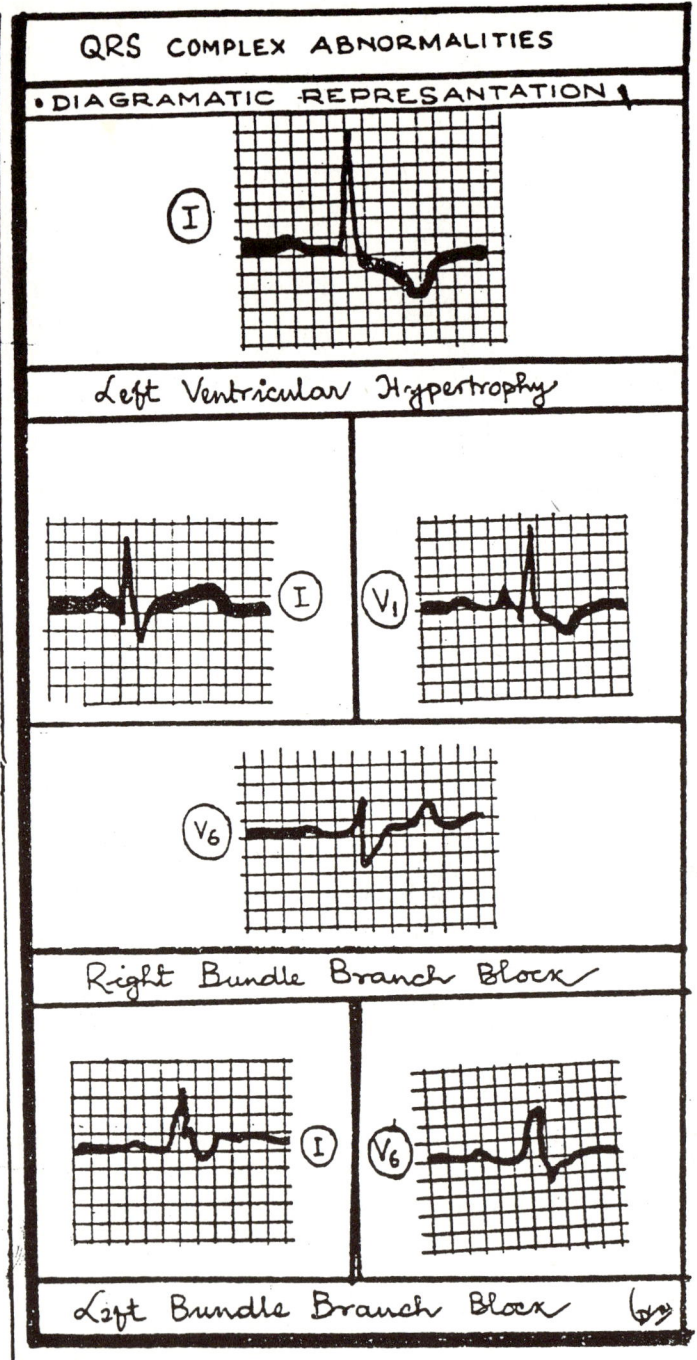

Fig. 3S : ECG showing Different abnormal QRS complexes.

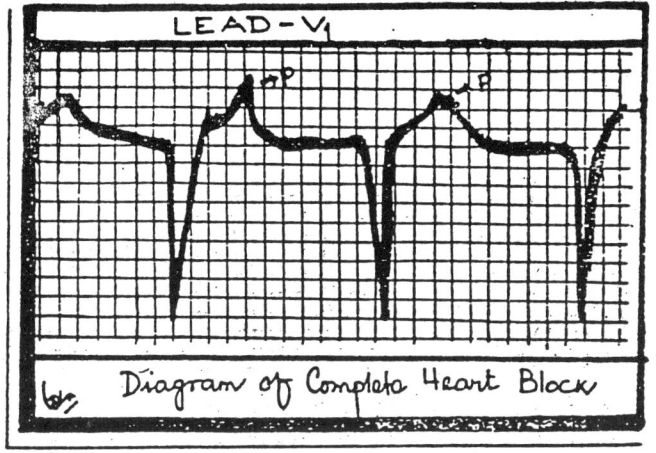

Fig. 3T : Another abnormal but common ECG finding.

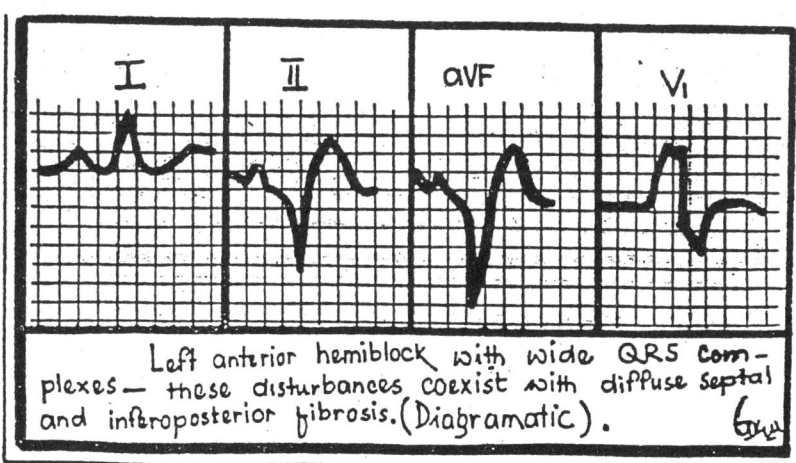

Fig 3U : Another abnormal ECG.

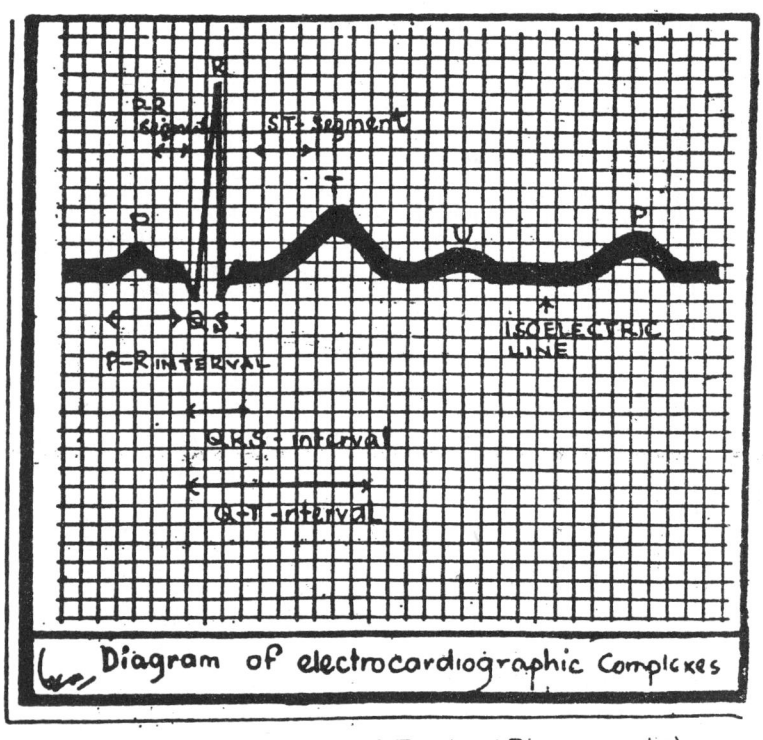

Diagram of electrocardiographic Complexes

Fig 3V : The Normal ECG Tracing (Diagrammatic)

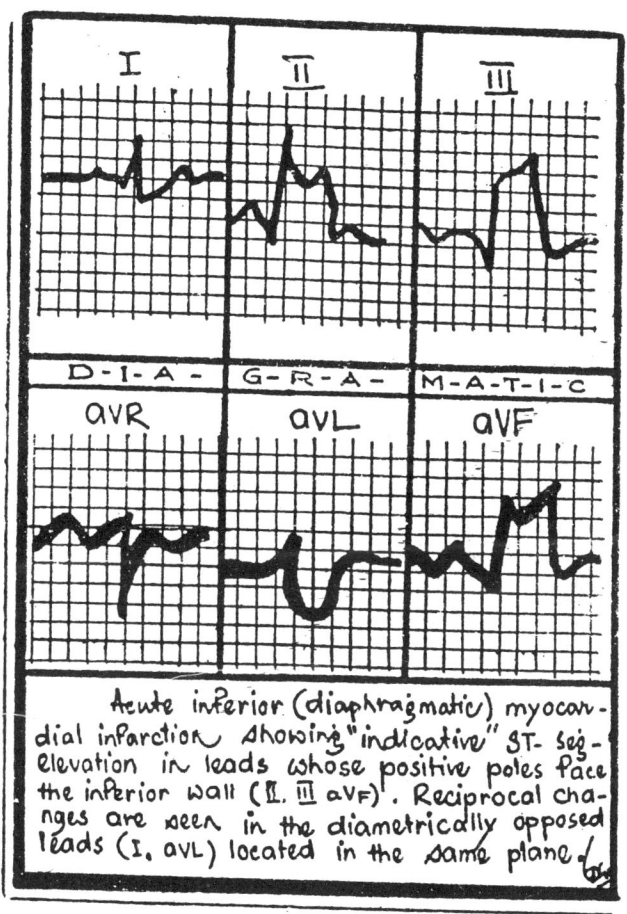

I   II   III

D - I - A -   G - R - A -   M - A - T - I - C

aVR   aVL   aVF

Acute inferior (diaphragmatic) myocardial infarction showing "indicative" ST-segment elevation in leads whose positive poles face the inferior wall (II, III aVF). Reciprocal changes are seen in the diametrically opposed leads (I, aVL) located in the same plane.

Fig 3W : ECG showing Inferior Interior Wall AMI.

(c) *Clubbing of the fingers and toes should be searched for*—they are seen in infective endocarditis, congenital cyanotic heart diseases, cardiac tumours e.g. left atrial myxoma and in post operative infections particularly in open heart surgery. Clubbing may be present only in the left hand in presubclavian coarctation and also in aneurysm of the arch of the aorta.

(d) *Note whether the patient is cyanosed or not.* Cyanosis due to cardiac causes in usually associated with clubbing of the fingers (i.e. central cyanosis). Peripheral cyanosis is found in acute left ventricular failure (e.g. due to acute myocardial infraction).

Differential cyanosis is a very important clinical finding— *Blue hands with red feet* are diagnostic of coarctation of the aorta with transposition of great vessels. *Blue feet with red hands* are diagnostic of patent ductus arteriosus with reversal of shunt due to pulmonary hype tension.

(e) *Examine the nail beds* for linear splinter haemorrhages and also look for tender Osler's node in the pulp of the fingers. These are found in infective endocarditis.

(f) *Examine the palms*, they may look pale and see whether they are moist or dry. Pallor is found in infective endocarditis and acute rheumatic carditis. Palmar erythema is one of the clinical features of hyperkinetic circulartory states. Warm an moist hands is found in thyrotoxicosis. Cold and moist hand is four l. in anxiety neurosis. Dry hand with thick and rough skir ,is found at times in hypothyroidism. Janeway lesions may be found in infective endocarditis.

(g) *Note digital pulsations* by gently holding t he pulps of the patient's fingers with those of your own. Prominent digital pulsations (Quincke's pulse) is commonl ' found in aortic regurgitation, thyrotoxicosis, patent ductus arteriosus, beriberi etc.

(h) *Look for the webbing of fingers, hypermobility of different joints* and arachnodactyly or long slender gracile spider-leg like fingers, as are found in Marfan's syndrome. Aortic regurgitation, dilatation of the aorta and various other congenital cardiac anomalies may be found in Marfan's syndrome.

Look for evidences of arthritis which might be rheumatic or rheumatoid or may be due to gout. In gout, gouty tophi may be found on hands, periarticular tissues and cartilage of the ear. Gout may be associated with pericarditis. Rheumatoid nodules may be the clue to apparently idiopathic pericarditis. In *active* rheumatic myocarditis rheumatic nodules may be found over the occiput, elbow or on the tendon sheath in front of the wrist.

Scleroderma affects the skin giving rise to a diffuse indurated feel of the skin of the fingers, hands and eyelids. It may be associated with pericarditis, cardiomyopathy, heart block, aortic valve diseases and systemic and pulmonary hypertension.

Xanthomata should be searched for over the eyelids, as nodules over the tendon sheaths or as orange yellow streaks on the palms of the hand. It is an important sign of hyperlipidaemia which is often associated with ischaemic heart diseases.

(i) *Search for syphilitic stigmata* in the pupil (Argyll Robertson pupil), condyloma late, features of tabes dorsalis etc.

(j) *Examine the arterial pulse*–its rate, rhythm, volume, tension, condition of the arterial wall, character, equality of the two sides and presence or absence of radio-femoral delay.

(c) Phaeochromocytoma.

(d) Conn's syndrome.

4. Neurological :

(a) Cerebral tumours.

(b) Pseudobulbar palsy.

(c) Bulbar poliomyelitis.

5. Vascular :

(a) Coarctation of the aorta.

(b) Renal artery stenosis.

6. Iatrogenic :

(a) Use of oral contraceptives.

(b) Prolonged steroid therapy (e.g. in bronchial asthma).

7.Pregnancy : Pre and post eclamptic renal cause.

III. *Symptoms*

Nothing typical : The symptomatic features are mostly psychogenic and follow the diagnosis of hypertension. These are – Headache, insomnia Irritability Lack of concentration, Weakness, Fatigue etc.

These may be due to cerebral artery sclerosis.

IV. *Signs*

1. Flushing of the face 2. Blood pressure; Systolic more than 150 mm Hg. Diastolic more than 90 mm Hg.

2. Initially this is intermittent but graually becomes persistent.

3. Opthalmoscopy reveals retinopathy which may be of the following grades :

Mild hypertension (Grade I) :

Diastolic pressure : 90-110 mm Hg

Tortuosity of the 3rd branch of central artery with engorged veins; A : V = 1 : 2 (diam); veins mildly depressed at AV crossing.

Moderate hypertension (Grade II) :

Diastolic pressure : 110-130 mm Hg

More tortuosity of the artery resembling cop per wire; there is arterio-venous nipping; A : V = 1 : 3.

| Severe hypertension (Grade III) : Diastolic pressure : 130-150 mm Hg | Features of Grade II+Silver wire appearance, vein not visible at AV crossing, A : V=1 : 4 or the arterioles may become fine fibrous cord, vein is dilated distal to AV crossing. Cotton wool exudates present. Flame shaped haemorrhage rarely, Hard exudates. |
| Malignant hypertension (Grade IV) : Diastolic pressure : above 150 mm Hg | Papilloedema in addition to the above changes. |

[Malignant hypertension is defined as marked elevation of blood pressure which is associated with :
   (i)   A diastolic pressure usually more than 150 mm Hg.
   (ii) Persistent or progressive uraemia.
   (iii) Papilloedema–confirmatory.]

5.   Apex beat : shifted down and out, heaving in character.

6.   Accentuated A_2, ejection click, ejection systolic murmur, S_2 paradoxically split and rarely aortic regurgitant murmur.

7.   In severe hypertension there is an S_3 due to hypertensive heart disease.

Hypertensive heart disease may lead to coronary atherosclerosis which in turn may ultimately lead to infraction.

Hypertensive heart disease may lead to left ventricular failure; this is known as hypertensive heart failure.

Decapitated hypertension is a condition when there is a sudden fall of systolic pressure from, say, 160 mm Hg to 130 mm Hg due to acute left ventricular failure diastolic pressure ramaining at about 110 mm Hg.

Divergent hypertension a condition in which there is *high systolic* and low diastolic blood pressure e.g. in aortic regurgitation, thyrotoxicosis, patent ductus arteriosus etc.

Effect on other systems :

A. Cerebrovascular–Sudden convulsion with unconsciousness, papilloedema. Paresis of the limbs;– these are all due to hypertensive encephalopathy. Cerebral haemorrhage, Cerebral thrombosis etc.

B. Renal manifestations; Chronic renal failure, acute on chronic renal failure. Urine examination reveals– albumin, RBC Pus cells, Blood and granular casts etc.

V. *Investigations*

1. Radiology–Enlargement of the left ventricle and widening of the arch of the aorta.

2. Electrocardiogram–Left ventricular hypertrophy with or without strain pattern.

3. Blood–biochemistry reflects the aetiological factors, or, with end organ damage e.g. those of the kidneys, there will be features of uraemia with an increase of creatinine level and a decreased creatinine clearance.

4. Intravenous pyelography (rapid sequence IVP) and /or retrograde pyelography reveals renal pathology.

5. Special blood tests e.g. estimation of (i) adrenaline and (ii) non-adrenaline–for suspected phaeochro-mocytomas.

6. Urine–Excertion of vanillylmandelic acid (VMA),

metanephrines and catecholamines to confirm phaeochromocytoma.

7. Split renal function test : to reveal renal artery stenosis.
8. Plasma renin activity (PRA) and renal vein renin assay from both sides.

VI. *Complications*

Acute	Chronic
1. Cerebral haemorrhage.	1. Angina pectoris.
2. Hypertensive encephalopathy.	2. Congestive cardiac failure
3. Subarachnoid haemorrhage.	3. Coronary artery disease.
4. Acute myocardial infraction	4. Chronic renal failure.
5. Acute left ventricular failure	5. Acute on chronic renal failure.

VII. *Management*

1. Weight reduction possible?
2. Physical exercise (e.g. regular walking gymnastic, etc.)
3. Change of eating habit–salt reduced (0, 5 gm salt/d)
   –Cholesterol reduced (vegetable oil instead of animal oil etc.
4. Reduction of restriction of alcohol consumption and smoking. If there is still a high blood pressure systolic over 150 mm Hg/elder pts, over 160 mm Hg and diastolic over 100 mm Hg–add.
5. Antihypertensive drug treatment.
   Avoid to rescript more than three different drugs.
   E. g. for step care treatment :
   1 Step :　diuretica (mostly elder pts.) of or e.g.
   　　　　　B-blocker
   　　　　　Regular BP measurement, it still hyper-
   　　　　　tension, than,
   2 Step :　–diuretica and B-blocker or

- diuretica and calcium antagonist or
- diuretica and ACE inhibitor or
- calcium antagonist and ACE inhibitor

ATTENTION : Never give B-blocker and calcium antagonists! Begain regular BP control, still hypertension present, than

3 Step : –diuretica, B-blocker and ACE inhibitor or – diuretica, calcium antagonists and ACE inhibitor control of BP regularly. There is still the possibility to try other combinations (see table).

Category	example	doses [mg/d]	side effect	contra-indication
a diuretics *Thiazid*	Hydrochlo-rothiazid	25-100	hyperglycaemia hyperuricemia hypokalemia	DIABETES renal failure, gout
Kalium saving	Amilorid	10-20	hyperkalemia, nausea vomiting diarrhoea	hyperkalemia severe liver-dysfunction, severe kid-neyinsufficiency
	Triam teren	100-200		
Henle-loop acting	Funosemid	20-40 (i.v.); 40-120(p.o.)	hypokalemia loss of Mg^{2+} Ca^{2+}, Cl hyperglycemia, hyperuricemia allergic reaction ototoxic	hypovolemia. renal failure with anuria, severe liver-dysfunction. hypokalemia
	Piretanid	3-9		
	Etacryn acid	50-150		
Aldosteron antagonist	Spirono-lactone	25-100	hyperkalemia gynecomastia impotence amenorrhoe.	renal failure hyperkalemia hypovolemia. natremia
		5-10	hyperkalemia	
B β - blocker	Atenolol (cardiose-lective	1× 50 200	bradicardia bronchospasm hyperglycemia sedation	bronchial asthma. congestive car-diac faiure.

category	example	doses [mg/d]	side effect	contra-indication
	metoprolol (cardiose-lective)	2-3×50 100	headache vertigo, gastro-intestinal dys-function	bradycardia. heart block shock situa-tion/metabo-lic acidosis
	Pindolo $(\beta_1+\beta_2;$ ISA)	3×5-10	rebound-effect	
	Propranol of $(\beta_1+\beta_2)$	2-4×10-80		
c. calcium antagonist	Nifedipin	3×5-20	ventricular fibrillation, tachycardia oedema, head-ache flush	pregnancy, aortic stenosis, heart failure, hypotension
	Diltiazem	3×60-120		
	Verapamil	3×40-120	bradycardia AV-block ↓ino-tropie	!never combine with β blocker
d. ACE-inhibitor	Captopril	2+12.5 50	cough. hyperkalemia	renal arterial stenosis (both sides), renal dysfunction. pregnancy, nursing period
	Enalapril	1+5-40		
e. Angio-tensin-II inhibitor	Losartan	25-50	vertigo, excessive BP reduction (when combined with diuretics). hyperkalemia	see ACE inhibitor
f.Vasodi-lator	Dihydra-lazin	3×12.5 50	angina pectoris, drug induced SLE (long term therapy >200mg/d), headache	! always combine with β-blocker and diuretics → reflactory tachycardia

category	example	doses [mg/d]	side effect	contra- indication
	Prazosin α_1 blocker	0.5-20	orthostatic collaps, vertigo	heart insuff, NYHAIV
g. central acting	clonidim (stimu- lates cen- tral α_2 re- ceptor	3+75- 300 μ g/d	bradycardia initial and rebound BP↑, sedation, dry mouth	sick sinus syndrome, bradycardia (lbe cautious in combining with beta- blocker or Verapamil
	α -Methyl- Dopa (see Clonidin)	500-1000	orthostatic dys- regulation, sede tion, Na^+-H_2O- retention	depression, pheochromo- cytoma, acute liver disease

VII. Management
a) Primary Hypertension :
   1. Weight reduction possible?
   2. Physical exercise→ regular walking gymnastic, etc.
   3. Change of eating hahit→ salt reduced (max. 6g/d) try KCL based salt → cholesterol reduced (vegetable oil and food etc.) →in diabetes, diet for it
   4. Leave hypertension promoting drugs.
   5. Reduction or restriction of alcohol, coffee con- sumption and smoking. If there is still a high blood pressure start.
   6. Antihypertensive drug treatment : Avoid to rescript more than three different drugs, think that the patient has to take them over a lot

of years perhaps the whole life. Routinious BP control is to be made, if possible by patient self control.

Step care treatment :

1st Step : **Monotherapy** with one of the basic drugs

β-blocker	Diuretics	Ca-anta-gonists	ACE inhibitor	$\alpha_1$blocker

Still no acceptable BP Extend to

2nd Step : **Doubletherapy**

Diuretics	and

β-blocker	Co-anta-gonists	ACE inhibitor	$\alpha_1$blocker

or

Ca-antagonists	and	β-blocker	ACE-inhibitor

ATTENTION : Never combine β-blocker with Verapamil!

3rd Step : Find out a combination which regulates the individual

hypertension of the patient best, for example ;

Diuretica	and	ACE-inhibitor	and	Ca-antagonists

In case of hypertensive emergencies :

(a)   Nitroprussid, 0, 5 to 8, 0 mg/kg/min continous intravenuous (i.v.) ATTENTION ! Blood pressure might come down to fast, intensive BP control necessary.

or (b) Diazoxid 150-300 mg i.v.

or (c) Trmetaphan, 1 to 45 mg/min i.v.

Other measures that are of help : Mannitol infusion in jet or Furosemid i.v. These drugs are rapid acting and have to replaced by a management shown in step 2 or 3 for long term treatment.

Surgical management according to the aetiology. These include—

1. Bilateral adrenalectomy.
2. Removal of the tumour in a case of pheochromo-cytoma.
3. In coarctation—end to end anastomosis or graft ing.
4. Renal artery garfting in renal artery stenosis.

ACUTE MYOCARDIAL INFRACTION

1. *Incidence*

More in males, below the age of 50 yrs. Beyond that age the incidences are nearly equal in both sexes. Exceptions,— young females, if they suffer from juvenile diabetes, hypertension, hypothyroidism, hyperlipidaemia etc. or if there is a prolonged use of contraceptive pills.

II. *Clinical features*

1. Precordial pain (usually severe) may be—
(a) Retrosternal, radiating to the ulnar aspect of the left arm.
(b) Across the chest radiating to the ulnar aspect of both arms.
(c) Localised at the jaw.
(d) Below the shoulder blades radiating anteriorly.
(e) Epigastric.

Character of the pain—squeezing, constricting, heavi-ness over the precordium or there may be a sense of impending death.

2. Associated features include—
(a) Profuse perspiration (cold sweat).
(b) Giddiness or even syncope (due to sudden hypo-tension or associated heart block).
(c) Frank features of cardiac asthma—severe breath-

lessness with ratting sounds in the throat, bilateral moist sounds. In the lungs, gallop rhythm with pulsus alternans.

(d)   Severe epigastric pain with vomiting, a sense of dysphagia and giddiness, resembling those of acute grastric perforation, acute heamorrhagic pancreatitis or acute pain of basal pleurisy.

3.   May be painless with none of few of the associated features.

III. *Clinical diagnosis*

1.   Patient is apprehensive, anxious and restless.

2.   Pallor of the face or even ashen gry appearance (due to low cardiac output which may again be due to peripheral circulatory failure).

3.   Rarely central cyanosis (if associated with left ventricular failure).

4.   Decbitus propped up (if associated with left ventricular failure).

5.   Extremities are cold and clammy.

6.   Pulse : Usually tachycardia but sometimes bradycardia if associated with heart block or reflex vegal stimulation.
        Rhythm may be irregular due to frequent ventricular premature beats, which is an aminous sign as these may herald ventricular tachycardia and/or fibrillation.

7.   Blood pressure : Both systolic and diastolic pressures are low. If systolic pressure is less than 90 mm Hg with cold and clammy extremities with marked cyanosis and oliguria–the condition is known as *cardiogenic shock*, which is a dreadful complication of myocardial infraction. However, sympathetic overactivity may lead to early transient hypertension.

Mechanism of cardiogenic shock–It is due to decreased coronary perfusion and peripheral circulatory failure. When the coronary perfusion is diminished, myocardial dysfunction occurs. This further reduces the perfusion and a vicious cycle sets in. Also peripheral circulatory failure produces splanchnic vasoconstriction giving rise to anoxia of the viscera which liberates lactic acid into the circulation resulting in metabolic acidosis, that is further responsible for the peripheral circulatory failure perpetuating the vicious cycle (Sodi-bi-carb prevents metabolic acidosis).

8. Jugular venous pressure : May be raised if associated with congestive heart failure.

9. Heart sounds : Usually muffled due to myocardial damage and an S_4 is very common and there may be an S_3 if heart failure sets in.
    After 1 to 2 days there may be a to and fro rough sound over the precordium mainly the left 4th intercostal space in the mid-clavicular line or over the pulmonary area. This is the *pericardial friction rub*. This is very common in an anterior wall myocardial infarction but rare in inferior wall infraction.

10. Body temperature within 36 hours the body temperature may rise to 102°F and this is due to a nonspecific reaction to the myocardial necrosis.

IV. *Investigation*

1, **ECG :** One of the basic diagnostic methods with 12 lead ECG.
    Peracute sign : high peak T wave is only seen during AMI (minutes) attack.
    acute sign : ST elevation in infract regions (hours).
    chronic sign : reduction of ST elevation and presence of (days to weeks) pathological Q wave.
    But be aware that ECG signs may be totally absent or minimized. Leads on the opposite of the infrac-

tion site may show ST depression, like in a mirror.

Infract region	Lead change in
anteroseptal	1, II, aVL, $V_1 - V_6$
inferior	II, III, aVF
septal	$V_1 - V_3$
lateral	$V_3 - V_6$.

2. Blood enzymes

(i) Creatinine phosphokinase (CPK) and CPK-MB (isoenzyme) rises after 6–10 hours of infraction.

(ii) Troponin T (and I), myocardial antigens rising earlier then CPK and are more specific, but not everywhere available.

(iii) Aspertal transaminase (AST) and lactte dehydrogenase (IDH) are released 2–4 days after infraction. There are not very specific.

(iv) Total and differential WBC counts : leukocytosis with a marked increase of polymorphs within 36 hours. Not AMI specific.

Mark if two of the following points are present start treatment without losing time !

1. characteristic clinical picture
2. ECG changes
3. characteristic enzyme increase in blood Fibrinolytic therapy

Several drugs are used today, the three most common are noted here.

Drug (Doses)	Dosis and effect
Streptokinase	1.5 mil units over 1h, with t ½ 80 min; allergenic and anaphylactic reaction possible, re-using should be avoided. Fast injection causes rapid fall of BP.

Tissue type plasminogen activator (t-PA) or recombinant-PA (rt-PA); Alteplase	10 mg bolus, 50 mg over 1h, then 40 mg over 2h later on. Give always heparin : first as 5000 U bolus then 1000 U/hiv. $t\frac{1}{2}$ 30 min; Due. to the selective activity directly on the thrombos location these drugs are less likely to produce systemic co-agulation disturbances.
Drug (Doses)	**Doses and effect**
Anisoylated plasminogen streptokinase activator complex (APSAC) I Anistreplase	30 units over 5 min. $t\frac{1}{2}$ 105 min; like streptokinase allergenic potence

Reperfusing the obstructed vessel, fibrinolytics have got their maximum effect within the first 4 hours. Still after 12-24 hours little benefit can be expected.

Because of the dangerous side effects as
(i) bleeding disorder
(ii) multiple microembolism
(iii) cardiac dyarithmias and
(iv) allergy
you have to follow strict **contraindications.**
1.   haemorrhagic diathesis
2.   Symptoms of peptic ulcer or GI bleeding
3.   recent cerebral stroke
4.   recent surgery and especially neurosurgery
5.   malignant and uncontrolled hypertension
6.   Prolonged cardiopulmonary resuscitation during this presentation.

V. *Management*

This is ideally done by admitting the patient in a coronary care unit (CCU) as early as possible where—

(i) The patient is put in a cardiac bed.

(ii)   Oxygen is given through a nasal catheter (or ventimask or if necessary at a high pressure) at the rate of 4–6 litres i.e., 300 to 600 bubbles per minute.

(iii)   To remove the anxiety and kill the pain—inj. morphine sulph—15 mg SC or IM to be repeated up to 60 mg or 2mg IV repeated as necessary.

or, Pethidine hydrocloride inj—100 mg stat IM with or without promethazine hydrochloride.

Or, inj, Pentazocine—which has minimum respiratory depressant effect, 40 mg IM. But this drug may increase LV. end diastolic pressure.

Or, Inj Diazepam—10 mg IV.

With this treatment the thrombotic obstracted coronararteria might be opened again. There is the chance to gain the stroken part of muscle back.

(v)   Anticoagulant theraphy is started with–

Inj Heparin—10,000 units stat, 7,500 units SC 6 hrly for 48 hours. It prevents thrombo-embolic episodes but never prevents further extenstion of the infraction. Along with the above, phenindione (DINDEVAN)–40 mg tablets 5 tabs stat and I tab BD given orally. Each dose of heparin should be given after determining the bleeding and clotting times.

Dindevan takes 48 hours for its onset of action and so the dose should be regulated by prothrombin index which should be kept within 50%.

Before starting an anticoagulant therapy a through history is taken to exclude any haemorrhagic disorders the presence of which contraindicates the use of the anticoagulants.

Heparin is withdrawn after 48 hours. Oral anticoagulant therapy is continued for 3-6 weeks and should be withdrawn gradually. A sudden withdrawal may precipitate another attack.

(N.B.–There is no uniform consensus of opinion regarding the merits of anticoagulant therapy in AMI.)

Oral anticoagulant therapy with aspirin acetylsalcylaci 100–160 m/d to lower the risk of a further myocardial infraction.

(vi)   B-adrenoceptor blockade with 50 mg atenolol : first intravenous and then a second dosage per os. Reduction of mortality in AMI patients.

In routine practice a 12 lead electrocardiogram is recorded.

The Leads more detailed :

Six limb leads divided into

(i) 3 standard or bipolar limb leads (Edberg leads):

Lead I– indicates potential difference between the left and the right arm.

Lead II– potential difference between the left leg and the right arm.

Lead III– potential difference between left by left arm

(iii) 3 augmented unipolar limb leads :

aVR

aVL

aVF

(V)   Complications of AMI e.g. (a) Cardiac arrhythmias, (b) Hypotension, (c) Cardiogenic shock etc. may appear and should be promptly diagnosed and treated detailed discussions of these are beyond the scope of this book and students are advised to consult larger text-books. IV infusions started with a "Polarising fluid" which consists of (i) One bottle of 5% dextrose solution and to this is added (ii) 2 amp of inj. potassium chloride (20 MEq of K in each amp) and (iii) 15 units soluble insulin.

The rationality of infusing polarising fluid remains controversial, but at least it helps maintaining an IV channel to readily combat the emergency problems of early complications of AMI.

If there is a fall of BP, 24 mg *dexamethasone* (Decadron) is added into the bottle. The drip is continued for about 2 days (or more if necessary) at the rate of 6 to 10 drops per *minute* (or more, depending upon the haemodynamic variables).

In cardiogenic shock, sodi-bi-carb 3.4% 100 ml/day and *dopamine* (intropin) 5-15 μg per kg body weight per minute, both by IV infusion, should be given. Dopamine, however, should never be mixed with any other solution and is given only in 5% dextrose solution.

Ventricular premature beats or ventricular tachycardia should be treated with *lignocatine* 250 mg IV stat given through the drip, but lignocatine may cause further fall of pressure. So DC shock is the treatment of choice, especially with VT and when there is haemodynamic compromise.

If there is a heart block that cannot be combated by steroids and atropine, immediately a bedside floating electrode catheter should be introduced into the right ventricle via a peripheral arm vein and connected with an external *temporary pacemaker.*

If the signs of ventricular failure appear, furosemide 40-80 mg IV stat and inj. *aminophylline* 0.25 gm in 10 ml

A slow 'y' descent is characteristic of right atrial outflow tract obstruction e.g. tricuspid stenosis. Huge pathological 'a' waves known as *cannon waves* appear when the atria contract against closed A-V valves. Irregular connon waves associated with varying intensity of first heart sound are seen in complete heart block, paroxysmal ventricular tachycardia etc. while regular cannon 'a' waves may occur with 1 : 1 atrioventricular relationship during VT or SVT or in junctional rhythms.

II. EXAMINATION OF THE HEART
Inspections :
General inspection of the chest with special reference to the shape. superficial veins, obvious bulgings, width of the subcostal angle, movement with respiration etc. should be done before proceeding to a detailed examination of the heart. The precordium is the area of the anterior surface of the chest that overlies the heart.

(i) Bulging of the precordium is very common in congenital and rheumatic heart diseases (but not in hypertension and coronary arterial diseases.) This is due to overaction of the heart, as a result of altered haemodynamics or due to enlargement of any chamber, inside a soft bony cage (i.e., before ossification). The chest becomes barrel shaped in chronic cor pulmonale (e.g. in emphysema), –the sternum becomes prominent and the anteroposterior diameter is increased due to the presence of the voluminous lung inside the chest.

(ii) Look for dilated and engorged superficial veins which may be present in superior vena caval obstruction. The direction of blood flow will be from above downwards.

(iii) Look for any retraction of the lower part of precordium e.g. in adherent pericarditis.
Systolic retraction of the back of the chest on the left side in the regions of 11th and 12th ribs is sometimes visible in adherent pericarditis (*Broadbent's sign*).

(iv) A depressed sternum may be the cause of a right ventricular outflow tract obstruction without any organic lesion in the heart (e.g. pectus excavatum).

(v) An accessory nipple (petolythelia) is found associated with some cases of systemic and pulmonary hypertension, cardiomyopathy and congenital heart diseases.

(vi) Next look for any pulsations over the precordium. Normally the apical impulse is visible in thin built persons in the left 5th intercostal space just internal to the midclavicular line. The apical impulse may be seen on the right side in dextrocardia. It may be displaced outward and downward due to left ventricular hypertrophy as occurs in aortic regurgitation, aortic stenosis, mitral regurgitation, patent ductus arteriosus, obstructive cardiomyopathy, ischaemic and hypertensive heart diseases, atrial septal defect (septum primum type) etc. Parasternal pulsations are seen in the left 4th and 5th space near the left parasternal line.
Pulmonary arterial pulsation in the left space is normally found in children with thin chests. In adults such pulsations are *pathognomonic* of hyperdynamic circulation through the pulmonary circuit, as occurs in atrial septal defect, patent ductus arteriosus and ventricular septal defect. Exaggerated pulsations of the *pulmonary artery* is

characteristic of pulmonary hypertension. A diffuse pulsation on the *right sternal edge* is suggestive of an aneurysm of the ascending aorta, that in the *suprasternal notch* suggests hyperkinetic circulatory state, aneurysm of the arch of the aorta, coarctation of the aorta and unfolded aortic arch in hypertension. Pulsations on the *lower right sternal edge* is due to enlarged right atrium, tricuspid stenosis, tricuspid atresia and Ebstein's disease. Abnormal pulsations to the left of the sternum may be caused by right ventricular or left atrial hypertrophy as occurs in mitral stenosis.

In this connection, it is worthwhile to mention that pulsations over the *epigastrium* may be found in hyperkinetic right ventricle or right ventricular hypertrophy; aneurysm of the abdominal aorta, transmission of the aortic pulsation by a tumour e.g. gastric carcinoma or due to the *pulsatile* liver of tricuspid incompetence. It might also be found at times during excitement in normal individuals. Carotid pulsations may be exaggerated and prominently visible in aortic regurgitation, thyrotoxicosis, aneurysm of the aorta, kinked carotid (more so on the right side) and hypertension and also during excitement, emotion and exertion.

(vii) Inspect the back below the level of the scapular angle for any visible pulsation (Suzman's sign) which is expected in coarctation of the aorta. The spine should be observed carefully for scoliosis or kyphosis as they may be responsible for the development of chronic cor pulmonale.

(viii) In massive pericardial effusion, a bulging is sometimes seen in the epigastrium. This is known as *Auenbrugger's sign.*

(ix) Systolic retraction : With each systole there is a retraction of the intercostal space at the apex. This is found in normal persons. In chronic constrictive or adhesive pericarditis there is retraction of ribs at the apex along with the retraction of the inter-costal space.

(x) Diastolic heart beat : In constrictive pericarditis a sudden thurst is seen and felt at the apex during diastole but no systolic impulse is there. This is known as diastolic heart beat. This is accompa-nied by a diastolic sound (pericardial knock) on auscultation and systolic retraction of the precordium. This is caused by sudden emptying of cervical veins is diastole. This is a pathognomonic sign of constrictive pericarditis.

Palpation

The patient should lie flat on the bed and the right palm is placed over the precordium Palpate the individual areas separately. The patient should be turned to the left to note the character of the *apex beat* more accurately, but never for its site. If the apex beat is not palpable in the dorsal position, *allow* the patient to sit up and lean forward and then locate the site. The patient should be turned to the left side to note three things–character of the apex beat, diastolic thrill and diastolic murmur.

(a) *Apex beat*–It is the downmost and outermost point over the precordium where a definite (and not necessarily the maximum) thrust can be felt.

During an examination of the apex beat the following points should be noted.

(a) Site–In a lean and thin person who has a tubular

chest, the apex beat may be in the left 6th space. Impalpable apex may be due to the apex beat lying under the rib, pulmonary emphysema, obesity, pericardial effusion and in elderly women with pendular breast. The apex beat may be displaced to the right in (congenital) dextrocardia or in acquired conditions of dextroversion. The extracardiac causes of shifting of apex beat to the right side are left sided pleural effusion, pneumothorax and hydropneumothorax and /or right sided pulmonary fibrosis and collapse.

The acquired dextroversion and congenital dextrocardia can be clinically differentiated by the fact that the trachea is deviated to the right in the former and remains central in the latter.

(b) Character–*Hyperdynamic* apex is a forceful and ill sustained one found in diastolic overloading of the left ventricle. This is observed in mitral regurgitation, aortic regurgitation, patent ductus arteriosus and ventricular septal defect. In these cases, the left ventricle receives the normal quota of blood together with the regurgitated blood of previous systole. The increased amount of blood dilates the left ventricle which forcibly pumps the blood into the systemic circulation. But the contraction is ill sustained because the left ventricle finds on obstruction to its outflow tract (because of patent valves or reflex vasodilatation of peripheral arterioles).

Heaving apex beat is a forceful and well sustained one, the finger being distinctly lifted for a moment. In this case the left ventricle is more hypertrophied than dilated (concentric hypertrophy) and is due to either (i) outflow tract obstruction as in aortic stenosis or obstructive cardiomyopathy or (ii) high peripheral vascular resistance as in systemic hypertension and coarctation of the aorta. All these result in overloading of the left ventricle.

The apical impulse may be tapping or slapping with a palpable loud first heart sound and is characteristically found in mitral stenosis and in any condition giving rise to hyperkinetic circulatory state with tachycardia.

Hypokinetic apex–The apical thrust is diminished and it is found in constrictive pericarditis, pericardial effusion, acute myocardial infraction, shock, myxoedema etc.

(2)   Feel for thrills in the mitral area. It is detected best when the breath is held in expiration. Thrills are purring sensations or vibrations felt on the precordium or over arteries and are caused by torrential and turbulent blood flow through a dis-eased valve or an abnormal opening. In other words, it is nothing but the palpable vibrations of low frequency associated with murmurs. If the thrill coincides with the apex beat, it is systolic and if it precedes the apex beat, it is diastolic. The thrill should always be differentiated from a friction fremitus which will disappear on holding the breath and also from fine contractions of pectoralis mus-cle in cold weather which will cease in a warm environment.

Thrills over the mitral area may be–

(a)   Systolic as in mitral regurgitation, atrial septal defect of septum primum type; some cases of obstructive cardiomyopathies and ventricular septal defect.

(b)   Diastolic as in mitral stenosis, best palpable with the patient in left lateral position, holding the breath after deep expiration. Presystolic thrills of organic mitral stenosis are found even in an early stage. It is best palpable *after* the patient performs some exercise (when the heart contracts more actively) and with the patient turned to the left. The diastolic thrill of Austin-Flint murmur is rarely palpable as also that of left artial myxoma.

(3)   Next palpate the lower left sternal edge with the fingers of the hypothenar eminence and–

(a)   Observe the character of the cardiac impulse. If it is heaving, it indicates right ventricular systolic overload. Right ventricular systolic overload may be produced by (i) right ventricular outflow tract obstruction as found in pulmonary stenosis and pulmonary atresia; or (ii) increased pulmonary vascular resistance in pulmonary hypertension of any aetiology. A hyperdynamic (forceful and illustained) right ventricular impulse indicates an eccentric hypertrophy of the right ventricle as it is dealing with an excessive volume of blood against a low peripheral resistance. This is typically found in atrial septal defect. In chronic cor pulmonale due to chronic bronchitis and emphysema, palpate the epigastrium for a right ventricular heave.

(b)   Search for thrills over the lower left sternal edge (usually systolic) and the possible causes are ventricular septal defect, infundibular pulmonary stenosis, tricuspid regurgitation, atrial septal defect of primum type etc. A continuous systolodiastolic thrill over this region indicates (i) coronary arteriovenous fistula or (ii) rupture of sinus of Valsalva into the pulmonary artery or into the right ventricle.

(4)   Palpate the pulmonary area for a detection of (i) the pulsations of the pulmonary artery, (ii) thrills and (iii) palpable 2nd heart sound.

(i)   Pulmonary artery pulsation may be palpable in

atrial septal defect, ventricular septal defect, patent ductus arteriosus, total anomalous pulmonary venous drainage, severe pulmonary hypertension (known as pulmonary heave) and idiopathic dilatation of the pulmonary artery.

(ii)   A systolic thrill over the pulmonary area is found in isolated pulmonary stenosis, two-thirds of the cases of atrial septal defect, high ventricular septal defect and Fallot's tetralogy.

A continuous thrill over the pulmonary area is characteristic of patent ductus arteriosus, aortopulmonary window and bronchopulmonary fistula or anastomosis.

(iii) A palpable 2nd heart sound over the pulmonary area is known as *diastolic shock*–characteristic of pulmonary hypertension of any aetiology.

(5)   Place the flat of the hand over the base of the heart and note whether there is any expansile pulsation. This indicates an aneurysm of the arch of the aorta.

(6)   Palpate the aortic area with the flat of the hand placed horizontally below the right clavicle, also covering a part of the sternum. A thrill over the aortic area is almost always systolic, indicative of congenital or acquired aortic stenosis.

Diastolic thrills over the base of the heart is not rare. It may be palpable in syphilitic or other varieties of aortic regurgitation and ruptured aortic cusps (e.g. in infective endocarditis). Systolic thrills over the carotid artery are found in aortic stenosis and is known as *carotid shudder*. It is very prominent in supravalvular aortic stenosis and may even be felt in the brachial arteries.

(7) Place your finger tips in the suprasternal notch. A suprasternal pulsation may be indicative of coarctation of the aorta, gross unfolding of the aorta, aortic regurgitation and aneurysm of the aorta. Also look for a tracheal tug.

(8) Place the ulnar border of the palm longitudinally over the right sternal edge. A pulsation in this region may be due to an aneurysm of the ascending aorta or rarely due to a huge right atrium caused by tricuspid atresia of Ebstein's disease.

(9) Feel for a pulsation over the back in the interscapular and infrascapular region. It is pathognomonic of dilatation of the collaterals in coarctation of the aorta (*Suzman's sign*). At times a systolic thrill over these collaterals may be present.

(10) *Pericardial* rub may be palpable over the precordium. It corresponds with heart beat and is neither influenced by nor related to respiration. It is found in various clinical conditions causing acute fibrinous pericarditis where the visceral and the parietal layers of the pericardium rub against each other with each contraction. It usually disappears when pericardial effusion develops. It is commonly found in tuberculous, acute rheumatic, viral pericarditis etc.

PERCUSSION

Although percussion of the heart become obsolete since the advent of the non-invasive investigative procedures, it may be used for the diagnosis of pericardial effusion, emphysema of the lungs and aneurysm of the arch of the aorta etc.

The surface marking of the borders of the heart has been described previously.

Percussion of the right border–Find out the level of the upper border of hepatic dullness along the right midclavicular line. Go one space above the liver dullness and keep the pleximeter finger parallel to the right border of the heart and apply light percussion on the right 3rd and 4th spaces. Go on percussing medially and put a mark on the point of dullness in each space. Join the skin marking with a slightly curved line with convexity towards the right.

The right border of the cardiac dullness may be increased in pericardial effusion, tricuspid stenosis, Ebstein's disease, aneurysm of the ascending or the descending aorta etc.

Percussion of the left border–First localise the apex by palpation and put a mark there; now start percussing the left border.

(i) Percuss the left 2nd, 3rd and 4th spaces from above downwards with the pleximeter finger placed 1/4 inch outside the lateral border of the sternum and note any change of resonance.

(ii) Now percuss along an arbitrary line that runs obliquely from the tip of the acromion process of the left side to the xiphisternum. The dullness will be normally obtained in the left 4th space.

(iii) Lastly percuss the chest, space by space from the anterior axillary line obliquely towards the apex from below upwards. This is the left border of the heart. The left border of cardiac dullness may cross the normal limit in left ventricular hypertrophy, pericardial effusion, ventricular aneurysm and in any condition giving rise to pulmonary arterial segment dilatation, such as in pulmonary hypertension, atrial septal defect, ventricular septal defect, patent ductus arteriosus poststenotic dilatation of the pulmonary artery, idiopathic dilatation of the pulmonary artery etc.

·Percussion of the base of the heart–Percuss the right second intercostal space, the midsternum and left second intercostal space starting from the right side. A dull note over the left 2nd space is observed in aneurysm of the arch of the aorta, massive pericardial effusion etc. Increase in the retrosternal dullness is also found in tumours of the anterior mediastinum.

Rotch's sign :– Dullness of the right 5th intercostal space and change of the cardiohepatic angle from a right angle to an obtuse angle are found in massive pericardial effusion.

AUSCULTATION

Place the chest piece over the apical impulse, then in turn over the pulmonary, aortic and tricuspid areas; then over the lower end of both sides of the sternum and also over other sites like the femoral artery, carotid artery etc. The anatomical landmarks of the different valves and the auscultatory areas have been already described.

During auscultation of the different areas. note the followings :

(a) First and second heart sounds :–their intensities, qualities and rhythms.

(b) Adventitious sounds e.g. murmurs, friction rubs or any added heart sound.

The murmurs are heard carefully to ascertain their timing (in *relation* to systole or diastole of the ventricles), intensity, character, site (whether localised or radiated) and alteration with respiration etc.

HEART SOUNDS : These are the sounds heard in one cardiac cycle and are –

I.   *Valve closure sounds*–The first and second heart

sounds are produced by the closure of the atrioventricular and semilunar valves respectively.

II.   *Valve opening sounds*–The opening snap of stenotic lesions of the atrioventricular valve is produced by the opening of the mitral valve (in mitral stenosis) or the tricuspid valve (in tricuspid stenosis).

III.   *Vascular vibration sounds*–They are known as ejection clicks and may be pulmonary and aortic. Nonejection systolic click (s) may be heard in mitral valve prolapse.

IV.   *Ventricular filling sounds*–The third heart sound, (or the protodiastolic or ventricular gallop) is classically a ventricular filling sound.

V.   *Atrial contraction sound*–The fourth heart sound (or the presystolic or atrial gallop) is a classical atrial contraction sound.

1. THE VALVE CLOSURE SOUND–

The first heart sound is *dull* and *prolonged*, best heard at the apex. It indicates the beginning of the ventricular systole. It is produced by the closure of the bicuspid (mitral) and tricuspid valves.

The second heart sound is best heard in the pulmonary and aortic areas and indicates the beginning of the ventricular diastole. It is *short* and *high pitched*, produced by the closure of the aortic and pulmonary valves, The aortic and pulmonary components are heard best over the aortic and pulmonary areas respectively.

Normally the mitral component of the first heart sound and the aortic component of the second sound are better heard than the tricuspid component of the first sound and the pulmonary component of the second sound respectively because the mitral and aortic valves are working against a high left ventricular pressure (100/0mm Hg) whereas the right sided valves are working against a low right ventricular pressure (20/0mm Hg).

Abnormalities of the First Heart Sound :

(A)   Alteration in the intensities of the first heart sound which depends upon :

(1)   Position of the valve cusps at the beginning of systole—

(a) If the valve cusps remain wide apart at the beginning of the systole due to a high pressure gradient between the atria and the ventricles (as in mitral and tricuspid stenosis) the first heart sound will be loud. First heart sound tends to be loud in *tachycardia* from any cause such as emotion. exercise, fever, anaemia, hyperkinetic circulatory states such as thyrotoxicosis, pregnancv etc. because of the same mechanism—

(b) If the valve cusps remain close to each other at the beginning of the ventricular systole or if they cannot appose closely on each other, the intensity will be muffled such as in mitral and tricuspid regurgitation. The sound tends to be faini in myocardial infraction, myocarditis, myocardial failure cardiomyopathy and also in hypothyroidism.

(2)   P. R. Interval—If the P. R. interval is short, the first heart sound becomes loud such as in tachycardia due to any cause.

First heart sound becomes muffled if the P. R. interval is prolonged as occurs in rheumatic carditis, digitalis toxicity etc. In heart block and Wenckebach's phenomenon, and in premature or ectopic beats, the first heart sound is of variable intensity.

(3)   Pliability of the valve cusps—If the pliability is lost,

the heart sounds will be diminished in intensity as occurs in calcification, fibrosis and rigidity of the anterior leaflet of the mitral valve even in presence of mitral stenosis.

(4)   Muscle mass of the ventricular pump–First sound *is booming* in intensity in hypertensive patients because of the increased muscle mass. If the rate of the left ventricular pressure pulse is rapid, S_1 will be accentuated.

(5)   Presence of fluid in the pericardial sac hinders the normal conduction of heart sounds and, therefore, intensity of the first heart sound is diminished in pericardial effusion. Presence of an emphysematous lung and increased thickness of the chest in obesity are also responsible for diminution of the intensity of the first heart sound.

Factors influencing the intensity of S_1 may be summarised as follows :

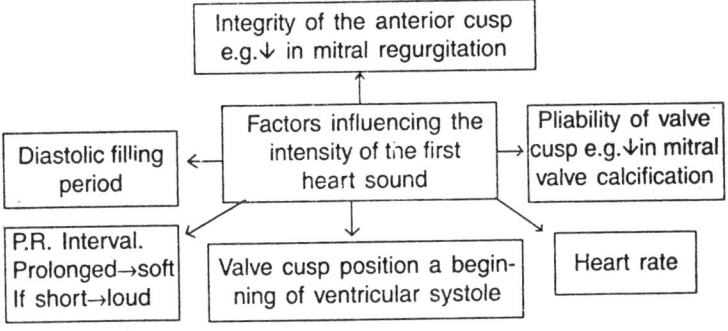

(B)   Splitting of the first heart sound

Normally there is a gap of 0.02 to 0.06 seconds between the closure of the mitral (M_1) and the tricuspid valves (T_1), *which cannot be clinically detected.* If the gap exceeds 0.06 seconds, it becomes detectable and is suggestive of *right bundle branch block.*

Normally M_1 precedes T_1 because the impulse starts from the left side and traverses towards the right. In mitral stenosis as the left atrium takes more time to empty, the *mitral valve* closes late and, therefore, M_1 and T_1 will fuse or M_1 will follow T_1 This is known as *reversed splitting* of the first heart sound. The tighter the mitral stenosis, the wider is the splitting. Physiological splitting of the first heart sound from slight asynchrony in ventricular contraction is a normal phenomenon. It can sometimes be detected on healthy individuals by listening at the lower end of the sternum with the breath held in expiration. The importance of the split first heart sound lies in its proper recognition and in differentiation from other extra heart sounds. *Pathological splitting of the first heart sound occurs in complete right bundle branch block.*

Splitting of the first heart sound must be distinguished from (i) The presystolic triple rhythm produced by atrial contraction sound (4th heart sound) and (ii) from a first heart sound followed by an ejection click as found in cases of aortic stenosis and pulmonary stenosis.

Presystolic triple rhythm (S_4) is found in patients with left heart disease with left ventricular hypertrophy, ischaemic heart diseases, hypertrophic cardiomyopathy, acute mitral regurgitation, delayed AV conduction even in the absence of clinically detectable heart diseases etc. It is absent in atrial fibrillation.

ABNORMALITIES OF THE SECOND HEART SOUND

(A) *Alteration in the intensity of character—*

The 2nd heart sound may be accentuated if there is a high pressure gradient between the ventricles and the great vessels as for example, the P_2 is accentuated in pulmonary hypertension and the A_2 is accentuated in systemic hypertension. Second sound has two components : – the aortic (A_2) and the pulmonary (P_2). A_2 is loud in systemic hypertension, aortic atherosclerosis, aortic dilatation caused by syphilis or atheroma, and is also accentuated in unfolding of the aorta because of the close proximity of the aorta with the chest wall.

A_2 may be ringing in syphilitic aortic aneurysm because the aortic cusps open against a dilated root and ascending aorta.

P_2 is loud in pulmonary hypertension due to mitral stenosis, primary pulmonary hypertension, pulmonary hypertension secondary to atrial septal defect, ventricular septal defect and patent ductus arteriosus. Loud P_2 may also be present in chronic lung diseases such as emphysema and massive pulmonary fibrosis and also in dilatation of the pulmonary artery.

Both A_2 and P_2 may be loud in a patient with thin chest wall or in co-existence of both systemic and pulmonary hypertension.

Factors influencing the intensities of A_2 and P_2 may be summarised as follows–

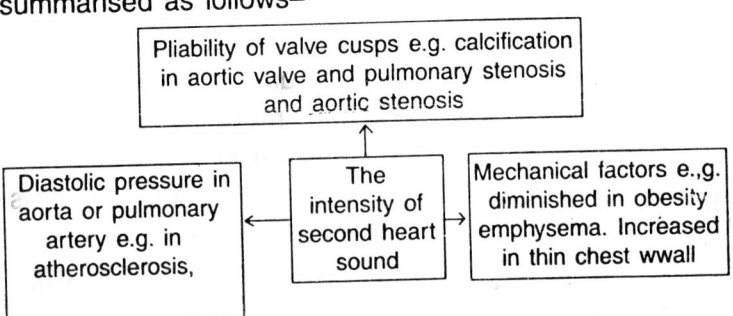

If there is calcification of the semilunar valve cusps, A_2 and P_2 will be of diminished intensity. This occurs in calcific, aortic and pulmonic stenosis.

In Fallot's tetralogy, the aorta is situated anteriorly and the pulmonic valve is stenosed and so the pulmonary second sound is *soft* or *inaudible*–thus the 2nd sound is single in this condition. Second heart sound is often single in moderate aortic stenosis because the two components (A_2 and P_2) merge and fuse with each other. In severe pulmonary stenosis the P_2 may become inaudible because it is very faint.

In common truncus arteriosus there is only one functioning valve and hence there is only one component of the second heart sound (i.e, the second heart sound is single).

In Eisenmenger's VSD or single ventricle, second heart sound is single as P_2 becomes synchronous with A_2.

Causes of single second heart sound : A single S_2 is heard when either the A_2 or the P_2 becomes inaudible or merge together and so the causes include :

(A)   *When the A_2 is inaudible :*
 (i) Diminished intensity in calcific aortic stenosis.
 (ii) Synchronous with P_2 in Eisenmenger's VSD or single ventricle.
 (iii) Concealed by
 (a) Loud P_2 in pulmonary area when there is pulmonary hypertension.
 (b) Loud holosystolic murmur of mitral incompetence or VSD.
 (c) Loud and prolonged ejection systolic murmur of pulmonary stenosis.

(B)   *When the P_2 is inaudible :*
 (i) Diminished intensity in Fallot's tetralogy, pulmonary atresia and rarely in pure pulmonary stenosis.

(ii) Diminished intensity may also be due to poor transmission caused by hyperinflation of the lungs.

(iii) Synchronous with A_2 {as in (ii) of (A) above.}

(iv) May be concealed by systolic murmur of aortic stenosis.

(C) When A_2 and P_2 fuse : vide supra.

(D) *Splitting of the 2nd heart sound*

Normally there is a gap of 0.03 second between the closure of the aortic and the pulmonary valves. If a normal person takes a deep breath and holds it, more blood comes to the right ventricle due to physiological suction. The right ventricle takes more time to eject this extra amount of blood into the pulmonary circulation. So the pulmonary component goes late and a small split of the 2nd sound is audible during inspiration, being known as *physiological splitting* of the 2nd sound.

Effect of posture on splitting of the second heart sound:–

In normal children and young adults expiratory splitting may sometimes be heard in recumbent posture. It should normally disappear on sitting or standing up. If it persists even after sitting or standing up it is *definitely pathological.* Normal physiological splitting may not be audible in presence of tachycardia, thick chest wall or emphysema lung.

Pathological splitting–Abnormally wide splitting of the second heart sound is due to either an abnormal delay in the pulmonary valve closure or a premature closure of the aortic valve.

Delay in *pulmonary valve closure* (P) may be due to (i) delayed activation of the right ventricle (as in right bundle branch block) or (ii) due to prolongation of the right ventricular systole. Prolongation of the right ventricular systole may be due to (a) ralative increase in right ventricular stroke volume (as in left to right shunt e.g. atrial septal

defect) or due to (b) right ventricular outflow tract obstruction (as in pulmonary stenosis) or due to (c) impaired right
ventricular function.

Early or premature *aortic valve closure* (P_2) may result
from decreased left ventricular outflow into the aorta as
occurs in mitral regurgitation and ventricular septal defect.

If the 2nd heart sound shows splitting both in inspiration
and expiration it is known as pathological splitting. It occurs
when the right ventricle deals with an enormous amount
of blood both in inspiration and expiration. The P_2 will be
significantly late (causing wide splitting) and this is found
in (i) *atrial septal defect and* (ii) *total anomalous pulmonary
venous drainage.* If the atrial spetal defect is a big one, an
already overdistended right ventricle cannot accommodate
the extra amount of blood from the left atrium via the right
atrium and as a result, wide and fixed splitting of the 2nd
sound occurs. Fixed splitting of the second heart sound is
also audible in (a) severe right heart failure, (b) massive
pulmonary embolism and (c) in conditions with impaired
right ventricular function as in cardiomyopathy.

Close splitting of the 2nd sound is an important sign of
ventricular septal defect as right ventricle receives an extra
amount of blood from the left ventricle through the septal
defect.

Reversed splitting of the 2nd sound is said to be present
when splitting is audible during expiration but absent during
inspiration. This happens when (i) the left ventricle takes
more time to eject the blood into the aorta or (ii) there is
a delay in the activation of the left ventricle. In these
conditions the aortic valve closes after the pulmonary valve
giving rise to audible splitting of the second sound on
expiration. During inspiration the increased venous return
to the right side of the heart causes a delay in the

pulmonary valve closure; so the A_2 and P_2 come very close to each other resulting in a single sound. This is the reverse of normal and hence called reversed or paradoxical splitting of the second heart sound. The common causes are (a) aortic stenosis, (b) systemic hypertension, (c) coarctation of the aorta, (d) left bundle branch block (e) myocardial infraction, (causing impaired left ventricular myocardial function) (f) severe aortic regurgitation and (g) patent ductus arteriosus.

Splitting of the second heart sound in expiration should be differentiated from (i) the opening snap of mitral stenosis, (ii) triple rhythm due to a third heart sound and (iii) from a pericardial knock which is found in early diastole in constrictive pericardities.

Causes of pathological splitting of the second heart sound
(A) Due to delayed pulmonary 2nd sound :
     (i) Atrial septal defect.
     (ii) Right bundle branch block.
     (iii) Left ventricular pacing or ectopic.
     (iv) Anomalous pulmonary venous return.
     (v) Pulmonary stenosis.
     (vi) Right ventricular failure.
(B) Due to abnormalities of left heart, causing early A_2 and / or delayed P_2 :
     (i) Ventricular septal defect.
     (ii) Mitral *incompetence.*
(C) Due to reversed splitting of the second sound :
     (i)   Electrical delay of A_2 :
        (a) Left bundle branch block,
        (b) Wolff-Parkinson-White syndrome.
        (c) Right ventricular pacing or ectopic.
    (ii) Mechanical delay of A_2 :
        (a) Aortic stenosis (outflow tract obstruction).
        (b) Systolic hypertension.
        (c) Aorto-pulmonary communication.

(d) Left Ventricular failure.

(e) Ischaemia of the left ventricular myocardium.

II. VALVE OPENING SOUNDS

The valve opening sounds are not heard in normal subjects because the atrioventricular pressure gradient is not so high as to open the mitral and tricuspid valves loudly. So an opening snap will be produced only when there is a *high pressure gradient between* the atrium and the ventricle. The best example is mitral stenosis. The opening snap is a sharp high pitched sound; best heard with a diaphragm chest piece, after deep expiration and is usually loudest between the apex beat and left sternal border. Its timing is early in diastole 0.06 to 0.10 second after A_2.

The opening snap is thus diagnositc of high atrioventricular pressure gradient as occurs in (i) organic lesions e.g. mitral stenosis, tricuspid stenosis, etc. or (ii) high flow across the AV valves e.g. posterior cuspal type of mitral regurgitation, ASD, VSD, PDA etc. The tricuspid opening snap is best heard on holding a deep breath. The absence of an opening snap in mitral stenosis may be due to rigidity of the anteromedial cusp caused by calcification, gross destruction of the valve cusps by fibrosis or infective endocarditis, or prevention of opening of the mitral valve cusps by the regurgitant blood coming from the aorta into the left ventricle in aortic valve incompetence.

Presence of an opening snap and a loud S_1 indicate a pliable mitral valve that would be readily amenable to mitral *comissurotomy* (valvulotomy), but experience has shown that although it signifies a mobile anterior cusp it by no means indicate that separation of the cusps will be easy.

The opening snap also denotes a significant mitral stenosis; tighter the stenosis, closer is the opening snap to the S. The opening snap. does not disappear after a successful mitral valvulotomy. It also denies the presence of significant aortic regurgitation or an anterior cuspal type of mitral regurgitation. Development of severe pulmonary hypertension in a case of tight mitral stenosis reduces the left atrioventricular pressure gradient and then the opening snap may be absent.

Opening snap must be differentiated from (i) wide splitting of the second heart sound, (ii) a third heart sound and (iii) pericardial knock. Though an opening snap may be present in tricuspid stenosis it is very difficult to hear and differentiate from a mitral opening snap; it is audible during deep inspiration and diminished after expiration.

III. VASCULAR VIBRATION SOUNDS (ejection click)

These are produced during the ejection phase of the ventricles when a sharp jet of blood comes out through a narrowed opening and strikes against the wall of the great vessels or when a jet of blood after crossing a high vascular resistance impinges on the wall of the great vessels. These sounds coincide with the maximal opening of the aortic or pulmonary valves.

An ejection click is a sharp, high pitched sound heard *immediately* after the S_1.

Aortic ejection click is best heard over the aortic area or in the apex. It is classically found in severe systemic hypertension, mild to moderate aortic stenosis, bicuspid aortic valve and gross aortic regurgitation.

Pulmonary ejection click is best heard over the pulmonary area and is found in early pulmonary stenosis, pulmonary hypertension, idiopathic dilatation of the pulmonary artery and Fallot's tetralogy. Some belive that the ejection click in Fallot's tetralogy is aortic in origin since an enormous amount of blood from both the ventricles enter the dextroposed aorta. A pulmonary click differs from an aortic click in *becoming quieter* or *absent with inspiration*, in contrast to all other right sided auscultatory events,–they accentuate with inspiration.

Non-ejection systolic clicks may be present in mitral regurgitation caused by a prolapse of the posterior leaflet of the mitral valve;–and may be multiple. Generally they occur later than systolic ejection sounds, but may be heard any time during systole. They are best audible at the apex as well as in the lower left sternal border. Such systolic clicks are the *commonest* physical findings in mitral valve prolapse (*Barlow's syndrome*) and may be associated with systolic murmurs;–hence also known as *click murmur syndrome*.

IV. VENTRICULAR FILLING SOUNDS OF THE THIRD HEART SOUNDS (S_3)

These are heard during ventricular diastole. The third heart sound (S_3) is heard during the rapid filling phase.

The S_3 is the vibratory sound produced as a result of sudden distention of the left or right ventricle by the rapid flow of blood from the respective atria during the early rapid filling phase of ventricular diastole. It occurs between 0.12 and 0.16 second *after aortic valve closure* (A_2). When the ventricle distends, the mitral valve cusps become taut and stretched by the papillary muscles and chordae tendinae between the mitral ring and the apex and the vibration sound is produced. S_2 is absent in significant mitral stenosis or tricuspid stenosis which precludes rapid ventricular filling.

Physiological S_3 is heard in children and young adults. If it is heard in persons over the age of 40 years it should be considered pathological and when triple rhythm is associated with tachycardia, it is called gallop rhythm.

Pathological S_4 (*or ventricular gallop, rapid filling gallop* or *Protodiastolic gallop*) may be heard loudest at the apex or near the sternum;–left sided S_3 is heard in systemic *hypertension* myocardial infraction, mitral regurgitation, thyrotoxicosis or cardiomyopathy causing left ventricular failure while the right sided S_3 is heard in massive pulmonary embolism, cardiomyopathy, tricuspid regurgitation etc.

A third heart sound in left ventricular failure will be heard in the middle of the diastole and hence the name diastolic gallop. The term gallop was given to this diastolic sound because of the usually associated tachycardia though." a gallop remains a gallop irrespective of the heart rate. "The diastolic gallop indicates diastolic overload and decreased myocardial contractility in a failing ventricle, and, therefore, is a bad prognostic sign.

V. ATRIAL CONTRACTION SOUND OR THE FOURTH HEART SOUND (S_4)

It results from and is simultaneous with the active atrial contraction against a raised and diastolic pressure of the right or the left ventricle and is either due to pulmonary hypertension and pulmonary embolism (causing right atrial S_4) or systemic hypertension and myocardial infraction (causing left atrial S_4). In a few normal persons an S_4 may be due to delayed atrioventricular conduction (i.e., prolonged P-R interval).

In complete heart block independent irregular S_4 may be audible, in the late part of diastole or in presystole. Addition of S_4 to the normal sounds also produce triple rhythm or (if associated with tachycardia produce) gallop rhythm called presystolic gallop rhythm. Often with the onset of cardiac failure S_4 *may be replaced* by S_3 or both may become audible.

Left sided S_4 are also audible in IHSS, aortic stenosis, other conditions associated with left ventricular outflow tract obstruction, coarctation of the aorta etc.

Left sided S_3 and S_4 should be searched for by the bell of the stethoscope, at the apex, with the patient in the left lateral position and breath held in expiration.

Quadruple gallop– Occasionally the third and the fourth heart sounds are heard separately giving rise to four audible sounds in one cardiac cycle. This is known as quadruple gallop. It is heard in some cases of hypertensive and thyrotoxic heart failure, and also in Ebstein anomaly.

*Summation gallop–*In some gallop rhythm the extra sound may be produced by superimposition of the S_3 on the S_4 i.e., by summation of the 3rd and 4th heart sounds. Such a cadance is called summation gallop. It is found most commonly in left ventricular failure due to systemic hypertension or acute myocardial infraction.

The *pericardial knock* is a sharp third heart sound which indicates the termination of the ventricular filling, occurring 0.10 to 0.12 second after A_2, and often audible in patients with constrictive pericarditis and is due to the restrictive effect of adherent pericardium on diastolic expansion of the ventricles.

VI. PERICARDIAL FRICTION SOUNDS

These are present both in systole and diastole. The pericardial rub is best heard inside the apex and over the pulmonary area. The character is rough and grating. It is better heard on holding the respiration. It may have three components, *presystolic, systolic* and *early diastolic.* The rub may be best elicited with the diaphragm pressed firmly to the chest wall with the patient upright and leaning forward and the intensity in increased by forced inspiration.

The pericardial friction rubs are heard in the following conditions :

(i) Acute fibrinous pericarditis of rheumatic origin.

(ii) Acute pericarditis of tuberculous origin.

(iii) Acute nonspecific pericarditis of viral origin.
(iv) Chemical pericarditis due to chronic renal failure.
(v) Reactionary or haemorrhagic pericarditis due to myocardial infarction.
(vi) Pyogenic pericarditis.
(vii) Malignant pericarditis in association with bronchogenic carcinoma.
(viii) Pericarditis associated with acute pulmonary embolism.

MURMURS

Definition–Murmurs are adventitious or abnormal cardiac sounds produced by circulatory sequences through the valves, great vessels of abnormal openings when there is an abnormal turbulence in the flowing blood. Bruits are sounds produced similarly in the peripheral arteries.

Classification

(A) (1) Ventricular regurgitant murmur.
     (2) Ventricular ejection murmur.
     (3) Ventricular filling murmur.
(B) Murmurs may be organic, where there is a structural defect in the heart; innocent, where the heart is normal and functional, where the murmur is due to an enormous blood flow in an already diseased heart.
(C) Murmurs are classified also according to their sequence with the systole and diastole i.e.
     (i) Systolic–when it coincides with the apex beat,
     (ii) Diastolic or (iii) Systolodiastolic or continuous.

(1) *Ventricular regurgitant murmurs.*

They are always systolic. If the blood regurgitates from the left ventricle into the left atrium through the incompetent mitral valve or from the left ventricle into the right ventricle through a ventricular septal defect, the murmurs are known as murmurs of mitral regurgitation and ventricular septal defect, respectively. Similarly, when blood regurgitates from the right ventricle into the right atrium through incompetent tricuspid valve during systole, the murmur is known as tricuspid regurgitation murmur. The regurgitant mumur starts immediately after the first heart sound and usually continues up to the second heart sound–hence they are known as *pansystolic murmurs*. They are usually associated with systolic thrills and coincide with the apex beat. In mitral regurgitation the murmur is conducted towards the back as the blood is flowing from an anterior (left ventricle) to a posterior chamber (left atrium). In ventricular septal defect the murmur is conducted towards the right side of the chest as the jet of blood is going from a left sided (left ventricle) to a right sided chamber (right ventricle). In tricuspid regurgitation the murmur is conducted from the left sternal edge obliquely upwards towards the right sternal edge because right ventricle is situated along the left sternal edge, whereas the right atrium along the right sternal edge.

The regurgitant pansystolic murmurs are always associated with a 3rd heart sound which is usually loud.

(2) *Ventricular ejection murmurs*

These murmurs are produced by the ejection of blood from the left or right ventricle into the aorta or pulmonary artery repectively during the rapid ejection phase of the ventricular systole. They are loudest during midsystole, start slightly after the 1st sound (following the ejection click) and stop before the onset of 2nd sound. Hence they are known as *midsystolic ejection murmurs*. They are usually associated with systolic thrills at the base of the heart and over the carotid or pulmonary arteries.

(a)   In aortic stenosis (congenital or acquired), obstructive cardiomyopathy, conditions giving rise to enlarged left ventricle with normal aortic ring (i.e., relative stenosis). Hyperkinetic circulatory states where an enormous amount of blood passes through a normal left ventricular outflow tract, an aortic midsystolic ejection murmur is produced.

(b)   A pulmonary ejection systolic murmur is produced in pulmonary stenosis and may be associated with a systolic thrill in the pulmonary area. In atrial septal defect an enormous amount of blood passing through the normal right ventricular outflow tract will produce a similar ejection systolic murmur of lesser intensity. This is known as functional ejection systolic murmur of atrial defect. The same mechanism explains the pulmonary ejection systolic murmur due to an anomalous pulmonary venous drainage.

(c)   An ejection systolic murmur in pulmonary hypertension with right ventricular enlargement is produced by flow of blood from the right ventricle into a dilated pulmonary, artery and may be heard over the pulmonary area.

(3) *Ventricular filling murmurs*

These murmurs are produced by (i) right or left atrial outflow tract obstruction or (ii) regurgitation of blood from the aorta or the pulmonary artery into the respective ventricles.

(a)   The murmur of atrial outflow tract obstruction is best heard in the *middle of diastole* as well as in *presystole*, There will be accentuation of the presystolic murmur because of the active atrial contraction in the last rapiu filling phase of the ventricle. These are classically found in mitral stenosis and tricuspid stenosis. The murmur in the former is *low pitched rumbling* in character. It is *localised* as the blood flows from a posterior to an anterior structure. It is usually accompanied by a diastolic thrill. The murmur of tricuspid origin increases with inspiration and this is known as *Carvallo's sign.*

Functional middiastolic murmurs occur when an enormous quantity of blood flows through a normal mitral valve, as occurs in PDA, VSD, hyperkinetic circulatory states or when a large amount of blood passes through the tricuspid valve as in ASD.

(b) When blood regurgitates back into the ventricles from the aorta or the pulmonary artery, a diastolic murmur is heard in *diastole* when the ventricles are in isometric relaxation phase. In this phase the atrioventricular valves are closed and so no blood is coming from the atria into the ventricles. They are less audible after middiastole as the blood coming from the artria into the ventricles will prevent the pulmonary and aortic regurgitations. However, in long standing aortic regurgitation the murmur may be long or *even holodiastolic*. The murmur is best heard over the left third intercostal space along the left sternal edge, which overlies the outflow tract of the left ventricle. This area is known as *Erb's point.* To differentiate between the diastolic murmurs of pulmonary and aortic regurgitation, look for the peripheral signs of aortic regurgitation (e.g. water hammer or high volume collapsing pulse, wide pulse pressure, dancing carotid arteries or Corrigan's sign capillary pulsation, Hill's sign, pistol shot sound or Traube's sign, Duroziez's diastolic murmur and de-Musset's sign) and try to find out if there is a right ventricular heave with accentuated P_2 suggestive of pulmonary incompetence. The murmur of pulmonary regurgitation caused by pulmonary hypertension (e.g. that due to mitral stenosis) is known as Graham-Steel murmur.

Hill's sign–Increase in the femoral arterial pressure of more than 20 mm Hg above the brachial artery pressure is known as Hill's sign. The normal difference is 20 mm Hg. The greater the incompetence the higher is the gap.

de-Musset's sign–To and fro nodding of the head along with carotid pulsation is known as de-Musset's sign.

Muller's sign–It is the rhythmical pulsatory movement of the uvula, found in florid aortic incompetence, caused by forceful arterial pulsation.

(4) *Continuous murmurs*

These are produced by the flow of blood from high pressure to low pressure vessels.

Causes–(1) Continuous murmur over the left 2nd intercostal space along the left sternal edge is audible in patent ductus arteriosus, pulmonary arteriovenous fistula, aortopulmonary window and bronchopulmonary anastomosis. The blood flows from the aorta into the pulmonary artery or from the bronchial artery into the pulmonary artery.

(2)   If it is heard below the left 3rd space along the left sternal edge. it is suggestive of coronary arteriovenous fistula or rupture of a sinus of Valsava into the right atrium, pulmonary artery.

The murmur of coarctation of the aorta is vascular in origin, and is late systolic in timing with spilling over into the diastole. When blood passes through the constriction, a late systolic murmur is produced and by this time the ventricle goes into the diastolic phase so that the murmur spills over into the early phase of diastole. When blood passes through the collaterals in coarctation of the aorta, a murmur can be heard over the dilated intercostal arteries in the interscapular and infrascapular regions. This is known as *Suzman's sign.*

N.B. – A continuous murmur e.g. that of PDA should be indentified carefully to differentiate it from a to and fro murmur e.g. that of AS and AR or VSD and AR.

(5) *Functional and innocent murmurs*

(a)   *Functional murmurs*–These occur in the absence of an organic heart disease at the site of production of the murmur. The examples include–

(i)   Systolic murmurs in the pulmonary area in ASD which is produced by an increased flow of blood through the normal pulmonary valve and not by the flow of blood through the septal defect.

(ii)   A middiastolic murmur at the lower sternal edge in ASD due to an increased flow of blood through the tricuspid valve.

(iii)   An apical, soft, low pitched, presystolic or middiastolic murmur in some cases of aortic regurgitation, when the regurgitant flow from the aorta along the ventricular wall impinges against the anteromedial mitral valve cusp–it produces a relative or functional mitral stenosis. This is the mechanism by which this *Austin Flint murmur* is produced. However, there are other theories about the genesis of the Austin Flint murmur.

(iv)   In mitral stenosis with severe pulmonary hypertension an early diastolic blowing murmur is heard along the left sternal border, produced by a functional pulmonary regurgitation, It is known as *Graham Steel* murmur.

(v)   An apical functional diastolic murmur may also be found in ventricular septal defect, patent ductus arterious, and mitral regurgitation because of torrential flow across the mitral valve.

(b)   *Innocent murmurs* are usually systolic murmurs arising in a normal heart and the causes of these are unknown. These are found in almost all children. The possible mechanisms are – (i) passage of a normal amount of blood through the pulmonary artery to the pulmonary vascular bed whose resistance is more than what is found in adults; and (ii) hyperkinetic circulatory states in children due to persistently high heart rate. As such, these murmurs disappear as age advances when the heart rate and pulmonary vascular resistance fall. At times innocent murmurs may only be heard after exercise. Innocent murmurs are best heard over the apical and pulmonary areas.

Haemic murmurs–This term is best avoided. It only indicates a murmur associated with hyperkinetic circulatory state producing increased amount of pulmonary blood flow in most cases. In some cases of severe anaemia there may be dilatation of the valve ring producing functional mitral regurgitation.

The following points are to be noted carefully when a murmur is detected on auscultation :

(i)   *Timing in the cardiac cycle* : Note carefully whether the murmur is systolic. diastolic or systolodiastolic. The timing is easily done during a slow heart rate but may be difficult during tachycardia. For timing of a murmur the apex beat or the carotid pulsation may be used. Apex beat coincides with S_1 and carotid pulsation occurs 1/10th second after S_1. A systolic murmur appears immediately after S_1 although there is a small gap if the murmur is midsystolic. A diastolic murmur appears immediately after S_2 or after an appreciable time interval but immediately before the S_1 (if it is presystolic). One should also note carefully whether the murmur is heard throughout the whole systole (pansystolic). or in the middle of diastole (middiastolic) and so on and so forth. At times it may be difficult to time a murmur. In such cases the timing of the murmur in the cardiac cycle should be found out by noting its. character. In most difficult circumstances phonocardiographic help is needed.

(ii) *Character of the murmur* : Various types of murmurs are heard of which the following are characteristic :

(a) Low pitched rumbling murmur of mitral stenosis.

(b) Soft blowing, high pitched early diastolic decrescendo murmur of aortic regurgitation.

(c) Continuous machinery (train through tunnel; Gibson's) murmur of patent ductus arteriosus.

(d) High pitched blowing murmur at the apex radiating towards the axilla in mitral regurgitation.

(e) Loud, rough and harsh systolic murmur beginning a little after S_1 with midsystolic accentuation (diamond shaped) and stoping just before S_2 heard in the aortic area in aortic stenosis. It is conducted upwards towards the carotid arteries, and sometimes best heard in the mitral area.

(iii) *Conduction of the murmur* : The direction in which the murmurs are conducted should be carefully noted. The murmur of mitral regurgitation is selectively conducted to the axilla and left infrascapular area of the chest. The murmur of mitral stenosis is localised to the apex. The direction of conduction or the absence of conduction characterises certain murmurs. The conduction depends on the loudness of the murmur; conductive nature of adjacent tissue, the direction of the blood flow that produces the murmur, and at times on the state of hypertrophy of the papillary muscles.

(iv) *Intensity of the murmur* : Murmurs have a wide variety of intensity ranging from very faint to very loud. The area of maximum intensity should be found out. It must be remembered that the intensity of a murmur is not always proportional to the haemodynamic disturbance. Thus a murmur of a small VSD may be much more intense than that due to large one. Arbitrarily the intensity of murmurs have been divided into SIX different grades, grade I to VI (vide infra). When a murmur is produced at a valve, the maximum intensity of the murmur will be heard at the particular point where that particular valve sound is best heard. For example, mitral stenosis murmur is best heard at the mitral area, aortic stenosis murmur is heard with maximum intensity at the aortic area etc.

(v) *Alteration of murmur with respiration* : The stroke

out put of the right heart increases during inspiration while that of the left gets reduced. So the murmurs originating in the right heart becomes more intense during inspiration, and accentuation of a tricuspid murmur with inspiration is known as *Carvallo's sign.* The murmur which becomes louder on expiration is of the left heart. A sustained Valsalva manoeuvre results in intensification of the murmurs of IHSS and prolongs or brings out that of mitral valve prolapse.

(vi) *Change of murmur with change of posture* : Murmurs should be studied both in the recumbent and in the upright (i.e., sitting or standing positions). The murmur of mitral stenosis is best heard in the mitral area with the patient recumbent and turned to a left lateral position; on the other hand, the murmur of aortic regurgitation is best heard in the aortic area of Erb's point with the patient sitting upright and leaning forward and the chest being held in a position of full expiration. The murmurs of mitral valve prolapse and IHSS are intensified on standing and *decreased or abolished* by prompt squatting.

(vii) *Behaviour of murmur during exercise* : Exercise increases the intensity of the faint murmurs or at times bring out an otherwise faint murmur to a prominence. Thus the diastolic murmur of mitral stenosis becomes louder and prominent after exercise. Isometric hand grip exercise accentuates the murmur of aortic regurgitation, but diminishes that of aortic stenosis and IHSS.

Remember that in children a transient systolic murmur may be heard after exercise–in most cases it is innocent.

Auscultation of special regions other than the heart

The results of the detailed examination of the heart, performed as advised above may direct the clinician to look for special signs specific for some diseases or conditions e.g. :

(1) Auscultation of the lung bases for crepitations should be done in cases with left heart enlargement. The crepitations are due to pulmonary venous congestion which leads to interstitial pulmonary oedema : and if sufficiently progressed, to alveolar oedema.

(2) The abdomen should be auscultated for systolic bruits over the renal artery, diagnostic of renal artery stenosis.

(3) Pistol shot sounds are present over the femoral artery in patients with high pulse pressure.

(4) Duroziez's murmur--It is the diastolic murmur heard over the femoral artery when one presses the femoral artery distally with the edge of the chest piece. This indicates arterial reflux in aortic regurgitation. *Duroziez's sign* : When the chest piece is placed over the femoral artery, a diastolic murmur is heard if the artery is pressed distally and a systolic one if the artery is pressed proximally. This is Duroziez's sign, one of the peripheral signs of aortic regurgitation.

(5) Auscultation over the lumbar region on the back may reveal a murmur due to blood flow through the constricted aorta in a subphrenic type of coarctation of the aorta.

(6) Auscultation over the shin bone may reveal a continuous murmur indicative of Paget's disease of the bones or peripheral arteriovenous fistula.

(7)   A continuous murmur over the jugular vein is known as *venous hum;* it is a common normal finding in children in an upright posture.

(8)   Systolic bruits may be heard over the thyroid in thyrotoxicosis.

(9)   A murmur may be heard over the closed eyes in a carotido-cavernous fistula.

ELECTROCARDIOGRAPHY

The electrocardiogram is the recorded magnified galvanometric deflections which reflect the electrical events of the heart. The waves produced are known as P. Q. R. S. T and U. This helps us (i) to understand the pathway of conduction of the excitatory wave, (ii) to detect hypertrophy of the ventricles even when its clinical or rediological detections remain elusive, (iii) to diagnose myocardial ischaemia or infraction and (iv) to record and analyse the arrhythmias. For a detailed account of electrocardiography the students are advised to consult specialised text-books, but if they comprehend the basic principles of electrocardiography they will be able to easily interpret the electrocardiogram.

In routine practice a 12 lead electrocardiogram is recorded; these leads are—

(a) Edberg lead ....

(A)   Six limb leads which are again divided into—

(a)   3 standard or bipolar limb leads.

Lead I–indicates the potential difference between the left and the right arms.

Lead II–Potential difference between the left leg and the right arm.

Lead III–Potential difference between the left leg and the left arm.

(b) Goldering leads...............................

(b) Augmented unipolar limb leads :

aVR–The exploring electrode is placed on the right arm.

aVL–The exploring electrode is placed on the left arm.

aVF–the exploring electrode is placed on the left leg.

NB–Remember that the limb leads are affected by the position of the heart within the chest.

(c) Wilson leads ....

(B) Six unipolar chest leads designated V_1 to V_6–

V_1–Right sternal border in the 4th intercostal space.

V_2–Left sternal border in the 4th intercostal space.

V_3–Between V_2 and V_4

V_4–Left 5th intercostal space on the midclavicular line.

V_5–Left 5th intercostal space on the anterior axillary line.

V_6–Left 5th intercostal space on the midaxillary line.

THE NORMAL ELECTROCARDIOGRAM

The waves produced in the ECG are P, QRS, T and U and indicate the depolarisation of the atria (P) and the ventricles (QRS) and repolarisation of the ventricles (T). The wave of atrial repolarisation remains buried in the QRS complex. The U wave is possibly caused by slow repolarisation of the Purkinje fibres.

The ECG is recorded on a specially prepared graph paper. The thin vertical lines or thin horizontal lines are 1 mm apart and represents horizontally 0.04 seconds and vertically 0.1 mV.

Normal Patterns

Normally in the standard limb leads, P, R, and T are positive waves and Q and S are negative waves.

It must be remembered that the deflection of waves in any lead will depend on the direction of the impulse relative to that particular lead.

P wave–First wave of electrocardiogram and represents the spread of impulse through the atria (atrial depolarisation). Its amplitude should not exceed 2.5 mm and width should be less than 0.11 sec. in duration.

P-R interval–P-R interval is atrioventricular conduction time and is measured from the beginning of the P wave to the beginning of the QRS complex.

Normally its duration is 0.12 to 0.20 seconds.

QRS interval–QRS interval denotes ventricular depolarisation and normal duration is 0.05 to 0.10 second.

Q wave–Q waves are absent in V_1 and V_2 and where present, it is less than 0.04 sec. in duration and less than 25% of R.

J point–This is the point where the QRS ends and ST begins.

ST segment–From the J point to the beginning of the T wave. Usually isoelectric but may be elevated up to 2 mm or depressed by 0.5 mm. Look for its shape; normally it curves smoothly and joins the proximal limb of the T wave. Its elevation or depression are in comparison to the T-P segment.

S wave–Represent ventricular repolarisation and usually rounded and slightly asymmetrical. It is inverted in a VR, may be upright, diphasic or inverted in III, aVL, V_1 and upright in all other leads. Normal height should not exceed 5 mm in standard leads and 10 mm in any precordial leads.

Q-T interval–It is measured from the beginning of the QRS to the end of the T wave. It represents the duration of the electrical systole. This interval is dependent on age, sex and heart rate.

U wave–Occassionally this is seen after the T wave. Its

significance is uncertain. U-wave coincides with the phase of super normal excitability during ventricular recovery. It is in this phase that most of the ventricular premature beats are seen to occur.

Electric heart axis

The normal electric. heart axis is between 30° to 90° You look in which standard limb lead. QRS in most positive, normally in 1 or 11.

Is e.g. III most positive, the axis is over, 90°, it is a right axis deviation.

Is e.g. III or aVF most negative the axis is under, 30°, it is a left axis deviation.

A slight right heart deviation might be seen physiologically in tall and thin but healthy people.

Abnormal Patterns

One should observe the shape, breadth and the height of each of the waves of PQRST complex.

(1) P wave :

    (a)   Broad and bifid–Left atrial hypertrophy (P-mitrale) ('P' more than 0.11 seconds).

    (b)   Tall and peaked–Right atrial hypertrophy (P-pulmonale ('P' more than 3 mm).

    (c)   Absent–AV nodal rhythms, S-A block, hyperpotassaemia (severe), atrial fibrillation (replaced by f wave).

    (d)   Inversion–Dextrocardia nodal rhythm.

    (e)   Difficult to identify–in extreme tachycardia e.g. paroxysmal atrial tachycardia.

(2) P-R interval :

    (a)   Prolonged–(i) Partial A-V block; first and second degrees.

    (ii) Giant left atrium in ASD of the septum primum type and mitral regurgitation.

(b) Shortened--(i) A-V nodal rhythm.

(ii) Atrial ectopic rhythm of lower origin.

(iii) Normally in infants.

(iv) WPW syndrome.

(3) QRS complex – Abnormalities of this complex may be found in ventricular hypertrophy, myocardial infraction, conduction defects etc.

(a) Prolonged QRS–intraventricular conduction defects, hyperpotassaemia, quinidine therapy etc.

(b) Low voltage QRS (height less than 5 mm in all three standard leads) found in–

Obesity, emphysema, anasarca, myxoedema, ischaemic heart disease, cor pulmonale, constrictive pericarditis etc.

(c) High voltage QRS--Seen in ventricular hypertrophy.

(4) ST segment–This segment is influenced by-Ischaemic heart disease, digitalis toxicity, myocarditis, potassium intoxication, acute pericarditis (concordant ST elevation), ventricular hypertrophy, intraventricular conduction defects etc.

(5) T wave–Normally the T wave is upright in leads I, II, V_2 to V_6; inverted in a VR and variable in leads II, aVL, aVF V_1 and V_2.

(a) Tall and peaked T waves are found in hyperkalaemia.

(b) Inverted T waves may be–

(i) Symmetrical in myocardial infraction (nontransmural).

(ii) Asymmetrical in L V-strain.

(6) Prolonged QT interval may be seen in–

Myocardial infraction, hypocalcaemia, quinidine and procainamide toxicity, myocarditis, congestive cardiac failure etc.

(7)   Shortened QT interval may be found in–
      Digitalis therapy, hypercalcaemia hyperpo-
      tassaemia.

(8)   U wave– Pronounced in potassium deficiency. In
      myocardial inschaemia and left ventricular strain
      its polarity is reversed i.e. inverted.

ECG changes in certain important clinical conditions

A. *Left atrial enlargement*

Broad an notched P wave (P-mitrale) usually best
seen in leads I and III. Notching is significant when
the distance between the two peaks exceed 0.04
sec.

In V_1, the P wave is characteristically wide, slurred
and diphasic in which the downward component
is most prominent.

B. *Right atrial enlargement*

(i)   Tall slender, peaked P wave in II, III and aVF
      (P- pulmonale).

(ii) P wave prominent, peaked diphasic or in-
      verted in V_1.

C. *Left ventricular hypertrophy*

(i)   R in V_5 or V_6 is 27 mm or more.

(ii) S in V_1 and R in V_5 or V_6 together 35 mm or
      more.

(iii) Ventricular activation time (intrinsicoid deflec
      tion or VAT) over 0.05 second in V_5 and V_6.

(iv) QRS greater than 0.13 sec. in V_5 and V_6.

(v)   ST segment depressed and T wave inverted in
      V_5 and V_6.

(vi) R in a VL more than 13 mm.

(vii) R in a VF more than 20 mm.

(viii) Left axis deviation (– 15° or more).

D. *Right ventricular hypertrophy*

(i)   R taller than S in V_1.

(ii)   Ventricular activation time (intrinsicoid deflec
        tion) over 0.03 second in V_1.

(iii)   Persistent S in V_5 and V_6.

(iv)   S-T segment depressed and T wave inverted
        in V_1 to V_3.

(v)   Right axis deviation (+110° or more); de-
        pressed ST segment and inverted T wave in
        II and III.

E. *Right bundle branch block (RBBB)*

(i)   RSR or rSR pattern in V_1 and V_2.

(ii)   Wide S wave in V_5 and V_6.

(III)   QRS interval 0.12 second or more.

(iv)   Ventricular activation time (intrinsicoid deflec
        tion 0.06 second or more in V_1 and V_2.

(v)   ST depression and T inversion in V_1 and V_3.

F. *Left bundle branch block (LBBB)*

(i)   Wide and slurred R in V_4 to V_6.

(ii)   Q absent in V_4 to V_6.

(iii)   QRS interval 0.12 second or more.

(iv)   Ventricular activation time (intrinsicoid deflec
        tion) more than 0.09 second in V_4 to V_6.

(v)   ST depression and T inversion in V_4 to V_6.

(vi)   Absence of Q, abnormal R with S T depres-
        sion and T inversion in lead I.

(vii)   In a VL a pattern similar to that seen in V_4
        to V_6.

G. *Acute myocardial infraction (AMI)*

(i)   Within a few hours after the infraction the ST
        segment becomes elevated with a convexity up-
        wards.

(ii)   Next to appear is the symmetrical T wave inver-
        sion ie. the peak of the T is midway between the
        beginning and the end. It occurs in hours to days.

(iii)   Abnormal Q waves appear. They are found usually before any gross T wave changes occur. At times instead of appearance of Q waves, there may be only a reduction of the voltage of R. Abnormal Q waves are usually permanent.

The above mentioned changes are found only in those leads which represent the area of the myocardium involved in infraction.

Following leads are to be examined for exact localisation of the site of infraction :

Anterior wall–I, aVL, V_1 to V_6.

Anteroseptal wall–I, aVL, V_1 and V_2.

Anterolateral wall–I, aVL, V_5 and V_6.

Inferior wall–II, III aVF.

Inferolateral wall–II, III aVF, V_5 and V_6.

H.   *First degree A-V block*

The P-R interval is prolonged to more than 0.2 sec. It indicates a delay in conduction through the A-V node or bundle of His.

I.   *Second degree A-V block*

It may be of two types–Mobitz type I or Wenckebach type and Mobitz II. *Wenckebach or Mobitz type I A-V block*–The PR interval is usually normal in the first beat. Then with each successive beat it gradually becomes longer and longer (while the PR interval becomes shorter and shorter) until one QRS is dropped indicating a complete failure of ventricular response to atrial activation. After that the next P-R interval is again normal and the same phenomena occurs over and over again. The site of block in proximal to the His bundle and within the A-V node. *Mobitz type II A-V block*–Here the PR and PP intervals are constant throughout but the ventricles fail to respond to atrial stimulation periodically either in a regular or an irregular fashion. The dysrrhythmia shows dropped beats regular e.g. with 2 : 1, 3 : 1 or 4 : 1 block or it may be irregular. Here the block is either in the His bundle or distal to it. Mobitz type II block is usually a more serious disorder than Mobitz type I block.

J. *Bifascicular Block.*
In this usually there is RBBB with left anterior or posterior hemi blocks (LAH or LPH) and the ECG shows—(i) Left (with LAH) or right (with LPH) axis deviations and (ii) Features of RBBB.

K. *Trifascicular Block.*
It is bifascicular block with PR prolongation.

L. *Complete Heart Block*
No impulse can pass through the A.V. node; the atria and the ventricles beat independent of each other. There is no definite relation between the P waves and the QRS complexes which are independent of one another. The artial rhythm is usually regular and the atrial rate is usually the average sinus rate. The ventricular rate is usually 40 per minute (varying between 20 and 60) and ventricular rhythm is also regular because the ventricle continues to beat in response to a pacemaker situated either in the A-V junction (nodal) or in the ventricular myocardium, producing idionodal or idioventricular rhythms respectively.

EXERCISE ECG—ECG in ischaemia is classically characterised by ST depression in leads with dominant R waves. Since the resting ECG may remain entirely normal in patients with IHD it may be necessary to document the ECG changes during and after exercise to demonstrate the ischaemia. During exercise the ECG may reveal *J point depression* increasing as the exercise progresses, with the ST *becoming entirely flat for* the first 80 msec of its duration and with further change may even be *negative or downsloping.* An important criterion is that 1mm or 0.10 mv or more of flat ST displacement in a standard lead indicates myocardial ischaemia. Where ST displacement is transient improving with cessation of exercise it is known as type I response and is of minor prognostic abnormality. Type II is a protracted ST depression provoked by mild exercise and constitutes a major prognostic abnormality, such as caused by severe multivessel disease or left main coronary artery disease.

TECHNIQUE OF PERICARDIOCENTESIS AND THE STUDY OF THE PERICARDIAL FLUID

A pericardiocentesis is done to–(i) attempt at establishing a diagnosis of pericardial disease, (ii) relieve acute cardiac tamponade, (iii) aid anaesthetic management of the perioperative decompensated patient needing pericardiectomy and (iv) study elevation of venous pressures.

If performed at the bedside, ECG monitoring essential.

Approaches are – (i) subxiphoid (ideal) and (ii) parasternal.

The patient is adequately sedated and 0.5 mg to 1 mg atopine given IV to prevent vasovagal reaction.

With the patient propped up to 45° " a point 2 cm below the tip of the xiphoid and just to the left of midline is locally anaesthetized. The needle (about 6 inch long and of small guage) is introduced under ECG monitoring and cautiously advanced towards the left shoulder. The resistance of the diaphragm and pericardium suddenly yields and as the needle touches the epicardium a scratch sensation is felt.

In the lateral thoracic approach the needle should be inserted just beyond the apex beat or in the left fifth intercostal space just internal to the lateral border of the cardiac dullness and directed backward and inward, towards the spine.

At first about 5 cc fluid is drawn out and allowed to clot if it is grossly haemorrhagic to exclude right ventricular puncture in which case the fluid readily coagulates.

When the pericardial space has been properly localised and LP needle of wider gauge is introduced along the same path and all possible fluid is removed.

In diagnostic pericardiocentesis air may be injected a. the completion of the procedure to aid in follow up radiological studies.

Following the procedure most patients should be observed for 24 hours in an intensive care unit.

Possible complications are—(i) laceration of a coronary artery, (ii) laceration of the right ventricle, (iii) right atrial or ventricular perforation, (iv) pneumothorax, (v) gastric or colonic perforation, (vi) arrhythmias, (vii) tamponade, (viii) systemic hypotension etc.

Assessment of the case is very important and should be done by carefully taking the history and performing the clinical examination and radiological studies because diseases like cardiomyopathy and fibroelastosis, may stimulate pericardial effusion. After pericardiocentesis, the pulse and the blood pressure are recorded at hourly intervals and any irregularity of the pulse is to be considered seriously.

The main therapeutic indications of pericardiocentesis are (i) cardiac tamponade—clinically characterised by the triad of low volume pulse, engorded neck veins and a quiet heart and (ii) evidences of considerable quantity of fluid in the pericardial cavity.

Similarly for diagnostic purposes in polyserositis, Meig's syndrome and if there is a strong suspicion of pericardial effusion on clinical grounds, this procedure is undertaken. Cases of amoebic abscess of the left lobe of liver bursting into the pericardium in the tropics have been diagnosed after a needle has been put into the pericardium.

The study of the fluid–macroscopic, microscopic, bio-chemical and pathological–is carried out as in cases of pleural and peritoneal fluids. Cholesterol crystals have occasionally been demonstrated in pericardial fluid of patients suffering from myxoedema.

RADIOGRAPHIC EXAMINATION OF THE HEART

Standard postero anterior and oblique views (both right and left) of X-ray chest are usually taken and if required, right anterior oblique (RAO) view with barium filled oesophagus is taken.

PA views–Cardiac silhouette is a flask shaped shadow between the two translucent lungs. Normally the cardiac apex is just internal to the midclavicular line.

The right border of the cardiac shadow is formed from above downwards by (i) the outer border of the superior vena cava with the ascending aorta and (ii) the convex outer border of the right atrium up to the diaphragm; the left border of the cardiac shadow is formed from above downwards by (i) the aortic kunckle, (ii) the pulmonary artery segment and then by (iii) the left ventricle up to the apex. If the left atrium is enlarged then in an overpenetrated film just internal to the right atrium another rounded border may be seen–that of the enlarged left atrium giving rise to a double contour of the right border of the heart. In left atrial enlargement an upward displacement of the left main bronchus is seen.

In the RAO view the barium filled oesophagus courses directly adjacent to the left atrium. This view is of particular importance for recognising compression of posterior displacement of the oesophagus by an enlarged left atrium.

In the left anterior oblique view of X-ray chest with the patient rotated to an angle of 50° or less the left ventricle is seen to overlap the spine when it is enlarged.

In the PA view an *enlargement of the ascending aorta* is seen in syphilitic aortitis with aneurysm, in aortic regurgitation and in aortic stenosis when poststenotic dilatation is present. Unfolding of the aorta is seen in atherosclerosis.

In mitral stenosis where the left atrial pressure is significantly high, engorged subpleural lymphatics are seen at the lung bases as horizontal lines. In radiographic finding these lines are called Kerley B lines. When the main branches of the pulmonary artery are engorged due to increased pulmonary blood flow it is called *pulmonary plethora*. When vascular markings in the lung fields are diminished it is called *pulmonary oligaemia.*

Fluoroscopy is used to see the (i) cardiac size (ii) pulsations of the different chambers and great vessels and (iii) to detect calcification of the cardiac valves, coronary arteries or pericardium etc.

Angiocardiography–The contrast media is injected via the catheter into the different chambers of the heart or into the great vessels and serial films are taken. When following an injection of the contrast media high speed X-ray motion pictures are taken it is called *cine angiography.* If the contrast media is injected selectively into a particular coronary artery and skiagrms taken, it is called *coronary angiography.* Angiocardiography, coronary angiography and cine angiography have helped in better understanding of the dynamic anatomy of the heart, cardiac valves and coronary arteries in normal conditions as well as in a variety of cardiac disorders. These procedures are very important in selecting the appropriate cardiac patients for surgical management. They help in accurate structural and functional diagnosis of complex cardiac lesions.

PHONOCARDIOGRAPHY

A phonocardiogram is a graphic display of the cardiac sounds and murmurs. It helps in proper and objective assessment of the auscultatory events and allows a perfect detection and understanding of the sequences of cardiac events so far as the heart sounds and murmurs are concerned. Its most important application is in the precise timing of cardiac sounds and murmurs especially in complex cardiac lesions.

ECHOCARDIOGRAPHY

This is a noninvasive method of examining the heart by utilizing ultrasound.

The frequency of the sound used in echocardiography ranges from 1 to 7 mega Hertz, i.e. 1 to 7 million cycles per second. Frequencies usually used in adults are 2 to 3 mega Hertz and those used in children are 3 to 5 mega Hertz. Sound waves of this frequency are produced by intermittently exciting a piezzoelectric crystal electronically. The waves of ultrasounu coming out of the transducer penetrate tissues and are reflected from the different structures of the heart back to the crystal in the transducer. A form of echo is provided by the reflected sound signals and the transducer receives if (when not transmitting) and sends out an electronic signal proportionate to the intensity of the echoes.

Echocardiography detects the motion of the solid struc- tures of the heart and by the standard frequency used, structures up to 8 inches from the surface can be exam- ined. Lower frequency ultrasonic beams are used in adults so that it penetrates well through the chest wall. Resolution of objects even only 1 to 2 mm apart is possible with this frequency.

The ultrasonic beams travel in a straight line through a homogeneous medium. But as it strikes the interface between two media of different acoustical properties it undergoes reflection and refraction akin to light. The reflected portion returns to the piezzoelectric element in the transducer and gives rise to an electric signal.

The different modes of display of the ultrasonic echoes received by the transducer are—

(i) **A Mode**–A stands for *amplitude*. Here the intensity of the reflected echo signal is displayed on the horizontal axis of the oscilloscope and the time required to travel from the transducer to the target and back is displayed on the vertical axis. With movement of the heart the echoes move up and down during the cardiac cycle. This mode of echo display system is now rarely used.

(ii) **B Mode**–B stands for *brightness*. This brightness is displayed on the z-axis of the oscilloscope and in this more practical method of recording echo motion the amplitude of the echo is converted to brightness and the returning *echoes* are displayed on the oscilloscope as dots rather than spikes. The distance from the transducer is plotted on the y-axis.

(iii) M Mode–M stands for *motion*. In this mode the ele- ment of time is introduced by sweeping the oscilloscope from the bottom to the top. In this mode of echocardiography time is recorded on the x-axis and the B mode echo signal is recorded on the y axis and thus the amplitude and the rate of motion of the moving objects can be recorded with great accuracy. An electrocardiogram is recorded simultaneously. The transducer is placed usually along the left sternal border on the third or fourth space and the beam of the ultrasonic wave is directed to the part of the heart to be examined. Usually the structures through which the beam travels and are reproduced on the oscilloscope from above downwards are–the chest wall, the anterior wall of the right ventricle, portion of the right ventricular cavity, the interventricular septum, a portion of the left ventricular, cavity, the mitral valve apparatus and the posterior left ventricular wall with endocardial and epicardial echoes. Other structures of the heart can also be visualized by suitably directing the beam of ultrasonic waves from the transducer.

(iv) Real-time–Cross-sectional or two dimensional (2D) echocardiography–This is a more advanced technique that provides information e.g. cardiac shape and lateral motion that are not available by the M-mode. This is also known as sector, scanner, in this a rapid and repeated scanning of a B mode echocardiographic tracing is done across a sector field at a rate that provides continuous image. Cross-sectional echocardiography helps to display transverse, sagittal or coronal sections of the heart and thus increases the scope of ultrasonic examination.

Echocardiography helps in the diagnosis of almost all the different morbidities of the heart but is especially helpful for mitral valve diseases, calcifications of the valve cusps, pericardial effusion, left atrial myxoedema, infective endocarditis (detection of vegetations), congenital heart diseases and cardiomyopathies.

DOPPLER ECHOCARDIOGRAPHY :

Now-a-days there are three types of Doppler echo :

(a) The oldest one is the PULSED Doppler, which is only able to record slow velocities of the blood corpuscle. This slow velocities give a hint to areas with thrombatic risk.

(b) CW-Doppler (continous wave D.) is able to screen high velocities, but not their direction.

(c) COLOUR Doppler is one of the newest investigations, enables the recording of high velocities and its direction. If the blood flews in direction towards the transducer it occurs a different colour as if it flews in the opposite direction.

With this investigation you can predict : congenital heart failure, congenital cranial aneurysm (through open fontanella of the newborn), heart valve failure (gradient estimation) and control of prosthetic valves.

Doppler is a server alternative to invasive diagnosis.

Radionuclide ventriculography.

Laen invasive then catheterization and also a very precise method estimating ventricular function and anatomy. Erythrocytes or albumine is labcled with technetium 99 No aview of myocardial perfusion thallium 201 is injected a bit before maximum exercise on an ergometer. Those exercise scans together with resting time scans taken 2-5 hours later detect reparfusion (ischaemic) regions and fixed defects (infraction).

SOME COMMON CARDIOVASCULAR DISEASES
CARDIAC VALVE DISEASES
1. MITRAL STENOSIS

I. *Aetiology* : 85% rheumatic, rest are congenital or associated with cardiomyopathy and very rarely associated with rheumatoid arthritis and Hurler's syndrome.

II. *Symptoms :*
1. Effort intolerance– sudden or insidious. Sudden when caused by pulmonary oedema.
2. Haemoptysis.
3. Angina pectoris, rarely which mey be due to–
   (a) Right ventricular hypertrophy–imbalance in blood supply and myocardial oxygen demand.
   (b) Atrial fibrillation due to cardiac ischaemia.
   (c) Discomfort due to costochondritis.
   (d) Associated coronary artery disease.
4. Easy fatiguability.
5. Palpitation resulting from–
   (a) Right ventricular hypertrophy.
   (b) Atrial fibrillation.
6. Dependent oedema and even anasarca.

III. *Signs :*
1. Malar flush, especially in fair-skinned individuals.
2. Small volume pulse.
3. Blood pressure-low.
4. Neck veins not engorged, but if there is pulmonary hypertension–gaint 'a' waves are found.
5. Apex beat–Normal in position, character is slapping or tapping. There is a diastolic thrill.
6. Parasternal heave and diastolic shock–when there is pulmonary hypertension.
7. Auscultation–S_1– short, sharp accentuated (not if the valve is calcified or if there is prosthetic valve). S_2–audible in mitral area.
   Opening snap (of Potain) : better heard after deep expiration.
   Murmur : mid-diastolic rumbling low pitched, localised to the mitral area, best heard after

expiration, on turning the patient to left lateral position and with the bell, in sinus rhythm, after exercising the patient, presystolic accentuation which disappears if there is atrial fibrillation, but may be audible rarely with a strong atrial contraction. S_2–in pulmonary area is split.

IV. *investigation :*
1. X-ray chest. PA and left lateral views.
2. ECG : P waves widened and notched (P mitrale). QRS complex shows verying degrees of right axis deviation in pulmonary hypertension, or P replaced by f waves in atrial fibrillation.
3. Echocardiographic : Left atrial enlargement; mitral valve situation (calcification, thickened etc); Doppler : less left ventricular at a diastolic input (degree estimation).

V. *Complications :*
1. Acute left atrial failure leading to pulmonary oedema.
2. Atrial fibrillation.
3. Systemic embolism usually due to atrial fibrillation.
4. Severe pulmonary hypertension.
5. Right heart failure and congestive cardiac failure.
6. Severe haemoptysis due to pulmonary infraction.
7. Infective endocarditis in 0.5% cases only. Percentage is low, since endocardial erosion is practically absent.
8. Dysphagia.

9. Ortner's syndrome : Hoarseness of voice due to involvement of left recurrent laryngeal nerve by–

(i) left atrial enlargement.

(ii) pressure of hilar lymph nodes

(iii) enlargement of pulmonary artery segment.

VI. *Treatment*

Mitral valvulotomy (comissurotomy)–clcsed or open types. The latter by open heart su:gery.

Indications for mitral valvulotomy

(1) Age between 20 and 40 years.

(2) Increasing breathlessness–from grade 1 to grade III cardiac disability status (NYHA).

(3) Severe haemoptysis.

(4) Clinical, radiological and electrographical evidences of progressive pulmonary hypertension.

(5) Associated with insignificant mitral and aortic regurgitations.

(6) Controlled congestive cardiac failure.

(7) Digitalised heart, with atrial fibrillation under anticoagulant cover.

(8) Treated cases of infective endocarditis with tight mitral stenosis.

(9) Damped mitral stenosis.

2. MITRAL REGURGITATION

1. *Aetilogy* (a) Organic :

(1) Rheumatic (commonest).

(2) Traumatic during mitral valvulotomy.

(3) Infective endocarditis.

(4) Congenital.

(5) Associated with collagen diseases, myocardial infraction and cardiomyopathies.

(6) Functional : Associated with left ventricular hypertrophy and dilatation (e.g. hypertension, severe anaemia, myocardial infraction complicated by left ventricular failure etc.)

II. *Symptoms*

1. Breathlessness on exertion ending in cardiac asthma due to left ventricular failure.
2. Palpitation due to an enlarged left ventricle.
3. Features of infective endocarditis e.g. (a) Fever, (b) Pallor, (c) Clubbing,(d)Splenomega -ly, (e) Microscopic haematuria, (f) Embolic episodes.

[Causative organisms are : Streptococcus viridans, Diphtheroids, Heamophilus.

A blood culture for these organisms is mostly positive. Clinically this endocarditis changes the murmur of mitral regurgitation into a musical one the *Seagull Murmur.* A ruptured chordae tendinae or a valve cusp acts as the string of the musical instrument.]

4. Features of congestive cardiac failure.

III. *Signs*

1. Low volume collapsing pulse.
2. Neck veins normal unless there is cardiac failure.
3. Apex shifted down and out, and usually forceful and illsustained.
4. Systolic thrill in the mitral area signifying an organic heart disease.
5. Right ventricular heave (rare).
6. Auscultation–S_1 muffled, S_2 normal S_3 due to left ventricular diastolic overload.

A pansystolic murmur, conducted towards the axilla (but to the base if the regurgitation is posterior cuspal).

IV. *Investigations*
1. Radiology–left ventricular enlargement with a prominent left atrium (Boat Shaped Heart).
2. Echocardiographic–Left atrial enlargement left ventricular enlargement (Echocardio Doppler is useful to foretell gradient of mitral regurgitation).
3. Electrocardiogram–Left axis deviation, left ventricular hypertrophy and rarely p-mitrale.
4. Cardiac catheterisation–Left atrium opacifies during the left ventricular contraction as shown by angiocardiography.

V. *Treatment*
Implantation of a valve prosthesis, under open heart surgery. It may be a cage prosthesis or a disc prosthesis. Also annuloplasty may be done.

VI. *Complications*
1. Acute left ventricular failure.
2. Infective endocarditis.
3. Congestive cardiac failure.
4. Arrhythmias e.g.–(a) Ventricular premature beat (b) Atrial fibrillation (c) Ventricular tachycardia.
5. There may be a giant left atrium with atrial fibrillation and pressure effects.
6. Prone to produce ball valve thrombus–leading to recurrent attacks of syncope.

3. AORTIC STENOSIS

I. *Aetiology*
Mainly congenital (unicuspid of bicuspid) and rheumatic. Atherosclerotic or calcific aortic stenosis

are mostly secondary to rheumatic aortic stenosis. Rest are due to obstructive cardiomyopathy. Rare causes are–SLE, rheumatoid arthritis, Hurler's syndrome.

II. Symptoms Mild or moderate aortic stenosis causes no symptoms.

Severe stenosis usually present with–

1. Angina pectoris (commonest) usually on effort.

2. Attacks of dizziness, blackout or even syncope due to reduced cerebral blood flow resulting from diminished cardiac output. Syncopal attacks may be severe and frequent. These symptoms appear with effort or even with a change of posture.

3. Dyspnoea and other features of left ventricular failure.

III. *Signs*

1. Facies–Dresden china pollar.

2. Cold extremities.

3. Anacrotic pulse, pulsus parvus et tardus.

4. Apex beat–shifted down and out, heaving in character.

5. A thrill (systolic) at the base of the heart conducted to the carotid artery. *Carotid shudder*–thrill in carotid artery with thrill at the base.

6. Auscultation–

Aortic area : A_2 diminished, single S_2 or a paradoxical split. Ejection systolic murmur–diamond shaped.

Ejection click–due to a sudden opening of the semilunar valve (this sounds like split 1st heart sound).

S at the mitral area.

IV. *Investigations.*

1. Radiology : Left ventricular hypertrophy, a poststenotic dilatation is common, an aortic valve calcification seen especially on fluoroscopy.
2. Echocardiographic : Left ventricular wall condition (thick enlarged, harmonious or nor har monious). Aortia valve cusps occurs as endease steretione eitheic ication and thickening of valve.
3. Electrocardiogram : Left ventricular hypertrophy usually with strain pattern.

V. Complications :
1. Sudden death due to ventricular fibrillation during physical in severe aortic stenosis; in 3 to 5% of patients during asymptomatic phase.
2. Acute left ventricular failure.
3. Congestive cardiac failure.
4. Infective endocarditis.
5. Arrhythmias (VT and VF).
   The mortality is 9% per year in adults with aortic stenosis.

VI. Treatment
Sp must be done heiere serious complication got in front.
1. Transventricular aortic valvotams.
2. Aortic valve prosthesia.
3. Infective endocarditis.
4. Atherosclerotic.
5. Aorta stenosis.
6. Marfan's syndrome.
7. Persistent truncus arteriosus.
8. Ankylosing spondylitis.

4. AORTIC REGURGITATION

I. Aetiology
1. Rheumatic,
2. Syphilitic,

3. Traumatic,
4. Infective endocarditis,
5. Aneurysm,
6. Atherosclerotic,
7. Persistent truncus arterious,
8. Marfan's syndrome and
9. Ankylosing spondylitis.

II. *Symptoms*
1. Throbbing sensation all over the body.
2. Palpitations.
3. Breathlessness.
4. Swelling of the body due to congestive cardiac failure.
5. Chest pain.
6. Excessive sweating.

III. *Signs*
1. de Musset's sign–bobbing of the head.
2. Quincke's sign or visible capillary pulsations.
3. Water hammer pulse.
4. Blood pressure–shows wide pulse pressure.
5. Neck–Corrigan's sign.
6. Suprasternal notch pulsation.
7. Pistol shot sound in the femoral artery.
8. Hill's sign : The blood pressure in tne lower limbs>60 mm Hg above that of the upper limb in severe aortic regurgitation.
9. Durozeiz's murmur and Duroziez's sign (i.e. a systolic murmur on proximal compression of the femoral artery and a diastolic murmur on distal compression).
10. Traube's sign is the double sound heard over the femoral artery with each cardiac systole.
11. Apex beat is down and out and forceful and illsustained.
12. A diastolic thrill in the aortic area and the lower left sternal area.

13. Rosenbach's sign is the hepatic pulsation witheach systole.
14. Gerhardt's sign is the pulsation of an enlarged spleen with each systole.
15. Landolfi's sign is the pupillary size changes with each systole.
16. Ascultation–S_1 audible and soft, S_2 (A_2) is loud and is followed by a diastolic decrescendo murmur which is high pitched, soft, blowing in character, heard in the left sternal border S_3 and Austin Flint murmur may be present (in severe regurgitation). S_4 in also often audible.

IV. *Investigations*

1. Radiology–Cardiac enlargement due to left ventricular dilatation. The aortic knuckle is prominent. An aortic valve calcification raises the possibility of a combined aortic stenosis.
2. Electrocardiogram–Left ventricular hypertro phy with tall precordial T waves.
3. Echocardiogram (and Doppler) : Degree pre diction of aortic regurgitation possible; left atrial ventricular dilation; mitral valve might fluttar in high frequency.

V. *Complications*

1. Acute left ventricular failure.
2. Infective endocarditis.
3. Congestive cardiac failure.
4. Cardiac arrhythmias.

VI. *Treatment*

Aortic valve prosthesis.
Protocol for the diagnosis of cardiac valve disorders and assessment of myocardial func tion

(i) History.
(ii) Physical examination.
(iii) Chest X-ray. PA view, left lateral view or other oblique views as may necessary.

(iv) Electrocardiogram

(v) Echocardiogram Doppler

(vi) Carotid pulse tracings especially in aortic valve disorders

(vii) Radionuclide ventriculography with or without echocardiography

(viii) Angiogram

(ix) Phonocardiography, if necessary

(x) Cardiac catheterisation in selected patients with pressure measurements, oxymetry and selective angiocardiography.

Points (vi) to (x) should only be done after serious reflection.

CARDINAL SIGNS OF SOME COMMON CARDIAC DISORDERS

I. Congestive cardiac failure

(1) Tachycardia and gallop rhythm.

(2) Engorged and pulsatile neck veins.

(3) Enlarged and tender liver.

(4) Dependent pitting oedema.

II. *Left ventricular failure*

(1) Gallop rhythm with tachycardia.

(2) Moist sounds at the lung bases.

(3) Pulsus alternans in severe failure.

Outline of treatment in left ventricular failure

(1) Bed rest in propped up decubitus.

(2) Morphine–15 mg IM stat for sedation and to cut off the Herring Breuer reflex. Other opioids e.g. pethidine or pentazocine, may be used. All these may be given IV if urgent *action is necessary.*

(3) O inhalation through a face mask if necessary.

(4) Aminophylline – 0.25 gm IV stat

(5) Furosemide–40-80 mg IV stat.

(6) If there is no history of digitalis in the previous 2 weeks digitalis intravenously followed by oral route.

(7) Antibiotics.

HYPERTENSION

I. *Definition*

This is a clinical condition in which the systolic blood pressure is more than 150 mm Hg and the diastolic one is more than 90 mm Hg in adult individuals.

II. *Types*

PRIMARY

1. Essential bengin (most common) : This is a multifactorial disorder. (If both the while if one of the perents is affected 35% risk of developing hypertension.

2. Essential malignant : Results from the untreated benign form. No organic cause has till date been found for primary hypertension. The possible theories are—

(a) Neurogenic : Due to sympathetic stimulation.

(b) Humoral : Due to liberation of renin resulting from renal ischaemia.

(c) Besides neurohumoral theories, electrolyte disturbances may be the causes in the genesis of primary hypertension.

SECONDARY

The occurs usually below the age of 30 years and an underlying cause is always responsible which may be—

D. Renal :
(a) Acute glomerulonephritis,
(b) Chronic glomerulonephritis,
(c) Chronic pyelonephritis.
(d) Polycystic kidney disease.
(e) Renal tumours.

3. Endocrine :
(a) Thyrotoxicosis.
(b) Cushing syndrome.

  (c) Phaeochromocytoma.
  (d) Conn's syndrome.
4. Neurological :
  (a) Cerebral tumours.
  (b) Pseudobulbar palsy.
  (c) Bulbar poliomyelitis.
5. Vascular :
  (a) Coarctation of the aorta.
  (b) Renal artery stenosis.
6. Iatrogenic :
  (a) Use of oral contraceptives.
  (b) Prolonged steroid therapy (e.g. in bronchial asthma).
7.Pregnancy : Pre and post eclamptic renal cause.
III. *Symptoms*
  Nothing typical : The symptomatic features are mostly psychogenic and follow the diagnosis of hypertension. These are – Headache, insomnia Irritability Lack of concentration, Weakness, Fatigue etc.
  These may be due to cerebral artery sclerosis.
IV. *Signs*
  1. Flushing of the face 2. Blood pressure; Systolic more than 150 mm Hg. Diastolic more than 90 mm Hg.
  2. Initially this is intermittent but graually becomes persistent.
  3. Opthalmoscopy reveals retinopathy which may be of the following grades :

Mild hypertension (Grade I) : Tortuosity of the 3rd branch of central artery with engorged veins; A : V = 1 : 2 (diam); veins mildly depressed at AV crossing.

Diastolic pressure : 90-110 mm Hg

Moderate hypertension (Grade II) : More tortuosity of the artery resembling cop per wire; there is arterio- venous nipping; A : V = 1 : 3.

Diastolic pressure : 110-130 mm Hg

Severe hypertension (Grade III) : Diastolic pressure : 130-150 mm Hg	Features of Grade II+Silver wire appearance, vein not visible at AV crossing, A : V=1 : 4 or the arterioles may become fine fibrous cord, vein is dilated distal to AV crossing. Cotton wool exudates present. Flame shaped haemorrhage rarely, Hard exudates.
Malignant hypertension (Grade IV) : Diastolic pressure : above 150 mm Hg	Papilloedema in addition to the above changes.

[Malignant hypertension is defined as marked elevation of blood pressure which is associated with :
  (i)   A diastolic pressure usually more than 150 mm Hg.
 (ii)   Persistent or progressive uraemia.
(iii)   Papilloedema–confirmatory.]

5.   Apex beat : shifted down and out, heaving in character.

6.   Accentuated A_2, ejection click, ejection systolic murmur, S_2 paradoxically split and rarely aortic regurgitant murmur.

7.   In severe hypertension there is an S_3 due to hypertensive heart disease.

Hypertensive heart disease may lead to coronary atherosclerosis which in turn may ultimately lead to infraction.

Hypertensive heart disease may lead to left ventricular failure; this is known as hypertensive heart failure.

Decapitated hypertension is a condition when there is a sudden fall of systolic pressure from, say, 160 mm Hg to 130 mm Hg due to acute left ventricular failure diastolic pressure ramaining at about 110 mm Hg.

Divergent hypertension a condition in which there is *high systolic* and low diastolic blood pressure e.g. in aortic regurgitation, thyrotoxicosis, patent ductus arteriosus etc.

Effect on other systems :

A.   Cerebrovascular–Sudden convulsion with unconsciousness, papilloedema. Paresis of the limbs;– these are all due to hypertensive encephalopathy. Cerebral haemorrhage, Cerebral thrombosis etc.

B.   Renal manifestations; Chronic renal failure, acute on chronic renal failure. Urine examination reveals– albumin, RBC Pus cells, Blood and granular casts etc.

V. *Investigations*

1. Radiology–Enlargement of the left ventricle and widening of the arch of the aorta.

2. Electrocardiogram–Left ventricular hypertrophy with or without strain pattern.

3. Blood–biochemistry reflects the aetiological factors, or, with end organ damage e.g. those of the kidneys, there will be features of uraemia with an increase of creatinine level and a decreased creatinine clearance.

4. Intravenous pyelography (rapid sequence IVP) and /or retrograde pyelography reveals renal pathology.

5. Special blood tests e.g. estimation of (i) adrenaline and (ii) non-adrenaline–for suspected phaeochro-mocytomas.

6. Urine–Excertion of vanillylmandelic acid (VMA),

metanephrines and catecholamines to confirm phaeochromocytoma.
7. Split renal function test : to reveal renal artery stenosis.
8. Plasma renin activity (PRA) and renal vein renin assay from both sides.

VI. *Complications*

Acute	Chronic
1. Cerebral haemorrhage.	1. Angina pectoris.
2. Hypertensive encephalopathy.	2. Congestive cardiac failure
3. Subarachnoid haemorrhage.	3. Coronary artery disease.
4. Acute myocardial infraction	4. Chronic renal failure.
5. Acute left ventricular failure	5. Acute on chronic renal failure.

VII. *Management*
1. Weight reduction possible?
2. Physical exercise (e.g. regular walking gymnastic, etc.)
3. Change of eating habit–salt reduced (0, 5 gm salt/d)
   –Cholesterol reduced (vegetable oil instead of animal oil etc.
4. Reduction of restriction of alcohol consumption and smoking. If there is still a high blood pressure systolic over 150 mm Hg/elder pts, over 160 mm Hg and diastolic over 100 mm Hg–add.
5. Antihypertensive drug treatment.
   Avoid to rescript more than three different drugs.
   E. g. for step care treatment :
   1 Step : diuretica (mostly elder pts.) of or e.g. B-blocker
   Regular BP measurement, it still hypertension, than,
   2 Step : –diuretica and B-blocker or

- diuretica and calcium antagonist or
- diuretica and ACE inhibitor or
- calcium antagonist and ACE inhibitor

ATTENTION :   Never give B-blocker and calcium antagonists! Begain regular BP control, still hypertension present, than

3 Step :   –diuretica, B-blocker and ACE inhibitor or – diuretica, calcium antagonists and ACE inhibitor control of BP regularly. There is still the possibility to try other combinations (see table).

Category	example	doses [mg/d]	side effect	contra-indication
a diuretics Thiazid	Hydrochlo-rothiazid	25-100	hyperglycaemia hyperuricemia hypokalemia	DIABETES renal failure, gout
Kalium saving	Amilorid	10-20	hyperkalemia, nausea vomiting diarrhoea	hyperkalemia severe liver-dysfunction, severe kid-neyinsufficiency
	Triam teren	100-200		
Henle-loop acting	Funosemid	20-40 (i.v.); 40-120(p.o.)	hypokalemia loss of Mg^{2+} Ca^{2+}, Cl hyperglycemia, hyperuricemia allergic reaction ototoxic	hypovolemia. renal failure with anuria, severe liver-dysfunction. hypokalemia
	Piretanid	3-9		
	Etacryn acid	50-150		
Aldosteron antagonist	Spirono-lactone	25-100	hyperkalemia gynecomastia impotence amenorrhoe.	renal failure hyperkalemia hypovolemia. natremia
		5-10	hyperkalemia	
B β - blocker	Atenolol (cardiose-lective	1× 50 200	bradicardia bronchospasm hyperglycemia sedation	bronchial asthma. congestive car-diac faiure.

category	example	doses [mg/d]	side effect	contra-indication
	metoprolol (cardioselective)	2-3×50 100	headache vertigo, gastro-intestinal dysfunction	bradycardia. heart block shock situation/metabolic acidosis
	Pindolo ($\beta_1 + \beta_2$; ISA)	3×5-10	rebound-effect	
	Propranol of ($\beta_1 + \beta_2$)	2-4×10-80		
c. calcium antagonist	Nifedipin	3×5-20	ventricular fibrillation, tachycardia oedema, headache flush	pregnancy, aortic stenosis, heart failure, hypotension
	Diltiazem	3×60-120		
	Verapamil	3×40-120	bradycardia AV-block ↓inotropie	!never combine with β blocker
d. ACE-inhibitor	Captopril	2+12.5 50	cough. hyperkalemia	renal arterial stenosis (both sides), renal dysfunction. pregnancy, nursing period
	Enalapril	1+5-40		
e. Angiotensin-II inhibitor	Losartan	25-50	vertigo, excessive BP reduction (when combined with diuretics). hyperkalemia	see ACE inhibitor
f. Vasodilator	Dihydralazin	3×12.5 50	angina pectoris, drug induced SLE (long term therapy >200mg/d), headache	! always combine with β-blocker and diuretics → reflactory tachycardia

category	example	doses [mg/d]	side effect	contra-indication
	Prazosin α_1 blocker	0.5-20	orthostatic collaps, vertigo	heart insuff, NYHAIV
g. central acting	clonidim (stimulates central α_2 receptor	3+75 300 µ g/d	bradycardia initial and rebound BP↑, sedation, dry mouth	sick sinus syndrome, bradycardia (lbe cautious in combining with beta-blocker or Verapamil
	α -Methyl-Dopa (see Clonidin)	500-1000	orthostatic dys-regulation, sedetion, Na^+-H_2O-retention	depression, pheochromo-cytoma, acute liver disease

VII. Management

a)   Primary Hypertension :

1. Weight reduction possible?
2. Physical exercise→ regular walking gymnastic, etc.
3. Change of eating hahit→ salt reduced (max. 6g/d) try KCL based salt → cholesterol reduced (vegetable oil and food etc.) →in diabetes, diet for it
4. Leave hypertension promoting drugs.
5. Reduction or restriction of alcohol, coffee consumption and smoking. If there is still a high blood pressure start.
6. Antihypertensive drug treatment : Avoid to rescript more than three different drugs, think that the patient has to take them over a lot

of years perhaps the whole life. Routinious BP control is to be made, if possible by patient self control.

Step care treatment :

1st Step : **Monotherapy** with one of the basic drugs

β -blocker	Diuretics	Ca-anta-gonists	ACE inhibitor	α₁blocker

Still no acceptable BP Extend to

2nd Step : **Doubletherapy**

Diuretics

and

β -blocker	Co-anta-gonists	ACE inhibitor	α₁blocker

or

Ca-antagonists

and

β -blocker	ACE-inhibitor

ATTENTION : Never combine β -blocker with Verapamil!

3rd Step : Find out a combination which regulates the individual

hypertension of the patient best, for example ;

Diuretica

and

ACE-inhibitor

and

Ca-antagonists

In case of hypertensive emergencies :

(a)   Nitroprussid, 0, 5 to 8, 0 mg/kg/min continous intravenuous (i.v.) ATTENTION ! Blood pressure might come down to fast, intensive BP control necessary.

or (b) Diazoxid 150-300 mg i.v.

or (c) Trmetaphan, 1 to 45 mg/min i.v.

Other measures that are of help : Mannitol infusion in jet or Furosemid i.v. These drugs are rapid acting and have to replaced by a management shown in step 2 or 3 for long term treatment.

Surgical management according to the aetiology. These include–

1. Bilateral adrenalectomy.
2. Removal of the tumour in a case of pheochromo-cytoma.
3. In coarctation–end to end anastomosis or graft ing.
4. Renal artery garfting in renal artery stenosis.

ACUTE MYOCARDIAL INFRACTION

1. *Incidence*

More in males, below the age of 50 yrs. Beyond that age the incidences are nearly equal in both sexes. Exceptions,– young females, if they suffer from juvenile diabetes, hypertension, hypothyroidism, hyperlipidaemia etc. or if there is a prolonged use of contraceptive pills.

II. *Clinical features*

1. Precordial pain (usually severe) may be–
(a) Retrosternal, radiating to the ulnar aspect of the left arm.
(b) Across the chest radiating to the ulnar aspect of both arms.
(c) Localised at the jaw.
(d) Below the shoulder blades radiating anteriorly.
(e) Epigastric.

Character of the pain–squeezing, constricting, heavi-ness over the precordium or there may be a sense of impending death.

2. Associated features include–
(a) Profuse perspiration (cold sweat).
(b) Giddiness or even syncope (due to sudden hypo-tension or associated heart block).
(c) Frank features of cardiac asthma–severe breath-

lessness with ratting sounds in the throat, bilateral moist sounds. In the lungs, gallop rhythm with pulsus alternans.

(d)   Severe epigastric pain with vomiting, a sense of dysphagia and giddiness, resembling those of acute grastric perforation, acute heamorrhagic pancreatitis or acute pain of basal pleurisy.

3.   May be painless with none of few of the associated features.

III. *Clinical diagnosis*

1.   Patient is apprehensive, anxious and restless.

2.   Pallor of the face or even ashen gry appearance (due to low cardiac output which may again be due to peripheral circulatory failure).

3.   Rarely central cyanosis (if associated with left ventricular failure).

4.   Decbitus propped up (if associated with left ventricular failure).

5.   Extremities are cold and clammy.

6.   Pulse : Usually tachycardia but sometimes bradycardia if associated with heart block or reflex vegal stimulation.
Rhythm may be irregular due to frequent ventricular premature beats, which is an aminous sign as these may herald ventricular tachycardia and/or fibrillation.

7.   Blood pressure : Both systolic and diastolic pressures are low. If systolic pressure is less than 90 mm Hg with cold and clammy extremities with marked cyanosis and oliguria–the condition is known as *cardiogenic shock*, which is a dreadful complication of myocardial infraction. However, sympathetic overactivity may lead to early transient hypertension.

Mechanism of cardiogenic shock–It is due to decreased coronary perfusion and peripheral circulatory failure. When the coronary perfusion is diminished, myocardial dysfunction occurs. This further reduces the perfusion and a vicious cycle sets in. Also peripheral circulatory failure produces splanchnic vasoconstriction giving rise to anoxia of the viscera which liberates lactic acid into the circulation resulting in metabolic acidosis, that is further responsible for the peripheral circulatory failure perpetuating the vicious cycle (Sodi-bi-carb prevents metabolic acidosis).

8.   Jugular venous pressure : May be raised if associated with congestive heart failure.

9.   Heart sounds : Usually muffled due to myocardial damage and an S_4 is very common and there may be an S_3 if heart failure sets in.
     After 1 to 2 days there may be a to and fro rough sound over the precordium mainly the left 4th intercostal space in the mid-clavicular line or over the pulmonary area. This is the *pericardial friction rub.* This is very common in an anterior wall myocardial infarction but rare in inferior wall infraction.

10. Body temperature within 36 hours the body temperature may rise to 102°F and this is due to a nonspecific reaction to the myocardial necrosis.

IV. *Investigation*

1,   **ECG :** One of the basic diagnostic methods with 12 lead ECG.
     Peracute sign : high peak T wave is only seen during AMI (minutes) attack.
     acute sign : ST elevation in infract regions (hours).
     chronic sign : reduction of ST elevation and presence of (days to weeks) pathological Q wave. But be aware that ECG signs may be totally absent or minimized. Leads on the opposite of the infrac-

tion site may show ST depression, like in a mirror.

Infract region	Lead change in
anteroseptal	1, II, aVL, $V_1 - V_6$
inferior	II, III, aVF
septal	$V_1 - V_3$
lateral	$V_3 - V_6$.

2. Blood enzymes

(i) Creatinine phosphokinase (CPK) and CPK-MB (isoenzyme) rises after 6–10 hours of infraction.

(ii) Troponin T (and I), myocardial antigens rising earlier then CPK and are more specific, but not everywhere available.

(iii) Aspertal transaminase (AST) and lactte dehydrogenase (IDH) are released 2–4 days after infraction. There are not very specific.

(iv) Total and differential WBC counts : leukocytosis with a marked increase of polymorphs within 36 hours. Not AMI specific.

Mark if two of the following points are present start treatment without losing time !

1. characteristic clinical picture
2. ECG changes
3. characteristic enzyme increase in blood Fibrinolytic therapy

Several drugs are used today, the three most common are noted here.

Drug (Doses)	Dosis and effect
Streptokinase	1.5 mil units over 1h, with t $\frac{1}{2}$ 80 min; allergenic and anaphylactic reaction possible, re-using should be avoided. Fast injection causes rapid fall of BP.

Tissue type plasminogen activator (t-PA) or recombinant-PA (rt-PA); Alteplase	10 mg bolus, 50 mg over 1h, then 40 mg over 2h later on. Give always heparin : first as 5000 U bolus then 1000 U/hiv. t $\frac{1}{2}$ 30 min; Due. to the selective activity directly on the thrombos location these drugs are less likely to produce systemic co-agulation disturbances.
Drug (Doses)	**Doses and effect**
Anisoylated plasminogen streptokinase activator complex (APSAC) I Anistreplase	30 units over 5 min. t $\frac{1}{2}$ 105 min; like streptokinase allergenic potence

Reperfusing the obstructed vessel, fibrinolytics have got their maximum effect within the first 4 hours. Still after 12-24 hours little benefit can be expected.

Because of the dangerous side effects as
(i) bleeding disorder
(ii) multiple microembolism
(iii) cardiac dyarithmias and
(iv) allergy
you have to follow strict **contraindications.**
1. haemorrhagic diathesis
2. Symptoms of peptic ulcer or GI bleeding
3. recent cerebral stroke
4. recent surgery and especially neurosurgery
5. malignant and uncontrolled hypertension
6. Prolonged cardiopulmonary resuscitation during this presentation.

V. *Management*

This is ideally done by admitting the patient in a coronary care unit (CCU) as early as possible where–

(i) The patient is put in a cardiac bed.

(ii)   Oxygen is given through a nasal catheter (or ventimask or if necessary at a high pressure) at the rate of 4–6 litres i.e., 300 to 600 bubbles per minute.

(iii)   To remove the anxiety and kill the pain–inj. morphine sulph–15 mg SC or IM to be repeated up to 60 mg or 2mg IV repeated as necessary.

or, Pethidine hydrocloride inj–100 mg stat IM with or without promethazine hydrochloride.

Or, inj, Pentazocine–which has minimum respiratory depressant effect, 40 mg IM. But this drug may increase LV. end diastolic pressure.

Or, Inj Diazepam–10 mg IV.

With this treatment the thrombotic obstracted coronarateria might be opened again. There is the chance to gain the stroken part of muscle back.

(v)   Anticoagulant theraphy is started with–

Inj Heparin–10,000 units stat, 7,500 units SC 6 hrly for 48 hours. It prevents thrombo-embolic episodes but never prevents further extenstion of the infraction. Along with the above, phenindione (DINDEVAN)–40 mg tablets 5 tabs stat and I tab BD given orally. Each dose of heparin should be given after determining the bleeding and clotting times.

Dindevan takes 48 hours for its onset of action and so the dose should be regulated by prothrombin index which should be kept within 50%.

Before starting an anticoagulant therapy a through history is taken to exclude any haemorrhagic disorders the presence of which contraindicates the use of the anticoagulants.

Heparin is withdrawn after 48 hours. Oral anticoagulant therapy is continued for 3-6 weeks and should be withdrawn gradually. A sudden withdrawal may precipitate another attack.

(N.B.–There is no uniform consensus of opinion regarding the merits of anticoagulant therapy in AMI.)

Oral anticoagulant therapy with aspirin acetylsalcylaci 100–160 m/d to lower the risk of a further myocardial infraction.

(vi) B-adrenoceptor blockade with 50 mg atenolol : first intravenous and then a second dosage per os. Reduction of mortality in AMI patients.

In routine practice a 12 lead electrocardiogram is recorded.

The Leads more detailed :

Six limb leads divided into

(i) 3 standard or bipolar limb leads (Edberg leads):

Lead I– indicates potential difference between the left and the right arm.

Lead II– potential difference between the left leg and the right arm.

Lead III– potential difference between left by left arm

(iii) 3 augmented unipolar limb leads :

aVR

aVL

aVF

(V) Complications of AMI e.g. (a) Cardiac arrhythmias, (b) Hypotension, (c) Cardiogenic shock etc. may appear and should be promptly diagnosed and treated detailed discussions of these are beyond the scope of this book and students are advised to consult larger text-books. IV infusions started with a "Polarising fluid" which consists of (i) One bottle of 5% dextrose solution and to this is added (ii) 2 amp of inj. potassium chloride (20 MEq of K in each amp) and (iii) 15 units soluble insulin.

The rationality of infusing polarising fluid remains controversial, but at least it helps maintaining an IV channel to readily combat the emergency problems of early complications of AMI.

If there is a fall of BP, 24 mg *dexamethasone* (Decadron) is added into the bottle. The drip is continued for about 2 days (or more if necessary) at the rate of 6 to 10 drops per *minute* (or more, depending upon the haemodynamic variables).

In cardiogenic shock, sodi-bi-carb 3.4% 100 ml/day and *dopamine* (intropin) 5-15 μg per kg body weight per minute, both by IV infusion, should be given. Dopamine, however, should never be mixed with any other solution and is given only in 5% dextrose solution.

Ventricular premature beats or ventricular tachycardia should be treated with *lignocatine* 250 mg IV stat given through the drip, but lignocatine may cause further fall of pressure. So DC shock is the treatment of choice, especially with VT and when there is haemodynamic compromise.

If there is a heart block that cannot be combated by steroids and atropine, immediately a bedside floating electrode catheter should be introduced into the right ventricle via a peripheral arm vein and connected with an external *temporary pacemaker.*

If the signs of ventricular failure appear, furosemide 40-80 mg IV stat and inj. *aminophylline* 0.25 gm in 10 ml distilled water IV are given and repeated if required. The role of digitalis in acute left ventricular failure complicating AMI is debatable, but may be given IV 0.5 mg stat and IV 0.25 mg every 6 hr after that.

Antibiotics may be needed for secondary infections.

Surgery–In pulmonary embolism (one of the commonest causes of death within 7 days) TERNDELENBURG'S OPERATION (pulmonary embolectomy(may be done in addition to the usual conservative measures.

Coronary dilators e.g. nitrates are now-a-days proving useful; 10 mg tab–1/2 tab given sublingually every 2 hours.

(vi) Emergency coronary artery surgery are the current modalities of treatment becoming established at sophisticated centres.

(vii) Gradual rehabilitation is attempted as the patient improves; attention is given to the control of diabetes mellitus, obesity, systemic hypertension, hyperlipidaemias, etc. and smoking and consumption of alcohol and caffeine containing beverages are discouraged.

Diet : This should be preferably liquid or semisolid for the first day and then fat restricted and protein rich food with restricted calories are resumed. As the patient improves he should be given solid fat free diet with a calorie value not exceeding 1300 calorie daily. The cooking media should be vegetable oils like soya-bean and sunflower oils. Carbohydrates are to be restricted as it is converted to cholesterol in the body.

If congestive cardiac failure is present, daily salt intake should not exceed 1–1.5 gm.

Other measures include–

1. The patient should be instructed not to smoke for the rest of his life because an excess of nicotine causes coronary vasospasm in addition to the other adverse cardiovascular effects.

2. Alcohol consumption should be stopped but very restricted amounts may be allowed, if at all necessary.

3. Limited physical exercise like walking in empty stomach, playing golf or squash to be advised. No exertion to be done immediately (1 ½ hrs) after meals.

4. Mental stress being one of the most important aetiological factors in coronary artery diseases the patient should be asked to lead an easy life.

ANGINAPECTORIS

This means an attack of central retrosternal discomfort (that may be oppressive, constricting or crushing in nature and not necessarily always a pain) of the chest, caused by a transient myocardial ischaemia, and which comes with exertion, after a heavy meal or during mental excitement and is relieved immediately by rest and or coronary vasodilators e.g. sublingual administration of glyceryl trinitrate. It is almost always caused by atherosclerotic coronary artery disease on which there may be a superimposed coronary artery spasm.

In contrast to the patient with AMI, that of angina pectoris remains calm and quiet and relatively immobile as exertion causes and aggravates the pain and rest classically brings about relief.

Angina decubitus and its management

If the pain comes even at rest but persists for a very short time (5 to 10 mins) it is known as 'ANGINA DECUBITUS' and the management includes rest for 3 weeks and frequent administration of glyceryl trinitrate or isosorbide dinitrate sublingually at intervals of 2 hours.

A short course of anticoagulant therapy is justified to prevent thrombo-embolic phenomenon.

Modern methods of treatment in angina pectoris and

angina decubitus consist of (i) localisation and assessment of the degree of obstruction (s), (ii) followed by coronary artery bypass grafting (CABG) employing a reversed saphenous vein graft, provided the myocardial function remains normal, or, (iii) sometimes a percutaneous transluminal coronary angioplasty (PTCA) may help in dilating the constricted segment. Of late, *nitroglyceine ointment* applied locally to the precordium has proved effective, especially in angina decubitus. IV *nitroglycrine* is also proving helpful in severe cases.

Beta blockers and calcium antagonists are also effective therapeutic against.

Administration of *Carbimazole*–15 to 30 mg daily in divided doses is one of the treatments of persistent angina which helps by reducing the BMR, lessening the need of tissue perfusion and this diminishes the oxygen demand of the myocardium. This is rarely used β adrenergic blockers e.g. *Propranolol* is also used in angina in a dose of 40 to 480 mg daily in 2 to 4 divided doses; the mechanism of action being–1. Reducing the oxygen demand of the cardiac muscle. 2 Slowing of the heart rate and thus preventing the ischaemia and cardiac arrhythmias. 3. Hypotensive effect particularly in hypertensive heart disease.

Sophisticated investigations for ischaemic heart diseases

(i) Coronary angiography.
(ii) Ventriculography.
(iii) Radio nuclide (e.g. thallium 201, technetium 99 m etc) uptake tests. These may be used in exercise testing too.

(iv)   Echocardiography.

(v)   Systolic Time Intervals (STI) and Apexcardiography.

(vi)   Haemodynamic and angiographic measurements—with ballon tipped (Swan-Ganz) catheter introduced into the pulmonary artery. Some of these have been discussed briefly earlier; but a detailed discussion of all remains outside the scope of this book and students are advised to consult textbooks of medicine or cardiology for further details.

The most modern treatment of acute Angina with impending acute myocardial infraction are :

1.   Sublingual administration of GTN Tablet under tongue.

2.   If no relief sublingual administration of Nefedepine to be crushed and under tongue.

3.   If there is no peptic ulcer Aspirin (300 mg) to suck.

4.   If no relief administration of Cyclomorphine or dimorphine injection sub-cut.

5.   Remove the patient to the nearest hospital with an ICCU where urgent administration of I.V. fibronolytic drugs like Streptokinase followed by I.V. Heparin Therapy.

6.   If there is no complication and no arrhythmia and heart failure, oral ACE inhibitor and Beta-blocker and oral Aspirin to be continued for six weeks.

APPENDIX TO CHAPTER III
GRADING OF MURMURS

The grading of murmurs, based on their intensities is as follows :

GRADE I—The murmur is very faint, audible only when carefully searched for with a good stethoscope in a quite room and with the patient holding his breath. Even then it is barely audible.

GRADE II–A faint murmur, still readily recognized.

GRADE III– Prominent, exactly not a loud murmur, but there is no thrill.

GRADE IV–A loud murmur, usually, associated with thrills.

GRADE V–Very loud murmur.

GRADE VI–Exceptionally loud mumur, such that it is audible even with the stethoscope just removed from its contact with the chest; without the stethoscope and with the examiner getting closer to the patient; and also when the chest piece is placed over the head of the patient or any part of the patient's body.

By convention, the murmur is usually recorded as, say, Grade 2/6, 3/6 or 5/6 etc. the denominator indicating the total number of grades.

GASTROINTESTINAL AND URINARY SYSTEMS

CHAPTER 3

The gastrointestinal system should be routinely examined in the following order–(i) the mouth, throat and oesophagus, (ii) the abdomen and (iii) ano-rectal examination.

EXAMINATION OF THE MOUTH

Lips–(a) Look for *herpes simplex*–These are painful vesicles on the outer surface of the lips commonly found in–

(i) Common cold, (ii) Influenza, (iii) Lobar pneumonia, (iv) Weil's disease, (v) Meningococcal meningitis, (vi) Malaria, (vii) After blood transfusion.

The herpes labialis often gives clue to the side and stage of lobar pneumonia e.g. right sided vesicles indicate a right sided lobar pneumonia. The vesicular stage of the herpes may indicate grey hepatisation and the denuded herpes suggests the stage of resolution of pneumonia.

(b) *Cheilosis*–It means cracking of the mucocutaneous junction of the lip. Caused by deficiencies of iron, niacin, riboflavin and pyridoxine or by a sudden change of climate (e.g, excessive cold). When associated with dysphagia in women, post-cricoid carcinoma should be suspected.

(c) *Angular stomatitis* (cheilitis) is the inflammation of the skin at the angle of the mouth and consists of superficial and reddish brown linear ulcers radiating from the angle of the mouth.

Causes : (i) Ill-fitted dentures. (ii) Vitamin deficiencies, especially that of riboflavine, (iii) Starvation. (iv) Iron deficiency anaemia and other debilitating diseases, (v) Occult candidiasis, (vi) Contact dermatitis etc.

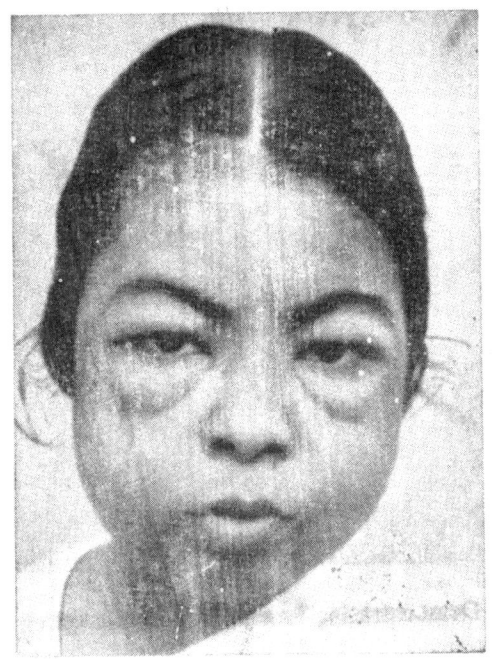

Fig. 4A : This was a case of membranous glomerulonephritis. Note the puffiness of the face and especially the Swelling of the eyelids,

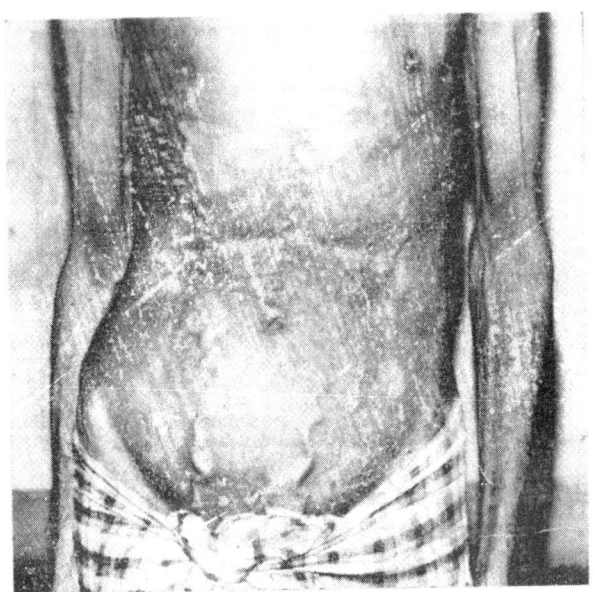

Fig. 4B : Inferior Vena Cava obstruction

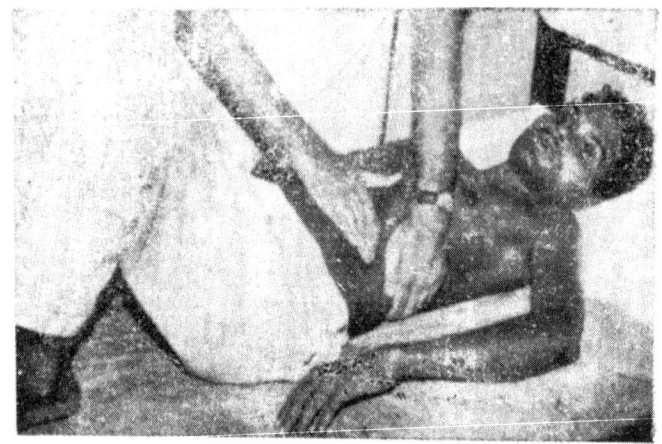

Fig. 4C : Demonstrating how to palpate the spleen

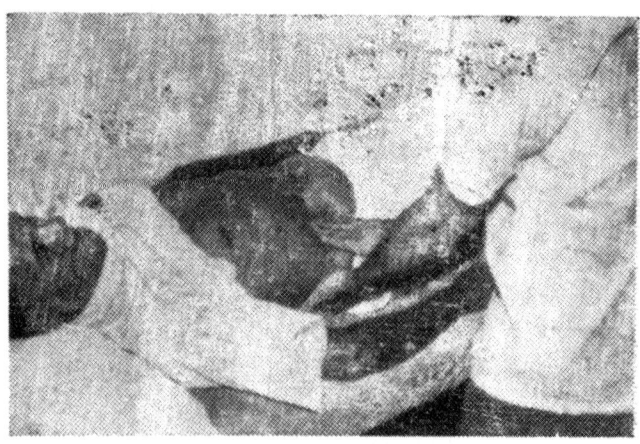

Fig. 4D : Demonstrating how to palpate
the kidney bimanualy

(d) *Colour of lip*–The lips may be blue due to cyanosis or methor sulphhaemoglobinaemia.

(e) *Cancrum oris*–gangrenous e.g. in chronic kala-azar.

(f) The mucous surface of the lips should be examined for *aphthous ulcers* and *retention cysts.* The aphtchous ulcers are painful, small and superficial with a whitish base surrounded by a red area of hyperaemia.

Cheek–The cheeks should be inspected with the help of a torch and look for–(i) Pigmentation that may be found in Addison's disease, haemochromatosis, polyposis of the colon (Peutz-Jegher syndrome), chronic arsenical poisoning etc. (ii) Koplik's spot around the opening of the parotid duct, found in measles. (iii) Cancrum oris. (iv) Haemorrhagic spots which may be due to (a) Haemophilia. (b) Purpura. (c) Hereditary haemorrhagic telantgiectasia (Rendu Osler Weber's disease).

Gum–Normally the gum is pink coloured. The lips should be retracted before examining the gum. With gingivitis the gums are not pinkish, bleed easily on slight pressure and may be swollen.

A blue line in the gum is found in lead poisoning. A bluish black or grey line of the gum may be seen in tartar on teeth and may be produced by *bismuth.* A wedge shaped slip of white paper is inserted between the gum and the teeth. The stippled line of lead poisoning will be rendered more distinct but discolouration due to tartar on the teeth will disappear. *Mercury* poisoning may also show as a darkline along the gingival margins.

Accumulation of food debris between the unhealthy gum and the teeth helps in the growth of commensal bacteria as well as the pathogenic organisms leading to the development of *pyorrhoea alveolaris.* The danger of pyorrhoea alveolaris are subsequent developments of : (i) Infective endocarditis. (ii) Rheumatic carditis, (iii) Aspiration pneumonia. (iv) Premature fall of teeth. Look for any *ulceration* of the gum. The ulcers of the gum are of the following types:

(i) Aphthous ulcers–These start as vesicles and ultimately rupture, are very painful and superficial with greyish edges and self-limiting.

(ii) Ulcers of Vincent's angina also known as acute necotizing gingivitis. Plaut Vincent's infection, trench mouth and fusospirochetosis–These are deep, clean cut ulcers with sharp edges associated with painful, bleeding gums and foulbreath. A swab from these ulcers will show fusiform bacilli (fusobacteria) and spirochaetes Borrelia vincenti) on dark ground illumination. Vincent's gingivostomatitis destroys interdental papillae, and produces halitosis.

(iii) Snail track ulcers of secondary syphilis.

(iv) Big ragged ulcers with or without sloughing may be due to acute leukaemias or agranulocytosis.

(v) Acute herpetic gingivostomatitis caused by herpes simplex virus is rather common in infants and children.

The gum may be *hypertrophied* in–

(a) Epileptics treated with sodium phenytoin, probably due to inhibition of collagen catabolism.

(b) Pregnancy.

(c) Leukaemias particularly acute monocytic leukaemia where there is also gum bleeding.

Lastly palpat for any tumour of the gum (epulis) and for any stone in the salivary gland.

Teeth–Count the number of teeth and note their colour. Normally there are 16 pairs of permanent teeth.

	M	P	C	I	Incisor	Canine	Premolar	Molar
Upper–	3	2	1	2	2	1	2	3
Lower –	3	2	1	2	2	1	2	3

Teeth may be less than normal in number due to–

(1) Traumatic loss, (2) Bad oral hygiene. (3) Extremes of age, (4) Delayed dentition as occurs in hypoparathyroidism and rickets. Teeth may become yellow and mottled with excessive use of tobacco and betels. *Fluorosis* also makes the teeth yellow and mottled. If expectant mothers after the first trimester of pregnancy or children up to 8 years of age are treated with *tetracyclines*, both the deciduous and permanent teeth of the child acquire permanent staining in the form of horizontal bands of yellow or grey colour.

Hutchinson's teeth–characteristic of *congenital syphilis*, the two central upper permanent incisors are broader near the gum than at the crown and there is a semilunar notch at the biting edge. The cross-sections of these incisors look rounded with inward sloping (inverted peg shaped). The lower teeth may close outside the upper ones causing an alteration of bite as is found in *acromegalic* patients with prognathism.

Breath–It is very important to smell the breath of a patient because some diseases give distinctive odour to the breath e.g. (1) Foul smelling (known as halitosis) present in gangrene of lung, lung abscess, bronchiectasis, pyorrhoea alveolaris, chronic pulmonary tuberculosis etc. (2) Sweetish or 'fruity odours' due to presence of acetone in expired air. This is encountered in diabetic ketoacidosis. (3) Garlic odour of breath in bismuth toxicity. (4) Pungent smell after administration of paraldehyde. (5) Mousy smell of hepatic failure. (6) Ammoniacal odour in uraemia.

Tongue–Ask the patient to protrude out the tongue. It may fail to protrude fully if there is a short frenum; known as tongue tie.

Note the following points–

(1) Hydration–(a) The tongue may exhibit minimum of secretion due to severe dehydration, after haemorrhage,

with administration of drugs like morphine or atropine, in mouth breathing, in uveoparotid fever (Heerfordt's syndrome, found in sarcoidosis) etc.

(b) Tongue may be excessively moist in heavy metal poisoning like arsenic, mercury, lead etc. in post-encephalitic Parkinsonism and also after administration of lozenges.

(2) Tremor–Fine tremors of the tongue is found in anxiety neurosis, thyrotoxicosis and chronic alcoholism. Coarse tremors of the tongue is characteristic of Parkinsonism. Coarse forward and backward movement of the tongue (also known as "trombone tongue") is characteristic of dementia paralytica.

(3) An apparent deviation of the tongue occurs in unilateral seventh nerve palsy. The tongue is deviated to the opposite side of the lesion in a case of upper motor neurone disease and to the same side of the lesion in lower motor neurone disease.

(4) Spasticity–characteristic of pseudobulbar palsy.

(5) Fasciculations, wasting and deep grooves or fissures in the tongue are observed in lesions of the hypoglossal nerve or nuclei e.g. progressive bulbar palsy or amyotrophic lateral sclerosis. This is lingual hemiatrophy; the tip deviates towards the side of lesion and the median raphe is concave towards the side of the lesion (see chapter 3 of part II).

(6) Colour–The tongue looks pale in anaemia. It may be blue in *central cyanosis*. The undersurface is examined to detect *jaundice*. An angry looking tongue with sores is characteristic of *niacin deficiency*. In chronic-superficial glossitis due to syphilis (syphilitic leucoplakia) the tongue surface is full of smooth and glazing patches. The tongue in typhoid fever is characterised by dryness of the surface with a central brown fur and red edges.

(7) Conditions of the papillae–A smooth of bald tongue due to generalised atrophy of the papillae is common in iron deficiency anaemia, sprue, pellagra, pernicious anaemia etc.

(8) Ulcers–A snail track ulcer over the dorsum of the tongue is highly characteristic of *secondary syphilis*. White patches with or without ulcerations are present in chronic superficial glossitis, Congenital fissures of the tongue and chronic superficial glossitis are differentiated clinically by the presence of normal papillae in the former.

The tongue may be ulcerated at the margins due to illfitted sharp dentures, short frenum etc. *Tubercular ulcers* are usually situated on the dorsum of the tongue whereas *malignant ulcers* can develop anywhere especially on the already existing leucoplakias. *Frenal ulcers* are frequently found in whooping cough and is occasionally due to persistent coughing.

(9) Size –The tongue may be large (macroglossia) or small (microglossia), Macroglossia is associated with acromegaly myxoedema, cretinism, primary amyloidosis, mongolism etc. Microglossia or glossal atrophy is seen in cerebral diplegia, pseudobulbar palsy and hypoglossal nuclear lesions as in amyotrophic lateral sclerosis, syringomyelia. etc.

(10) Taste sensation–Vide examination of the nervous system.

Palate –Ask the patient to open his mouth and see the colour, degree of the arch and presence of cleft, if any. Note also the movements by asking the patient to say 'Ah'. It does not move in palatal palsy as in diphtheritic polyneuritis or bulbar paralysis. The degree of anaemia and jaundice can be assessed by the colour of the soft palate. The high arched palate may be found in Marfan's syndrome, mongolism or in association with some congenital heart diseases (see Sick Children). Congenital cleft in the palate is an occasional finding. Pinhead petechial haemorrhagic spots are often found over the hard palate in glandular fever. In herpes zoster of the maxillary division of the trigeminal nerve, vesicles are found on one side of the hard palate which progress to painful oral ulcers.

Tonsils – These are usually slightly enlarged up to the age of 12 years. The septic tonsils are very big and red with liberation of pus on squeezing. The septic tonsils are the predisposing factors of rheumatic fever and acute glomerulonephritis.

Tonsils should be inspected after depressing the tongue with the help of a tongue spatula.

The patches *of faucial diptheria* are greyish white membranes confined to the tonsils and they cannot be easily removed. Oozing of blood occurs after removal of the membrane.

In thrush i.e. candidiasis–the plaques are curdy white and can be easily removed without any bleeding.

The white or yellowish grey patches of follicular tonsillitis are easily removed and on removal leave behind a sound surface which does not bleed.

Fauces –These are examined with the help of a torch after depressing the tongue with a tongue spatula. Note the colour, texture and any discharge from the mucosa. The posterior pharyngeal wall looks congested and granular in heavy smokers and orators. Look for cherry red spots on the pillars of the oropharynx, diagnostic or infectious mononucleosis.

Pharynx–Normally on its surface small adenoid swellings are seen–these are much increased and the mucous membrane of the pharynx become congested in chronic pharyngitis while it may bulge inwards in retro-pharyngeal abscesses.

EXAMINATION OF THE OESOPHAGUS

Ask the patient to swallow water as well as solid food and note if there is any difficulty in swallowing.

The oesophagus is 10 inches long and extends from the level of the cricoid cartilage up to the 9th thoracic spine. There are two sphincters in the oesophagus—pharyngooesophageal and oesophagocardiac. A difficulty in swallowing is known as *dysphagia*. The dysphagia may be due to lesions in the bulb (e.g. bulbar palsy) or due to any local pathology, e.g. due to poor salivation. Paresis of the tongue or painful conditions of the mouth or pharynx. Besides, dysphagia may be due to—(1) Involvement of the *upper part* of the oesophagus—(a) Kelly-Patterson syndrome or Plummer-Vinson syndrome—This type is also known as sideropenic dysphagia. In oesophageal dysphagia the feeling is as if the food is lodged at the end of the throat or behind the sternum. *Mechanism*—Iron in the body is stored up in the epithelial cells. In severe iron deficiency states, the iron stored in the epithelial cells of the mucous membrane of oesophagus is used up to maintain haemoporesis as a last resort. The epithelium is thereby denuded and the Auerbach's piexus becomes exposed to irritants and food particles. Reflex spasm occurs during the passage of food bolus.

(b) Benign strictures e.g. due to ingestion of corrosives.

(c) Pressure from outside e.g. carcinoma of the thyroid. retropharyngeal abscess, caries spine etc.

(d) Pseudobulbar palsy.

(e) Carcinoma oesophagus, upper part.

(2) *The middle part* of the oesophagus may be narrowed by the pressure of bronchogenic carcinoma, aneurysm of

the aorta, congenital aortic ring, enlarged left atrium (in mitral stenosis), caries spine etc. The lumen is also narrowed by malignant strictures of the oesophagus, carcinoma oesophagus middle third etc.

(3) *The Lower part* of the oesophagus plays an important part in the etiology of dysphagia as it is the site for cardiospasm, carcinoma oesophagus, scleroderma, hiatus hernia etc.

Normally the food bolus takes 6 seconds to reach the stomach after deglutition.

N.B. *Dysphagia lusoria* is a very rare condition due to compression of the oesophagus by an aberrant right subclavian artery.

Besides the routine clinical examination of the relevant systems, a routine blood examination, a straight X-ray of chest, screening of the chest, Ba-swallow X-ray of the oesophagus and oesophagoscopy and biopsy must be done in order to find out the cause of dysphagia.

EXAMINATION OF THE ABDOMEN

Anatomical subdivisions and landmarks–For the purpose of localising the sings and symptoms, structures and organs within the abdomen in relation to the anterior abdominal wall; the abdomen is subdivided into *nine regions* by two horizontal and two vertical lines or planes.

The vertical line on either side is drawn vertically upwards from the midpoint of the line joining the anterior superior iliac spine and the symphisis pubis or the midinguinal point. The upper horizontal line lies at the level of the lowest points of the chest wall i.e. joining the tips of the tenth costal cartilages on either side. The lower horizontal plane or line lies at the level of the highest points of the iliac crests as seen from the front.

The upper section is subdivided into the *right* and the *left hypochondric* and *epigastric* regions; middle section **into** *umbilical* and *right* and *left* lumber regions and the **lower** section into *hypogastrium (or suprapubic region) and right and left iliac* regions.

The intraabdominal structures and organs in relation to these arbitrary subdivisions should be kept in mind and are as follows—

(1) *Right hypochondrium*–right lobe of the liver, gall bladder, hepatic flexure of the colon, upper part of the right kidney and the right suprarenal gland.

(2) *Epigastrium pylorus of the stomach*– a part of the liver; the pancreas, the aorta and the duodenum.

(3) *Left hypochondrium*–the spleen, the tail of the pancreas, the splenic flexure of the colon the upper part of the left kidney, the left suprarenal gland and a part of the stomach.

(4) *Right lumber region*–the lower part of the right kidney, the ascending colon, parts of the duodenum and the jejunum.

(5) *Umbilical region*–the omentum, the transverse colon, parts of the jejunum and the ileum.

(6) *Left lumbar*–the lower part of the left kidney, the descending colon, parts of the jejunum and the ileum.

(7) *Right iliac*–the lower end of the ileum, the caecum, the appendix, right ureter, the right ovary in the female and the right spermatic cord in the male.

(8) *Hypogastrium*–the urinary bladder, the enlarged or gravid uterus and coils of the ileum.

(9) *Left iliac*–the sigmoid colon, the left ureter, the left ovary in the female and the left spermatic cord in the male.

The above anatomical recapitulations will help the student of medicine to correlate symptoms and signs in relation to the regions of the abdominal wall, with the organs and structures underneath. In hiatus hernia a portion of' the stomach enters into the thoracic cavity due to a laxity of the oesophageal hiatus of the diaphragm. It occurs usually in obeses subjects aggravated by a raised intraabdominal pressure (e.g. pregnancy) and kyphoscoliosis. Symptoms are mainly due to acid reflux. Heart burn on stooping or lying down, lower sternal pain, dysphagia, haemorrhage and pallor are the main symptoms.

INSPECTION

The patient should be lie flat on his back, quite straight. The legs are extended. Extended, the arms should lie parallel to the body. A broad daylight is preferable and inspect the abdomen from the foot end of the bed. A systematic examination is to be done following these guidelines–

(i) The general contour of the abdomen should be first described--whether normal, scaphoid or distended. The *scaphoid* abdomen is commonly found in cases of undernutrition, tuberculous peritonitis, extreme degrees of dehydration etc.

The abdomen may be distended due to the presence of fluid in the peritoneal cavity, pregnancy, acute intestinal obstruction, intraabdominal tumours, obesity, full bladder, acute dilatation of the stomach etc. The flanks appear full if there is free fluid in the peritoneal cavity. The localised swellings should be inspected in relation to the conventional areas of the abdomen.

(ii) Inspect the general condition of the skin for any striae or excessive *shininess* or pigmentation at the creases. *White striae* are commonly met with when an obese person suddenly loses weight or in women following pregnancy, after paracentesis of the abdomen in a case of ascites, thyrotoxicosis, diabetes mellitus etc.

Purple striae are characteristic of Cushing's syndrome and prolonged corticosteroid therapy. After repeated pregnancies broad silvery lines called striae gravidarum are seen in the abdominal wall.

(iii) Observe for any alteration in the position of the umbilicus, whether it is inverted to everted, whether there is any bluish discolouration or any sinus over it.

A blue discolouration around the umbilicus is known as *Cullen's sign* and is due to extravasated blood coming forwards from the retroperitoneal space and the sign is seen in cases of ruptured kidney, leaking abdominal aneurysm, acute pancreatitis (which also causes a green discolouration in the loins–*Grey-Turner's sign*) and occasionally in ruptured ectopic gestation. An inverted umbilicus may be found in obesity and in bowel obstructions. An everted umbilicus is found in any conditions giving rise to increased intra-abdominal tension as occurs with an adynamic bowel e.g. Hirschprung's disease in which the abdomen becomes enormously tense and tympanitic with umbilical eversion and marked widening of the subcostal angle.

The umbilical sinuses are produced as a result of malignant or tuberculous peritonitis, Meckel's diverticulum and persistent urachus. The black rash of acanthosis nigricans may be seen around the umbilicus in addition to axillae, neck, groins and nipples and is associated with intraabdominal adenocarcinomas in nonobese adults in the majority of cases.

Distended veins around the umbilicus (caput medusae) are characteristic of portal hypertension syndrome. It may also be found if there is a persistent patency of recanalisation of the umbilical vein. A red, raw angry looking tissue may at times be seen at the umbilicus which might be due to,

(i) chronic infective granuloma of the umbilicus, (ii) umbilical adenoma or Raspberry tumour, or a (iii) secondary
carcinoma (primary being situated in the stomach, colon,
ovary or breast).

An umbilical abscess or nodule may be a clue to an
obscure abdominal pain, though the lump itself is painless
usually, e.g. that due to chronic abdominal infection like
tuberculosis and pneumococcal peritonitis.

Endometriosis of the umbilicus also look raw and red but
it bleeds at each menstrual cycle.

(iv) Note the movement of the abdomen with each
respiration. Normally the abdomen bulges during inspiration and goes back during expiration, the order being
reversed in a diaphragmatic palsy. The movement may be
diminished as a whole in perforative peritonitis and tuberculous peritonitis.

(v) Look for visible peristalsis and pulsations, if any. A
left to right visible peristalsis indicates *reflex pylorospasm*
or *organic pyloric stenosis.* Pylorospasm is produced by
inflammation of the 1st and 2nd parts of duodenum or of
the gall bladder as they are supplied by the 9th thoracic
segment. Organic pyloric stenosis may be produced by
fibrosis in chronic duodenal or peptic ulcer diseases,
carcinoma of the stomach affecting the pyloric antrum or
may be due to congenital hypertrophic pyloric stenosis. If
the stomach is grossly, dilated, a visible peristalsis will be
seen passing down to the suprapubic region and then
again ascending to the right side of epigastrium. When
dilated to such an extent, the stomach may hold even two
litres of fluid–and on shaking the abdomen a splashing
noise is produced. This is the *succusion splash.*

Obstruction of the *transverse colon* is diagnosed by
distension of the midpart of the abdomen and a right to left

visible peristalsis. A visible peristalsis in the middle part of the abdomen around the umbilicus in a zigzag fashion is diagnostic of *small intestinal obstruction.*

An *epigastric pulsation* may be visible in right ventricular hypertrophy, a tumour overlying the abdominal aorta, aneurysm of the abdominal aorta and may be present normally in thin built persons.

(vi) Superficial veins are engorged in portal hypertension and inferior vena caval obstruction. The engorgement can be unmasked by asking the patient to sit up and to hold the breath in deep inspiration or by vigorous coughing.

Portal vein obstruction	*Inferior vena cava obstruction*
1. Direction of flow is away from the umbilicus.	1. Direction of flow of the veins below the umbilicus is towards the superior vena cava i.e., towards the umbilicus.
2. Ascities precedes oedema.	2. Oedema precedes ascites.
3. Spleen is enlarged.	3. Spleen is not enlarged.
4. Varicosity is present in the paraumbilical vein (Cruveilheir-Baumgarten syndrome)	4. Varicosity affects the veins of the lower limbs especially those of the calfmuscles.
5. Haematemesis from rupture of the oesophageal varices and bleeding per anum from the haemorrhoids are common.	5. None of these occur.
6. Portal venous pressure is high.	6. Femoral venous pressure is high.

Next look for any hernia that may be–(a) inguinal on one or both sides (b) umbilical or paraumbilical (c) epigastric (small hernia due to extrusion of portions of the extraperitoneal fat) (d) incisional, protruding through an incision site of post-operation or (e) femoral hernia.

PALPATION

The patient lies on his back with the head and shoulder's supported by a pillow and the knees drawn up to relax the abdominal muscles. The clinician stands or sits on a tool to the right of the patient.

Warm your hands by rubbing each other if they are cold. Gently place the right hand first over the left iliac fossa and palpate it. Subsequently pulpate the left lumber. Left hypochondrium epigastrium, right hypochondrium, right lumbar, right iliac fossa hypogastrium and umbilical regions. Palpation should always be done by the flat of the hand and finger movements must be gentle and from the metacarpophalangeal joints. *Superficial palpation* should be done to get the following informations :

(1) *Consistency or feel of the abdomen*–The normal feel of the abdomen is elastic. Rigidity is a sign of peritonitis or any localised infection. Doughy feel is obtained in tuberculous peritonitis. Abdominal guarding is due to contraction of the abdominal muscles. It occurs reflexly as a part of a defense (protective) mechanism which may be localised (e.g. over an inflamed organ) or generalised (as in peritonitis).

(2) *Tenderness*–It indicates an inflammation of the peritoneum or a stretching of the capsule of intra-abdominal organs as a result of inflammation or enlargement. Ask the patient to show the site of pain by his index finger (*Pointing sign*).

In peptic ulcer, particularly in chronic duodenal ulcer, the tenderness corresponds with the area shown by the pointing finger.

(3) *Any Localised lump*– If it is superficial, do the rising test;–ask the patient to raise the head from the bed and see whether the lump becomes more superficial (perietal (swelling) or disappears (intra-abdominal swelling). During superficial palpation try to locate the lump in relation to the area of the abdomen.

4) *Fluid thrill*–The patient lies flat on the bed with thighs flexed. The ulnar border of the right hand of the patient is placed vertically on the middle to prevent transmission of vibrations by the abdominal wall. Place your left palm on one flank and sharply tap the other flank with the right hand. If there is any enlargement of a local organ tapping should be done from that side for better conduction. To have a fluid thrill there must be at least 2 litres fluid in the peritoneal cavity under tension. Fallacy of the test :–It may be positive even in conditions where there is no free fluid in the peritoneal cavity such as obesity, ovarian cyst, encysted ascites and also in paralytic ileus. In ascites the bulging is mainly lateral whereas in an ovarian tumour it is an anteroposterior bulging of the abdominal wall. The dullness in the ovarian tumour is central and does not change with the position of the patient.

(5) *Divarication of the recti*– Sometimes even in healthy individuals separation of the rectus muscles are found to produce a wide gap, the abdominal viscera being palpable distinctly, only separated by a thin abdominal wall. This is called the divarication of the rectus muscles and is common in those with chronically distended abdomen e.g. in long standing huge ascites.

(6) *Direction of blood flow in prominent abdominal veins*– It is examined if the abdominal veins are prominent. A promi-

nent abdominal vein is selected and made more prominent by making the patient sit up and cough, if possible. Standing on the right side of the patient place the index fingers of both the right and the left hands on the vein side by side; the left index finger being placed above that of the right. Empty a portion of the vein by milking the two fingers in two directions i.e., the left index finger drawn upwards and the right downwards. Each end of the emptied vein is sealed with the pressure of the finger. One of the fingers is then removed and the rate and rapidity at which the vein fills up is noted. The same procedure is repeated, removing the finger at the other end. The rate and rapidity of filling of the vein indicates the direction of the blood flow. The direction of the flow of blood in prominent abdominal veins in portal venous obstruction and in inferior vena cava obstruction has already been discussed.

Deep Palpation

Now the abdomen is palpated more deeply with the flat of the hand as well as with the fingers. The patient should be asked to breath quietly with the head turned to the left side. During palpation of the liver, spleen and the kidneys, the patient should be asked to take deep breaths by mouth.

(i) Palpate the different areas for detection of any mass. The organs or the portions thereof that occupy the different anatomical regions have been discussed earlier.

If a mass is felt, the points to be described are – *site, size, shape, consistency, margin; surface, movement with respiration, pulsatile or not, ballotable or not, tenderness, condition of the overlying skin etc.*

(ii) During each expiratory phase of respiration, gradually apply pressure on the abdomen and then suddenly take off the hands and look for an expression of agony in the patient's face, if there be any. This is known as *rebound tenderness* found in peritonitis from any cause viz, appendicitis.

Sometimes a sharp pressure over the left iliac fossa elicits a pain over the appendix due to pressure exerted by gas on the wall of the inflammed caecum. This is known as *Rovsing's sign* found in acute appendicitis.

(iii) *Palpation of the liver*

Sit by the side of the patient and place the two hands side by side in the right subcostal region (Fig 4-2). The hands should lie flat on the abdomen lateral to the rectus abdominis, fingers pointing towards the ribs. If any resistance is encountered, the hands should be moved down-

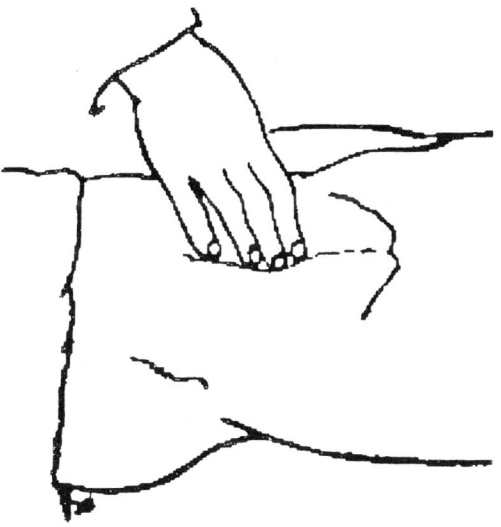

Fig. 4-1 :   *Palpation of the liver–Conventional mathod*

wards till there is no resistance, The patient is then asked to inspirate deeply and at the height of inspiration, the fingers are pressed firmly upwards and inwards. A palpable liver is felt as a sharp regular border riding beneath the fingers. The whole process is repeated from the lateral to the medial regions to find out the edge of the liver.

The liver can also be palpated by the conventional method (Fig 4-1). Ask the patient to turn his head to the left and breath regularly. Place the right hand firmly and flatly over the right iliac fossa and slightly press it inwards and upwards during the phase of inspiration. The radial border of the right hand should be kept parallel to the lower border of the liver and on the outer side of the rectus muscle to avoid its upper septum. Keep the hand steady when the patient takes a deep breath by mouth. In this way go on palpating upwards. At the height of deep inspiration, the tip and the radial margin of the index finger should slip over the lower border of the liver, if it is palpable. Trial is made at different levels before concluding that the edge cannot be felt.

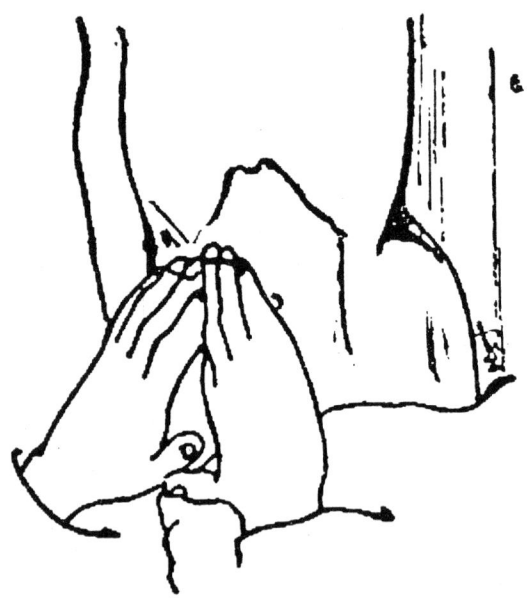

Fig. 4-2 : Palpation of the liver–Better method

The edge of the liver can be felt in normal children and *emphysema*. The enlargement of the liver in the epigastrium should be noted in the usual way as a routine. A simple anatomical variation of the liver, the Riedel's lobe, is a downward tongue-like projection from the right lobe and is more-frequent in women;–occasionally it gives rise to diagnostic difficulty. It is usually freely mobile and may be mistaken for a movable kidney or if situated closer to the midline, for a gall bladder lump, It is usually palpable in the right upper quadrant of the abdomen. If the liver is palpable, note–

(a)   The degree of enlargement expressed by the number of fingers placed between the costal arch and the lower border of the liver or by the number

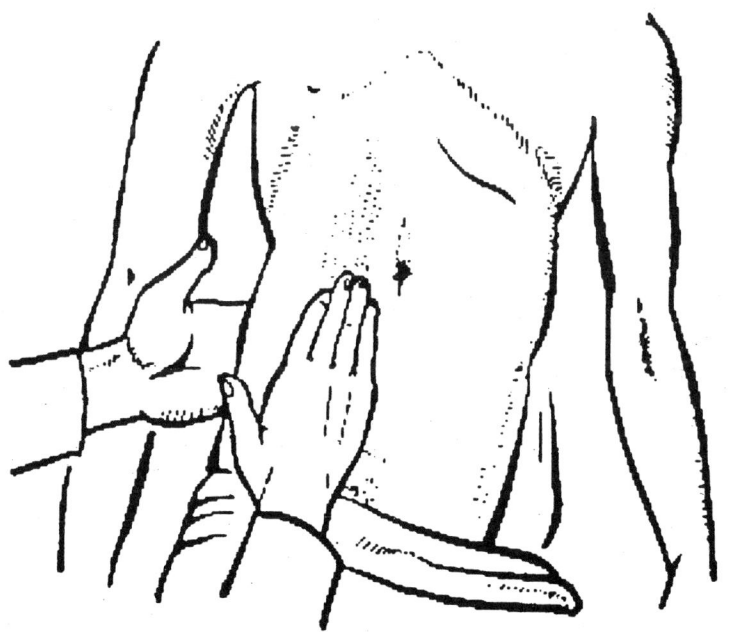

Fig. 4-3 : Bimanual palpation of the liver

of inches or centimeters below the costal margin up to the lower border of the liver. Note that a *palpable liver* is not necessarily an enlarged one; to confirm the latter the upper border of the liver dullness should be detected.

(b)   The consistency–This may be soft, firm or hard. An enlarged liver of soft consistency is found in congestive cardiac failure, fatty liver, infective hepatitis, acute malaria and early stages of amyloid disease.–

A *firm* liver is due to chronic kala-azar, Hodgkin's disease, infective hepatitis, Weil's disease, amoebic hepatitis, early stage of cirrhosis, intrahepatic cholangitis etc.

A *hard* liver is characteristic of carcinoma and secondary deposits in the liver; but may also be seen in chronic malaria, chronic myeloid leukaemia, cirrhosis of the liver etc.

(c)   The surface–A *smooth* surface of the enlarged liver is found in congestive cardiac failure, chronic malaria, kala-azar, infective hepatitis, amoebic hepatitis, Weils' disease, chronic myeloid leukaemia etc. *Finely irregular* surface is characteristic of portal cirrhosis in the early stage. A grossly *irregular* liver with nodules is a clinical finding in post-necrotic cirrhosis, carcinoma of the liver, secondary deposits in the liver and gumma liver.

(d)   Any tenderness–This is due to stretching of the capsule because of enlargement of the liver or an inflammation causing perihepatitis. A tender liver is commonly seen in congestive cardiac failure, amoebic hepatitis, infective hepatitis, Weil's disease and occasionally in carcinoma of the liver.

(e)   The margins–A hard or a firm liver usually shows a sharp margin whereas a soft liver has a rounded margin

(f)   Any pulsation–Sitting in a low chair beside the patient place the right hand on the anterior abdominal wall over the liver and the left hand over the costal arch in the back (Fig 4-3). Now ask the patient to hold breath after deep inspiration. Note if there is any *expansile pulsaion* and also decide whether it is systolic or presystolic. Systolic and presystolic pulsation of the liver are the characteristics of tricuspid incompetence and tricuspid stenosis. respectively. Haemangioma of the liver is also pulsatile, Hepatic pulsations may be transmitted from an enlarged right ventricle or from the aorta in thin built subjects, but then they are not expansile.

(g)   The movements with respiration–Normally the liver moves 1 to 3 cm downwards with deep inspiration and may be particularly conspicuous in athletes and singers.

(h)   The upper border of the liver dullness–This is mappd out by percussing the chest downwards along the right midclavicular line. Find out the lower edge by light percussion moving upwards from the umbilicus towards the costal margin. A *small liver is clinically* detected by this method only. The upper border of the liver dullness may be *obliterated* or *lowered* in (a) emphysema, (b) right sided pneumothorax, (c) perforated peptic ulcer, due to accumulation of gas under the diaphragm, (d) cirrhosis of the liver, due to shrinkage, (e) pneumoperitoneum, (f) Hirschprung's disease etc.

The upper border of the liver dullness may be raised by (a) amoebic liver abscess, (b) subdiaphragmatic abscess, (c) basal pneumonia and (d) right sided pleural effusion. On deep inspiration the upper border of the liver dullness goes down in the diseases mentioned above except in pleural effusion where it remains unchanged.

N.B.– In presence of huge ascites the liver is palpated by the method of *dipping* i.e., the tip of the fingers are sharply and quickly but gently thrust into the abdomen to displace the fluid and feel for the edge of the liver.

Enlargement of the liver (hepatomegaly), may be mild, moderate, or huge.

Causes of (*mild hepatomegaly*) (1-2 fingers) are : (a) infective hepatitis, (b) early congestive cardiac failure, (c) acute malaria and kala-azar, (d) serum hepatitis, (e) ascending cholangiohepatitis, (f) amyloidosis, (g) septicaemia or pyaemia. (h) haemolytic anaemias etc.

Moderate hepatomegaly (2-5 fingers)–Found in chronic malaria, chronic kala-azar post-necrotic cirrhosis, pre-cirrhotic liver, amoebic liver abscess, chronic myeloid leukaemia, Hodgkin's disease, hydatid cyst of the liver and acquired haemolytic anaemia.

Huge hepatomegaly (more than 5 fingers)–Found in chronic malaria, chronic kala-azar, post-necrotic cirrhosis, carcinoma of the liver, chronic myeloid leukaemia and myelosclerosis.

Jaundice associated with hepatomegaly occurs in infective hepatitis, ascending cholangic-hepatitis, haemolytic anaemias, carcinoma of the liver, Weil's disease, chronic malaria and post-necrotic cirrhosis with hepatocellular failure.

The combination of *hepatomegaly* and *ascites* may be due to hepatic cirrhosis carcinoma of the liver, cirrhosis of the liver with tuberculous peritonitis, chronic myeloid leukaemia, abdominal Hodgkin etc. *Budd-Chiari syndrome* causes acute tender gross hepatomegaly with intractable severe ascites

Lymphadenopathy with hepatomegaly occurs in Hodgkin's disease, chronic lymphatic leukaemia, infective hepatitis and many other conditions where there is generalised lymphadenopathy (see chapter I). The liver is moderately enlarged and associated with *rise of temperature* in–(i) infective hepatitis, (ii) amoebic hepatitis and amoebic liver abscess, (iii) acute malaria, (iv) acute kala-azar. (v) Hodgkin's disease, (vi) Weil's disease, (vii) septicaemia and pyaemia, (viii) hydatid cyst of the liver when secondarily infected etc.

Predominant enlargement of the left lobe of the liver might be due to (i) liver abscess (amoebic), (ii) primary hepatoma, (iii) secondary deposits or (iv) hepatic syphilis (gumma).

The left lobe may be severely *atrophied* and is not uncommonly detected at postmortem, the usual cause being interference with the left branch of the portal vein when the degeneration occurs at birth and atrophy persists into the adult life. Rare causes in later life are—compressions of the left hepatic duct or the left branch of the hepatic artery or the left branch of the portal vein by malignant diseases.

It must be remembered that the palpable liver may occasionally be due simply to a downward displacement of the liver without any hepatomegaly and this might be caused by a right sided massive pleural effusion, empyema or pneumothorax; pulmonary emphysema and severe kyphoscoliosis.

N.B.–A liver palpable below the umbilicus is commonly caused by (i) malignant deposits, (ii) polycystic disease, (iii) Hodgkin's disease, (iv) amyloidosis, (v) congestive heart failure, (vi) gross fatty change etc. Rapid change of the liver size may occur with–(i) correction of congestive heart failure, (ii) relief of cholestatic jaundice, (iii) control of severe diabetes, (iv) control of fatty liver etc.

In hepatopsis or wandering liver the organ leaves its normal situation and can be moved laterally or rotated manually about a horizontal axis–patients usually present with a dragging pain and heaviness in the hepatic region.

(iv)   *Gall bladder*

This pear shaped saccular organ is situated in a fossa on the visceral surface of the liver. It is about three inches long and weights about $1\frac{1}{2}$ ounces. Its fundus is rounded and projects beyond the inferior margin of the liver. At the level of the tip of the ninth costal cartilage and the outer border of the right rectus muscle the gall bladder comes in contact with the anterior abdominal wall.

The organ is felt as a pear shaped, smooth, tense swelling projecting beneath the right costal margin in the direction of the umbilicus only when it is distended. A pyriform swelling situated just outside the right rectus muscle, moving freely from side to side around a point opposite the 9th costal cartilage and moving freely with respiration is the classical feature of a gall bladder swelling. In order to palpate the organ, the patient is asked to take a deep breath and at the same time the hand is moved upwards under the costal margin. During palpation note for the gall bladder tenderness and Murphy's sign.

Murphy's sign–If a continuous gentle pressure is exerted over the right hypochondrium while the patient takes a deep breath, there will be a catch in the breath at the height of inspiration. To elicit the Murphy's sign place your hand over the right costal margin with the thumb resting at the junction of the tip of the ninth costal cartilage and the lateral border of the right rectus muscle. The

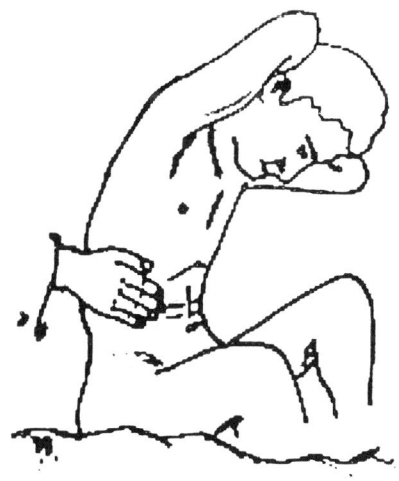

Fig. 4-4 : Elicitation of Murphy's sing.

patient is then asked to take a deep inspiration when the descent of the diaphragm causes the gall bladder to strike against the examiner's thumb and just at that moment, the patient feels a sharp pain and there is a catch in the breath before the zenith of inspiration. This is *Moynihan's* method of eliciting the Murphy's sign.

In some cases of acute cholecystitis subcutaneous oedema may be demonstrated by carefully comparing the appearances of the skin and the subcutaneous tissues above the tip of the 8th and the 9th ribs on the right side with that of the left side. This right sided subcutaneous oedema is called *Leake's oedema test.*

Sometimes in acute inflammation of the gall bladder an area of hyperaesthesia may be demonstrated between the 9th and the 11th ribs posteriorly on the right side–this is the *Boas' sign.* A distended gall bladder in the presence of jaundice is probably not due to a gall stone impacted in the common bile duct; in cholelithiasis, previous episodes of cholecystitis have already made the gall bladder fibrotic and small which, therefore, cannot distend. This is *Courvoisier's law.* In such cases the cause of the palpable gall bladder along with obstructive jaundice is probably carcinoma of the head of the pancreas.

An enlarged gall bladder had to be distinguished from a visceroptotic right kidney. The latter can be displaced towards the pelvis and has to resonant colon anteriorly.

(v)   *Spleen*

The spleen lies behind and below the 9th, 10th and 11th ribs with its long axis along the direction of the 10th rib. Its posterosuperior end lies $1\frac{1}{2}$ inches lateral to the 10th thoracic spine and its anteroinferior end extends anterioly up to the midaxillary line. The spleen moves with respiration and very rarely with deep inspiration may be normally palpable. It beomes palpable when it enlarges to about thrice or more its normal size. *Palpation of the spleen :* Preliminary preparation of the patient is the same as that during palpation of the liver. The examiner should stand on the right side of the patient. Ask the patient to take deep breaths by mouth. Place the left hand over the edge of the left costal margin (i.e., over the 9th, 10th and 11th ribs on the lateral side) and flank; firmly press medially and forward so that the ribs and the lateral abdominal wall are brought a little forward and medially. Now palpate the spleen with the right hand, starting from the right iliac fossa, going gradually more towards the left hypochondrium.

The spleen, as already stated is not normally palpable and needs to be enlarged to about 3 times its usual size to become palpable. A *just palpable spleen* offers a great difficulty in detection which may be overcome by turning the patient to the right side (i.e., in the right lateral position) and then palpating the spleen with the help of the finger tips of the right hand placed loosely under the costal arch. Here the hooked fingers of the examiner's right hand are placed under the left costal margin and the patient is asked to take deep breaths. A just palpable spleen touches the finger tips at the height of inspiration.

The following findings should be noted in case a palpable spleen is found–situation, margin, splenic notch size, shape, consistency (i.e., soft, firm or hard), surface, tenderness, movement with respiration, any palpable splenic rub or fremitus (found in cases of perisplenitis) and whether the fingers can be insinuated between the costal margin and the enlarged spleen.

A palpable spleen should be differentiated from a kidney swelling by the following points :

Splenic swelling	Kidney swelling
1. The spleen enlarges downwards, forwards and to wards the right iliac fossa. It has a tendency to buldge forward.	1. The kidney enlarges downwards towards the respective iliac fossa. It has a tendency to buldge into the loin.
2. The margin is sharp.	2. The margin is rounded.
3. The spleen has a notch on the anterior border.	3. There is no palpable notch.
4. The fingers cannot be insinuated between the costal margin and the spleen and an enlarged spleen cannot be pulsed back into the loin.	4. Fingers can be insinuated easily between the costal margin and the kidney and there is a fullness of the loin (at the back) due to the enlargement of the kidney.
5. The fingers can be insinuated between the sacrospinalis and the subcostal margin on the back.	5. In the back the fingers cannot be insinuated between the kidney lump and the erector spinae muscle as there is no space.
6. Percussion note is dull over the spleen.	6. A band of colonicresicres onance is found over the kidneys
7. It is not palpable bimanually and is not ballotable.	7. It is bimanually palpable and ballotable.
8. Renal angle is not tender.	8. Renal angle may be tender.

Other swellings or enlargements which should be differentiated from an enlarged spleen are—enlarged left lobe of the liver, rolled up carcinomatous or tuberculous omentum, carcinoma of the body of the stomach, malignant left suprarenal tumour and carcinomatous mass involving the splenic flexure of the colon.

Mild enlargement ot the spleen (I finger) may be found in enteric fever, infective endocarditis, acute malaria, acute kala-azar, haemolytic anaemias, miliary tuberculosis, acute leukaemia, infectious mononucleosis, in a few per cent cases of idiopathic thrombocytopenic purpura, infective hepatitis etc. *Moderate enlargement of the spleen* (2-5 fingers) found in chronic malaria, chronic kala-azar, portal hypertension, Hodgkin's disease, congenital haemolytic anaemias, chronic myeloid and lymphatic leukaemias, sarcoidosis, non-Hodgkin (lymphocytic) lymphomas, haemochromatosis, chronic active hepatitis, sarcoidosis etc. *Huge splenomegaly* (5 fingers or more) is characteristic of chronic myeloid leukaemia, chronic malaria, chronic kala-azar, myelofibrosis, myelosclerosis, tropical splenomegaly syndrome, primary polycythaemia, portal hypertension, thalassaemia major, in children Gaucher's and other lipid storage diseases etc. Enlargement of the *spleen and the lymph nodes* may occur in chronic lymphatic leukaemia, Hodgkin's disease, miliary tuberculosis sarcoidosis, non-Hodgkin's (lymphocytic) lymphoma, infectious mononucleosis etc. In fact any condition which causes generalised lymphadenopathy may cause splenomegaly.

Ascites may be present along with splenomegaly in portal hypertension syndrome, chronic myeloid leukaemia, lymphoma etc.

Rise of temperature may be associated with splenomegaly in enteric fever, infective endocarditis, kala-azar, acute malaria, infective hepatitis, miliary tuberculosis, acute leukaemias, crisis in haemolytic anaemias etc.

The combination of *hepatomegaly and splenomegaly* is a common clinical finding and usually occurs in chronic malaria, kala-azar, chronic myeloid leukaemia, heamolytic anaemias, myelofibrosis, myelosclerosis, infective hepatitis, post-hepatitic cirrhosis with portal hypertension.

Hypersplenism– This often accompanies splenomegaly and is characterised by an enlarged spleen, anaemia leucopenia and/or thrombocytopenia in addition to hyperactivity of the bone-marrow. Splenectomy often reverses the condition. Though hypersplenism may be present in most splenomegalic states, *splenomegaly does not always cause hypersplenism*.

Besides the bedside clinical methods of detecting splenomegaly, the best method is *scanning* of the spleen by introducing IV a colloid tagged with technetium 99m. The latter is taken up by the RE cells and helps in visualizing the size, shape and defects of spleen.

(vi)   *Kidneys*

The kidneys lie on either side of the dorsolumbar vertebrae; their upper poles roughly corresponding to the upper border of the 12th thoracic vertebra; the left kidney being placed slightly higher than the right. Kidneys are about 10 cm in length. The hila lie opposite the space between the transverse processes of the 1st and 2nd lumbar vertebra.

Method : Sit on a low chair on the right side of the patient who lies on his back with the knees flexed. To palpate the right kidney place the left hand over the renal angle and press the loin forward. The fingers of the right hand are placed over the lower hypochondrium and upper lumbar regions of the abdomen and pressed backward, upward and inward. Ask the patient to relax the abdominal muscles and take a deep breath when a firm mass with a rounded lower pole may be felt lying in the posterior abdominal wall. Now give a sharp tap by the left hand on the back and as the kidney is *ballotable*, the right hand should feel it following which the kidney falls back on the posterior abdominal wall which will be felt by the left hand. The left kidney is best palpated from the left side; the clinician's right hand being placed posteriorly.

Following points should be noted : situation, size, shape, (kidneys are ovoid in shape), margins (rounded), ccnsistency (normally resilient feel), surface (irregular in polycystic kidney), movement with respiration and *tenderness over the renal angles*. Tenderness of the renal angles may be found in acute pyelonephritis, stone, renal tuberculosis, hypernephroma and perinephric abscess. The kidneys may be palpable in cases of *dropped kidney*. In *normal thin built* persons the lower pole of the right kidney may be palpable. But the left kidney is rarely palpable unless enlarged or displaced.

The movable kidney can be easily restored to its original position by manipulation. A movable right kidney is often mistaken for a distended gall bladder. The distended gall bladder can only be temporarily pushed back and always comes forward rapidly.

Both kidneys are enlarged in polycystic disease and in bilateral hydronephrosis due to obstruction of the urinary tract at the level of the bladder or below it. *One kidney may be enlarged* in unilateral hydronephrosis hypernephroma. Wilm's tumour and in a large solitary cyst of the kidney.

Shape of the kidney may vary due to congenital defects in development, e.g. in horse-shoe shaped kidney.

The kidney mass should be differentiated from : enlarged spleen, perinephric abscess, retroperitoneal tumours, tumours of the bowel, pancreatic cyst and Riedel's lobe of the liver (if present).

(vii)   Left iliac fossa, right iliac fossa and hypogastrium should be palpated deeply with both hands–the left being placed over the right.

Deep palpation in the left iliac fossa may reveal a freely movable, tender, rope like structure in a case of intestinal amoebiasis, irritable colon syndrome etc. A scyballous mass, tumour or any other lump may be palpated in this way.

A lump in the right iliac fossa may be palpated in cases of appendicular abscess, amoeboma of the colon, iliocaecal tuberculosis, Crohn's disease, carcinoma of the caecum or ascending colon carcinoid tumour etc.

Palpate the splenic and the hepatic flexures in the left and the right hypochondria respectively.

A lump due to faecal accumulation occurs more often in the left iliac fossa than elsewhere and it pits on pressure and may disappear after administration of a high enema.

Palpate the hypogastrium for any tumour of the bladder or uterus. Tenderness. over the hypogastrium may be found in bladder stone, cystitis and acute retention of urine.

(viii) *Miscellaneous swellings* within the abdomen should be looked for. They are often due to lymphoglandular enlargement found in tabes mesenterica, Hodgkin's and non-Hodgkin lymphomas, leukaemias etc.

The *testes* should be examined for any tumour e.g., seminoma which metastasises by lymph vessels and as such. mesenteric glands may become enlarged.

(ix) One must perform a digital examination of the rectum to note the condition of the sphincter, presence of scybala, stricture or growth. In the male the prostate, the seminal vesicles and the trigone of the bladder may be recognised by this technique; in the female, the uterus and the pouch of Douglas can be examined. The anus should be examined for haemorrhoids, fistulae, fissures or growths.

Lastly palpate the hernial sites, i.e., the inguinal, the umbilical and the epigastric regions. Hernias of the abdominal wall become prominent in the erect position or after coughing.

PERCUSSION

(1) General percussion–It should be done to detect any alteration in the tympanitic note of the abdomen.

(2) Shifting dullness–*First of all palpate the liver and the spleen.* If they are enlarged avoid percussion over them. Go on percussing on the midline from the epigastrium to about the midpoint between the umbilicus and the symphysis pubis. Now change the direction laterally to that side where there is no enlargement of organs. When you get a dull not turn the patient to the other side keeping the fingers in the same position; wait about a minute for the intestine to float up and then percuss again. The dull note obtained previously will have changed to a resonant one and the resonant area near the midline will be dull. *Shifting dullness and fluid thrill, together of singly make the diagnosis of ascites certain.* However, they can be elicited in only half of the cases of ascites and absence of either or both does not exclude ascites.

A fluid thrill can be elicited when a large amount of ascitic fluid has accumulated. One hand is placed flat on the patient's flank. An assistant (or the patient) is asked to put the side of his hand firmly on the midline of the abdomen. When the other flank is flicked or tapped, a shock wave is transmitted to the palpating hand. The patient's or assistant's hand prevents any ripple from passing through the fat of the abdominal wall.

Common causes of ascites are :

(1) Hepatic–Portal hypertension syndrome, carcinoma

of the liver, hepatic vein thrombosis (Budd-Chiari syndrome).

(2) Cardiac–Chronic constrictive pericarditis, congestive cardiac failure.

(3) Renal–Nephrotic syndrome.

(4) Nutritional–Malabsorption syndrome, famine oedema.

(5) Haematological–Severe anaemia, Hodgkin's disease, chronic myeloid leukaemia.

(6) Lymphatic–Filariasis.

(7) Infection–Tuberculous peritonitis, pyogenic peritonitis.

(8) Malignancy – Malignant peritonitis.

Percussion of the individual organs like liver, spleen, kidney, stomach bladder etc. should next be performed. *Heavy percussion* should be done starting about the second rib and gradually going downward until *impairment* is detected. The upper limit of the liver dullness forms an almost horizontal line around the chest. The upper border of the right lobe is at the level of the 5th rib, 2 cm medial to the right midclavicular line while the upper border of the left lobe corresponds to that of the 6th rib on the left midclavicular line. The lower border of the liver is defined by *light percussion* from below upward.

The percussion note over the left hypochondrium is tympanitic because of air in the stomach. The fundus of the stomach is normally situated in Traube's space. As such any growth in the fundus of the stomach will produce a dull note on percussion over the Traube's space (vide Respiratory system). Enlargement of the liver and the spleen should be confirmed by percussion. In a case of ruptured spleen the area of splenic dullness increases.

Percussion note over the lumbar region i.e., over the kidney is resonant owing to the presence of gas in the colon.

Bladder in percussed from the umbilicus, downwards, on the midline.

AUSCULTATION

Auscultation of the abdomen is an invaluable clinical method of diagnosis in many abdominal and extra-abdominal disorders. The chest piece of the stethoscope should preferably be placed to the right of the umbilicus and the auscultation might reveal–

(1)   *Increased* peristaltic sounds in acute intestinal obstruction and an otherwise *silent* abdomen with the sounds of pulsations of the abdominal aorta only is characteristic of paralytic ileus.

(2)   Peristatic sounds may also be *increased* in nervous diarrhoea, Crohn's disease, carcinoid tumour etc.

(3)   *Succussion splash* induced by vigorous shaking of the trunk in pyloric stenosis and paralytic ileus. It may also be detected by placing the stethoscope on the abdominal wall and quickly depressing the abdominal wall by the free hand. A succussion splash may be *normally* found one to two hours after a meal.

(4)   *Friction rubs* over the liver and spleen with the movements of respiration are characteristic of perihepatitis and perisplenitis. The commonest cause of the former is a liver biopsy. It may also be audible over the surface of splenic infracts.

(5)   *Foetal heart sounds and uterine souffle* (which is

a systolodiastolic murmur) are important clinical signs of pregnancy.

(6) *A soft systolic murmur over the lumbar region* on deep pressure with the chest piece is *diagnostic of renal artery stenosis.* In this case a systolic murmur may also be present in the renal angle. *A systolic murmur* over the abdomen is a common clinical finding in coarctation of the abdominal aorta.

(7) A *presystolic gallop* is often present over the epigastrium in corpulmonale.

(8) *Pansystolic murmur* over the epigastrium or the tricuspid area increasing with inspiration (*Carvallo's sign*) is diagnostic of tricuspid incompetence.

(9) In aortic regurgitation, a *splashing sound* is often heard over the stomach if the patient drinks a glass of water. This is due to the splashing of stomach (partially filled with water) by the booming aorta.

(10) *Auscultopercussion* helps to delineate the outline of the stomach in cases of acute dilatation of the stomach and pyloric stenosis. This is done by placing the chest piece over the left hypochondrium and simultaneous percussion of the stomach by another clinician in the direction away from the chest piece. Note the character of the sounds and put markings over the skin where there is a change of character. Another method may be employed where the percussion is replaced by scratching the skin with the help of match sticks. This should be done in straight lines directed away from the chest piece.

(11) A *venous hum* may be heard on or below the

xiphisternum or at the umbilicus in *congenital hypoplasia of the portal venous system with patent umbilical vein* or may be due to a *dilated paraumbilical vein in* cirrhosis of the liver. This is known as Cruveilhier-Baumgarten syndrome.

Clinical signs in diseases of the stomach and duodenum

(1)   Pointing sign–Indicates the area of maximum tenderness in duodenal ulcer.

(2)   Unilateral rectus rigidity–An important sign of inflammation of the stomach or the duodenum such as chronic duodenal ulcer.

(3)   Visible peristalsis–Ask the patient to drink a glass of water before he or she lies down. Look for visible peristalsis which may be induced by sharp tapping over the abdominal wall. A left to right peristalsis is found in pyloric stenosis.

(4)   Succussion splash–Characteristically found in pyloric stenosis and acute dilatation of the stomach.

(5)   Percussion of Traube's space–Dull if there is a growth in the fundus.

(6)   Auscultopercussion–*vide supra.*

ANO-RECTAL EXAMINATION

Students should remember that the examination of the gastrointestinal system remains incomplete without a rectal examination. The physician might miss a very prognostically grave disease e.g. a carcinoma of the rectum if he avoids this part of the exmination. One should do a per-rectal examination with the patient in any of the following positions :

(1)   Left lateral–In this position the right leg should be flexed while the left leg is extended. The buttocks should be placed over the edge of the bed. (2) Knee elbow. (3) Dorsal. (4) Lithotomy.

EXAMINATION–Inspection

First inspect the region of the anus. Note the presence of discharges–blood or pus, condylomas, external haemorrhoids, protrusion of the internal haemorrhoids, anal fissure, prolapse of the rectal mucosa, external opening of anal fistula etc.

Digital palpation

The petient is asked to open his mouth and breathe quietly. Wearing a glove in the right hand, smear the right index finger with petroleum jelly. Now gently and slowly introduce the finger into the rectum starting with the pulp of the finger. Following are the conditions that can be diagnosed by digital palpation :

(i)   In the rectum–Apex of an intussusception, distended rectum (i.e., ballooning) in intestinal obstruction, internal opening of anal fistula, rectal polyps, carcinoma and stricture of the rectum.

(ii) Outside the rectum–ischiorectal abscess, pelvic appendicitis, salpingo-oophoritis, aneurysm of internal iliac artery, enlarged prostate, seminal vesicles etc.

After withdrawal of the index finger inspect it for blood, pus or mucus.

Proctoscopy and sigmoidoscopy

The patient is placed in the left lateral position with the left leg extended and the right leg flexed. A lubricated proctoscope with an obturator is gently introduced to its full depth per rectum very carefully and slowly. The obturator is then removed and the interior of the rectum and the anus is inspected carefully as the instrument is withdrawn slowly. For better visualisation a torch may be focussed at the sites of the mucous membrane that is being inspected. By this process about 3 inches of the rectum and the anal canal is visualised. It is particularly helpful in the diagnosis of *haemorrhoids.* If more of the lower part of the large gut needs to be visualised, sigmoidoscopy should be done. The lubricated sigmoidoscope is introduced into the colon per rectally. As the instrument is longer than a proctoscope its use demands experience and some skill. A lighting arrangement is attached with the sigmoidoscope. It is a safe procedure and is useful in the *differential diagnosis of diarrhoea caused by colonic pathology* and also in the diagnosis of *polyps* and *malignancies.* At times a biopsy is also taken through the sigmoidoscope. With its help about 8 to 9 inches of the colon can be inspected.

PARACENTESIS ABDOMINIS

In paracentesis abdominis free fluid is withdrawn from the peritoneal cavity usually by means of a trocar and canula.

Indications :

(1) Diagnostic–The colour and the character of the fluid is studied to determine the cause.

(2) Therapeutic–To reduce the intra-abdominal pressure when the patient feels distressed due to breathlessness, palpitation etc.

Contraindications :

During the procedure of paracentesis if the patient starts having cardiorespiratory distress the manoeuvre must be stopped immediately.

Method :

(a) Ask the patient to empty his bladder before the procedure to prevent an accidental puncture of the bladder by the trocar.

(b) Then make the patient sit at the edge of the bed, supported with a back rest. A rubber sheet is placed over the patient's lap.

(c) The site of puncture is just outside the midpoint of the line between the umbilicus and the anterior superior iliac spine to prevent any damage of the abdominal viscera. Before selection of the site the abdominal organs should be examined avoid an injury to the *spleen* or the *liver* in cases of huge splenomegaly or hepatomegaly respectively and the uterus in a case of pregnancy.

(d) The selected site is sterilised with iodine and spirit.

(e) Anaesthetise the site of puncture by 2% lignocaine.

(f) Put an abdominal binder above the umbilicus in order to maintain a steady external pressure over the abdomen.

(g) Puncture the abdominal wall by the trocar and canula. Initially a resistance is met with which is due to the subcutaneous tissue, fascia and muscles. The resistance suddenly disappears when the abdominal cavity is reached.

(h) The fluid comes out of the canula like a jet and collected in a tumbler.

(i) Samples of the fluid are stored in sterile test tubes for subsequent biochemical and pathological examinations.

(j) After removal of 2 to 3 litres of fluid the trocar is reintroduced into the canula and both are now removed together from the abdominal cavity.

(k) Seal the puncture site with Tinc. Benzoin and apply dressings.

N.B.–For small samples of fluid and also for a continuous slow drainage a wide bore needle may be used in place of a trocar and canula.

Complications :

(1) Sudden cardiorespiratory distress or shock caused by blood polling in the acutely decompressed systemic veins of the abdomen.

(2) Introduction of infection.

(3) Precipitation of hepatic encephalopathy because of the mechanisms as in (l) above.

Investigation of a sample of ascitic fluid :

The fluid withdrawn may be an exudate or a transudate.

A *transudate* is formed by the passive transudation of fluid into the peritoneal cavity and is commonly found in cirrhosis of the liver, nephrotic syndrome and severe anaemia. The fluid contains protein less then 2.5gm%, cells not more than 250/cmm in cirrhosis and less than 1000/ cmm in congestive cardiac failure which are endothelial cells and culture and animal inoculation tests are negative.

An *exudate* is formed by the inflammatory reaction of the peritoneum itself due to infection, chemical irritation or malignancy. Exudates are commonly found in Koch's peritonitis, pyogenic and malignant peritonitis and it may be serous, purulent or haemorrhagic. The *protein content* is more than 2.5gm% and *sugar* is less than normal. Sp. gr is more than 1016, spontaneous coagulation occurs on standing (due to a high protein content), cells are more than 1000/ cmm (mostly lymphocytes) in Koch's peritonitis and more than 1000/ cmm (mostly polymorphonuclear cells and pus cells) in pyogenic peritonitis. In 20% of neoplastic peritonitis more than 10000 cmm RBC's are present. Bacteriological examination of a smear, culture, and animal inoculation tests are to be carried out.

(A) *Physical character* :

(1) Appearance :

(a) In ascites due to cirrhosis of the liver, nephrotic syndrome, congestive cardiac failure and severe anaemia the fluid will be *clear and straw coloured.*

(b) *Opalescent* or even clear fluid may be obtained in Koch's peritonitis.

(c) *Haemorrhagic* fluid may be due to malignancy or Koch's infection.

(d) *Chylous* fluid may be turbid, milky or creamy due to presence of thoracic or intestinal lymph. It results from lymphatic blockage caused by trauma. tumour, filariasis, tuberculosis etc. The turbidity of such a fluid tends to disappear on addition of fat solvents like ether or chloroform. Rarely congenital abnormalities of lymphatic vessels or nephrotic syndrome may produce chylous ascites.

(e) *Turbid of frankly purulent fluid* is due to pyogenic infections.

(f) Rarely *mucinous* ascitic fluid may be due to pseudomyxoma peritonei or gastric or colonic colloid carcinoma with peritoneal implants.

(2) Specific gravity–If the specific gravity is below 1016 the fluid is a transudate and this is commonly found in ascites due to cirrhosis of the liver, nephrotic syndrome, congestive cardiac failure etc. In Koch's peritonitis, pyogenic infections and malignant peritonitis, the specific gravity is more than 1016 (exudate).

(3) Spontaneous coagulation–Fluid of high specific gravity may clot on standing due to its high protein content.

(B) *Chemical examination* :

(i) Protein more than 2.5gm% in exudates.

(ii) In transudates the protein content is less than 2.5 gm%

(iii) Sugar grossly reduced in ascitic fluid due to pyogenic and Koch's peritonitis. But in the ascitic fluid of cirrhosis or congestive cardiac failure the sugar content will not be altered.

(C) *Cytological examination* :

In transudates the cell count is not more than 250/ cmm and are mostly endothelial cells.

In Koch's peritonitis the cell count is more than 1000 cmm and are mostly lymphocytes.

In pyogenic peritonitis the cell count is more than 1000./ cmm they are mostly polymorphs.

In haemorrhagic ascities due to malignancy the centrifuged deposit is stained specially to detect malignant cells.

(D) *Bacteriological study* :

   (i)   A smear prepared from the centrifuged deposit of the ascitic fluid when stained with Gram's stain may show gram-positive cocci or gram-negative bacilli in cases of pyogenic peritonitis. The type of the organism may be confirmed by further culture, biochemical reactions and animal inoculation tests.

   (ii)   Centrifuged deposit smeared and stained by Ziehl-Neelsen's method may show acid fast bacilli. The diagnosis may be confirmed by culture and animal inoculation tests.

   (iii)   If the fluid is milky white in character, the centrifuged deposit should be examined by ordinary coverslip preparation or staining by Leishman's method. The slides may show Microfilaria.

INVESTIGATIONS FOR LIVER DISEASES
(A) LIVER FUNCTION TESTS

These are done to :

   (i)   confirm whether the liver cells are diseased or not;

   (ii)   detect whether there is parenchymal disease or obstruction of the biliary tree (cholestasis) or both;

   (iii)   assess the degree of severity or liver damage and,

   (iv)   indicate the prognosis of the patient.

Note all the tests are routinely done.

Commonly done tests are :

(1)   *Serum bilirubin*–Normal value is 4–1.8 μmol/ litre (0.2–1.0 mg 100ml). Unconjugated and conju-

gated factors are estimated. *Unconjugated* hyperbilirubinaemia occurs in haemolytic anaemias early stage of infective hepatitis, Glibert's syndrome etc. *Conjugated* hyperbilirubinaemia occurs in later stages of infective hepatitis and in obstructive and cholestatic jaundice.

(2) *Plasma proteins,* particularly serum albumin and globulin. Serum albumin (normal 35.45 G/litre) is reduced in chronic liver disease e.g. cirrhosis, while serum globulin is increased (>30 G/litre) increase in gamma globulin peak can be detected by plasma protein electrophoresis.

(3) *Serum enzymes* :
(i) Alanine aminotransferase, ALT (GPT or SGPT). Normal value–3-30 units/L.
(ii) Aspartate aminotransferase AST (GOT or SGOT). Normal value–5-40 units/L.
Both are increased in hepatic cell damage. AST is more than ALT in secondary deposits or infiltrations; the reverse is seen in acute hepatitis, chronic active or persistent hepatitis and cirrhosis of the liver.
(iii) Serum alkaline phosphatase : Normal value is 20-100 U/L or 3-13 KA/100 ml. It is moderately raised (up to 250 u/litre) in hepatocellular damage but greatly raised in biliary obstruction, *Extrahepatic conditions* where alkaline phosphatase may be raised are metastatic tumours of bones, Paget's disease, hyperparathyroidism pregnancy and rickets.
(iv) Other enzymes : (a) 5' nucleotidase–rasied in biliary obstruction (b) γ-glutamyl transpeptidase (GGT), an enzyme of the liver cells rises in liver

diseases and also after taking cetain drugs and alcohol.

(4) *Prothrombin time :* Impairment of synthesis of coagulation factors like II, VII, IX and X (vitamin K dependent factors) results in prolongation of the prothrombin time. It indicates both the severity of damage and the prognosis of the patient, especially in infective hepatitis.

(5) *Urine urobilinogen* : Normal value is 1-2 mg/ day and increased excretion occurs in haemolytic diseases and parenchymal diseases of the liver e.g. viral hepatitis, cirrhosis, congestive cardiac failure, hepatic malignancy etc.

Decreased excretion occurs in cholestasis. Difficulty arises in interpretation of the results when both parenchymal disease and cholestasis are simultaneously present.

(6) *Urine bilirubin* : Responsible for the smoky appearance of the urine which should be differentiated from haemoglobinuria and myoglobinuria. It indicates excretion of conjugated bilirubin in the urine.

(7) *Bromsulphthalein* (BSP) *excretion test*–5 mg of BSP per kg body weight is injected IV and the blood concentrations are measured after 45 minutes and 2 hours. BSP is found almost completely (except about 2%) to albumin, carried to the liver and excreted in bile after conjugation with glutathione. Normal blood concentration after 45 minutes will be less than 5 per cent; this is a *sensitive but non-specific test*. False results may be obtained in old, febrile or hypoalbuminaemic patient and is valueless in presence of jaundice.

Hypersensitivity reaction to the dye may limit its use.

(8) *Serum lipids* : Serum total cholesterol (normal 130 to 230 mg/ 100ml) and cholesterol esters are measured. In cholestasis total cholesterol level is increased. There is a rise in low-density lipoprotein level of the plasma, whereas the high density fraction is reduced. An abnormal low-density lipoprotein, lipoprotein X is an important marker or cholestasis.

Other tests that are infrequently done :

(1) Lactate dehydrogenase (LDH)–Not a specific test but the serum level is moderately elevated in acute viral hepatitis and in cirrhosis of the liver.

(2) Alpha fetoprotein (AFP) : Marked increase or rising serum level occurs in hepatoma. Increased serum levels may be found in acute viral hepatitis, chronic hepatitis, gastric carcinoma, ovarian or testicular embryonal tumours, pregnancy, ataxia, telangiectasia etc.

(3) Detection of hepatitis B surface antigen (HBsAg) by haemaglutination and radioimmunoassay methods. It is present in type B hepatitis; sometimes in cirrhosis, chronic hepatitis, hepatic carcinoma and carriers of type B hepatitis virus. Carriers who are HB_3 Ag positive are much more infective than those who are not.

(4) IgM detection of anti-HAV for diagnose H hepatitis A.

(5) Igm_2 anti HCV to discover acute infection with hepatitis C virus.

(6) Igm_2 anti-HDV to find out if there is a superinfection or coinfection with hepatitis D virus upon a hepatitis B.

(7)   IgM anti-HEV to detect acute hepatitis E.

(8)   Serum ceruloplasmin level –Decreased in Wilson's disease (Normal 30-60/100 ml).

(9)   Serum iron, iron binding capacity and serum ferritin concentrations– for detection of *haemochromatosis*–higher values are found.

(10) Leucine aminopeptidase and isocitrate dehydrogenase levels in, serum are increased in hepatic parenchymal damage.

(11) Plasma cholinesterase level *falls* in hepatocellular diseases.

(B) RADIOISOTOPE SCAN

Radioactive isotopes that emit gamma rays are injected IV; these are selectively extracted by the liver which is followed by external radiation scanning of the upper aodomen by a gamma camera. Liver scans are of 3 types– (i) Colloidal (ii) HIDA or PIPIDA and (iii) gallium.

(i) Colloidal scan employs colloidal gold 198 Au or 99m Tc sulfur colloid which are taken up by kupffer cells and demonstrates filling defects greater than 2-3 cm diameter, so is *falsely negative in smaller diffuse metastatic deposits while falsely positive in cirrhosis* because of distroted lobular architecture.

(ii) In HIDA or PIPIDA scans the iminodiacetic dye is taken up and excreted by hepatocytes and so a *liver abscess* or *hepatoma* produces a reduced uptake area known as a hole.

(iii) Gallium scan employs radioactive 67 Ga that is taken up by neoplastic and inflammatory cells selectively and so shows a 'hot spot' in *hepatoma* or *liver abscesses*. The HIDA or PIPIDA hepatic scans are of great value in the diagnosis of *acute cholecystitis* when the dye may fail to enter the gall bladder thus showing cystic or common bile duct obstruction.

(C) ULTRASOUND

This is done by moving a probe (that emits ultrasonic pulses) across the liver and its surrounding areas and echoes are received with a transducer, amplified and then displayed. Cysts abscesses, dilated intrahepatic bile ducts and metastases are suitably demonstrated.

(D) CAT SCAN

By computerized axial tomography cross-sectional images of the liver can be obtained and different lesions can be diagnosed.

(E) NEEDLE BIOPSY

This is an established, state and reliable method. The material obtained is subjected to histopathological study. It may be done with the Vim-Silverman or the Menghini needle :– inserted through an intercostal space using local analgesia and sedation. *Best results* are obtained in patients with *diffuse liver diseases.* Complications are bleeding, abdominal pain, shoulder pain and rarely biliary peritonitis. It is contra-indicated in patients with suspected hydatid disease, haemorrhagic diatheses, deep obstructive jaundice, ascites etc. It is also contra-indicated in un-cooperative subjects, but in them it may be done by a *transvenacaval* approach, entering the liver through the hepatic vein.

(F) SELECTIVE ANGIOGRAPHY OF THE COELIAC AXIS AND HEPATIC ARTERY

This invasive procedure is not used frequently. Abnormal vascular patterns in isolated lesions e.g. in *hepatoma* can be demonstrated where other procedure have failed.

Some important laboratory tests in common hepatic disorders–

(i) *Acute hepatitis* – ALT AST ↑, ALT > AST; Alkaline phosphatase N or mild ↑; Albumin N, γ-globulins usually N, IgM slightly ↑ in viral hepatitis; bilirubin variable.

(ii) *Chronic hepatitis*–AST may be N, ALT > AST; Alk phosphatase ↑ or N γ-globulins all ↑ especially IgG; Bilirubin N or variable; Albumin N or ↑.

(iii) *Cirrhosis*–AST > ALT or ALT or both N : Alk phosphatase ↑ or N; Albumin ↓; γ-globulin all ↑ especially IgA; Bilirubin N; Prothrombin time may be pronlonged (Vit K does not help),

(iv) *Biliary cirrhosis*–ALT, AST variable; Alk phosphatase ↑↑; Albumin usually N; γ globulin IgM↑; Conjugated bilirubin↑.

(v) *Total biliary obstruction*–ALT, AST variable; Alk phosphatase ↑↑; Albumin γ-globulin usually N; Conjugated Bilirubin ↑↑; PT pronlonged and responds to Vit K.

INVESTIGATIONS FOR DISEASES OF THE GALL-BLADDER AND BILE DUCTS

(A) *Straight X-Ray* : It may show–

(i) Stones in the gall-bladder or bile ducts (10% cases)

(ii) Soft tissue shadow of the inflammed gall-bladder.

(iii) Rarely gas in the biliary tree due to *fistulous* communications with intestine or in *emphysematous cholecystis* occurring as a complication of diabetes mellitus.

(iv) Pancreatic calcification, if present, will be demonstrated.

(B) *Oral Cholecystography* : An iodine containing substance (Telepaque tablet) is given orally the night before the investigation. After absorption from the intestine it is excreted by the liver and concentrated in the gall-bladder, thus rendering it opaque.

Normal gall-bladder is seen as an ovoid homogeneous opacity which is absent in case of a nonfunctioning gall-bladder.

Radiolucent stones and rarely a tumour may be seen a filling defects. Also anatomical variations and failure to contract in response to a fatty meal be demonstrated.

N.B.–In case of a nonfunctioning gall-bladder, the investigation is to be repeated with a double dose of the contrast media.

(C) *Intravenous Cholangiography* : This is performed by administering Iodipamide Methyglucamine (Biligrafin) intravenously. The bile ducts and any pathology thereof e.g. dilatation, stones etc. can be demonstrated. As in cholecystography it cannot be performed on -a jaundiced patient.

(D) *Percutaneous Transhepatic Cholangiography* (PTC): It is nontraumatic procedure because a five gauge (FR 22, 25) needle is used and can be performed even in the presence of obstructive jaundice provided prothrombin time and platelet count are normal. As in intravenous cholangiography, pathology in the biliary tree can be demonstrated. Almost all patients other than young children tolerate this procedure well. The needle should be incrementally withdrawn through the liver whilst contrast injection is screened.

(E) *Endoscopic Retrograde Cholangiopancreatography* (ERCP) :

This is a very useful application of fibreoptic endoscope. A fibreoptic duodenoscope is introduced and the duodenal papilla is identified. Biopsy and brushing of the papilla are taken for cytological and histological examinations. Then the ampulla of Vater is cannulated by a fine bore catheter and a radio-opaque dye is injected into the pancreatic and biliary ducts. Any abnormalities of these ducts are therefore, well demonstrated. The procedure is very useful in suspected pancreatic diseases and obstruction of the main bile ducts. Complication rate is extremely low in the hands of an experienced operator and pancreatitis and cholangitis remain the main problem.

(F) *Operative T-tube Cholangiography.*

(G) *Ultrasonography* : A non-invasive procedure, it can demonstrate dilated biliary tree caused by mechanical obstruction and can also detect gall stones. It is particularly useful in pregnancy.

INVESTIGATIONS FOR DISEASES OF STOMACH AND DUODENUM

Gastric intubation– Intubation is done both for *therapeutic* and *diagnostic* purposes. Either an original rubber Ryle's tube or a disposable plastic tube of about 16 gauze is used. These tubes have bulbous ends containing a solid metal olive to make it heavy as well as radio opaque. There are 4 marks on the tubing to show the position of the tip of the tube from the incisor teeth : mark 1 at 40 cm and the tip is at the *cardiac* end of the stomach; mark II at 50 cm and the tip inside the *stomach;* mark III at 57 cm and the tip is at the *pylorus* and mark IV 65 cm and the tip is inside the *duodenum.*

The different uses are :

A. *Diagnostic*–(i) Gastric acid studies and measurement of secretory functions (ii) Diagnosis of gastric diseases (by occult blood, mucus, exfoliated malignant cells and poisons in the analysis of gastric contents) (iii) Diagnosis of extra-gastric diseases e.g. Mycobacterium tuberculosis in the gastric lavage of children to diagnose pulmonary tuberculosis (as children cannot cough out sputum).

B. *Therapeutic*–(i) Gastric lavage (2 sodi bicarb etc.)

(ii) Gastric decompression e.g. in acute dilatation of the stomach.

(iii) Feeding and administering drugs to a comatose patient. Before the study of gastric acid the position of the tip should be confirmed by X-ray screening–it should be in the most dependent part of the stomach.

Fractional test meal–An overnight fast should follow a light evening meal. In the morning remove the resting juice by manual suction (first sample). Then give the patient a test meal of oat meal gruel, barley water of 7% alcohol. Next suck out manually 6.8 ml of the gastric juice every 15 minutes till 12 samples are drawn. *All the samples are studied for total acid. free acid, blood, bile or mucus.* This is the fractional test meal study. In addition, if malignancy is suspected malignant cells can be searched for by special staining and microscopy (exfoliative cytology).

Definite variations of gastric secretions occur among normal subjects and patients of gastric and duodenal ulcers. But the wide range of secretion to each group makes the differences between individuals of little value. As such, fractional test meal is an obsolete procedure, and only of historical value.

Gastric acidity is studied–

(i) To demonstrate *achlorhydria* in patients of pernicious anaemia, gastric carcinoma (18%) and chronic gastritis etc. Achlorhydria is defined as the failure of the stomach to produce a juice of pH less than 7 even after a maximal stimulus by parenteral. *histamine* (0.04 mg/kg body weight) or *pentagastrin* (6μg/kg body weight) see MAO below).

(ii) To demonstrate gross elevation of the basal acid output (BAO) as occurs in *Zollinger-Ellison syndrome.*

(iii) In surgical practice to *decide the type of operation* to be done in a particular case of peptic ulcer.

(iv) *To verify the completeness of a vagotomy* by Hollander's insulin test.

(v) In the *diagnosis of atrophic gastritis* and *gastric carcinoma.*

Basal Acid Output (BAO) : After an evening meal the patient is not allowed to eat, drink or smoke any more. In the morning a tube is inserted into the stomach and the position of its tip in the most dependent part of the stomach is confirmed fluoroscopically. All the resting fluid is removed completely by manual syringe suction and this first aspirate is discarded. The patient is asked to expectorate out any saliva or sputum. During the next *one hour* the gastric juice is aspirated and a total of four samples are taken out by manual suction–this is the *basal secretion* in which basal acid output is measured. So basal secretion is the juice obtained in the morning after an overnight fast, from an unstimulated stomach. If reflects the *vegal plus the hormonal factors* acting on the gastric mucosa. This is usually measured for one hour. In normal individuals the basal secretion is only a few millilitres containing up to 10 mEq HCl. The volume of the basal secretion is *high in duodenal ulcer* and *much higher in Zollinger-Ellison syndrome* and BAO may be as high as 500 mEq/hour.

Maximal Acid Output (MAO) : After the basal secretion has been measured for 1 hour either subcutaneous histamine (0.04 mg per kg body weight) or subcutaneous or intramuscular pentagastrin $6 \mu g/kg$ body weight is given. This causes a maximum acid output which *cannot be increased* further by increasing the dose of the stimulant. The gastric juice is then collected for 1 hour and the *total acid secreted is the maximum acid output* (MAO). In normal individuals the maximum value reached is about 20 mEq/hour in females and 24m Eq/hour in males. In patients with Zollinger-Ellison syndrome much higher values are found and in cases of duodenal ulcer values from 20-110 mEq/hour may be found.

The maximun acid output is *proportional to the 'Parietal cell mass'.* If the stomach so stimulated fails to produce a juice of pH less than 7, *achlorhydria is said to be present.*

N.B.–Other diagnostic procedures that help in confirming the diagnosis of *gastrinoma* (i.e. Zollinger-Ellison syndrome) are–(i) Ba-meal radiography, (ii) Demonstration of increased serum gastrin levels by radioimmunoassay which even in fasting state is almost always greater than 200pg/ml, while in a normal subject is about 60 pg/ml and in one, with typical duodenal ulcer not more than 160 pg/ml. Other provocative tests include (iii) *Calcium infusion test* and (iv) *Secretin infusion test* and of these the last one is of greatest diagnostic value.

The Insulin (Hollander) test :

Insulin causes hypoglycaemia and stimulates the vagus nerve to secrete gastric acid. In complete vagotomy this fails to occur. So measurement of gastric acidity following hypoglycaemia after insulin injection can test whether vagotomy had been complete and is particularly useful in recurrence of duodenal ulcer following vagotomy. The procedure is as follows : The blood sugar level should fall to below 45 mg/dL. It is measured both before and after administration of 15 units of soluble insulin slow IV, (or 2 units/10kg) following which gastric aspiration is done for 120 mins and the patient is watched to avoid hypoglycaemic coma. If the acid secretion rises to 20 mEq/L or more above the basal level, vagotomy had been incomplete.

II. *Plain X-ray* : Plain X-ray of the abdomen is taken both in the supine, and erect postures to detect gas under the diaphragm (commonly on the right side) which confirms perforation of a gastric or duodenal ulcer.

III. *Barium Meal* : Passage of radio-opaque barium sulfate is observed by fluorescent screening and films are taken. The followings are looked for–

Gastric Ulcer : Barium filled crater as a rounded deposit or as a projection from the wall.

Duodenal Ulcer   (i) Stellate appearance of mucosal folds.

(ii) Deformity of the duodenal cap.

(iii) No definite crater may be seen.

Pyloric Stenosis : Grossly enlarged stomach emptying slowly

Polypoid Carcinoma : Filling defects.

Infiltrating Carcinoma : (i) Rigid conical shape of the stomach.

(ii) Absence of peristalsis.

(iii) No ulceration.

IV. *Endoscopy and Biopsy* : Flexible fibreoptic gastroscope and duodenoscope are used for visualization of oesophagus, stomach and duodenum for taking biopsy specimens for cystological and histological examinations.

INVESTIGATION FOR DISEASES OF SMALL AND LARGE INTESTINES & PANCREATIC FUNCTION TESTS

(1) *SMALL INTESTINE*

(a) **Estimation of Faecal Fat**–This is useful for demonstrating steatorrhoea (see Pancreatic Function Test).

(b) **Barium Meal Follow-through**– *In malabsorption*– Abnormal transit time to colon, dilatation, narrowing, flocculation which is known as *moulage sign* etc.

In Crohn's disease–Narrowing with proximal dilatation, mucosal abnormalities e.g. skip lesions, cobblestone appearance, small ulcerations occurring on small irregular nodules which may extend to produce longitudinal ulcers and transverse fissures; irregular thickening and fibrosis leading to stricture formation that may be multiple : and loss of mucosal detail and rigidity of involved segments due to submucosal oedema and stenosis : *Kintor's string sign* caused by gross narrowing of terminal ileum lumen due to thickened walls–a long continuous thin column of barium with irregular edges resembling a frayed piece of string. Beside these, fistulae and sinuses may be demonstrated.

Neoplasms–Filling defects

Small bowel diverticula.

(c) **Small intestinal Biopsy**–A spring loaded capsule (the Crosby capsule, which is 7 mm in width and 1.5 cm in length and contains a cutting blade to cut out small pieces of intestinal mucosa when negative suction is applied via the attached tube) is used. The patient swallows this capsule and when it has reached the desired site of the small intestine, its position is checked by X-ray screening. After the biopsy tissue has been cut out, the capsule is removed and the biopsy specimen is examined microscopically without delay. It is particularly important in the investigation of *malabsorption syndrome*. One of the important findings is flattenning of the vill which may be virtually absent with elongation of crypts.

(d) **Endoscopy, Endoscopic Biopsy and Gastro-camera technique :** With the help of a conventional gastroscope or a flexible fibreoptic gastroscope it is possible to visualise the whole of the oesophagus, stomach and duodenum. It is also possible to see the orifices of the bile and pancreatic ducts. The procedure can be carried out rapidly and safely. Through a channel in the same instrument it is possible to introduce a biopsy forceps or brush to obtain the specimen for the cytological examination. In some instruments a proximal camera is attached with which photographs of the inner mucosal walls can also be taken.

(e) **Ultrasonography**–Noninvasive test to find pancreatic tumors or defects due to necrotic lesions.

(2) LARGE INTESTINE, RECTUM AND ANAL CANAL

(a) **Proctoscopy–** Piles, opening of an anal fistula, polyps and anal fissures can be seen.

(b) **Sigmoidoscopy–**Ulcers, polyps, carcinomas, proctitis are visualized and biopsy can be taken.

(c) **Barium enema–** Carcinomas, polyps diverticular disease, fistulae and colonic obstructive lesions can be demonstrated. In ulcerative colitis the earliest features are *irritability and incomplete filling* because of concomitant inflammation : fine ulcers of early stages give way to *deeper ulcers* with progression of disease and *polypoid defects* may appear. In chronic ulcerative colitis the features are shortening of the gut, narrowing of lumen, *rigidity, loss of haustration* and *tubular appearance–*the pipe stem colon.

N.B.– If the lumen becomes eccentric, a carcinoma should be suspected.

(d) **Coloscopy–**With the help of a *fibreoptic instrument* it is possible to inspect the whole of the colonic mucosa and take biopsy specimens. At times pedunculated polyps can be removed via a coloscope without going for a laparotomy.

TESTS FOR PANCREATIC DISORDERS

(a) STOOL should be examined for :

   (i) Estimation of faceal fat in 24 hours. If it exceeds 7 gms in 24 hours with a diet containing 100 gms fat it is suggestive of steatorrhoea of pancreatic origin.

   (ii) Presence of undigested meat fibres *(creatorrhoea)* indicates deficiency of proteolytic enzymes of the pancreas.

   (iii) In chronic pancreatic disorders excretion of nitrogen will be more than 2.4 gm in 24 hours.

(b) Blood should be sent for estimation of *serum*

amylase which exceeds 1000 Somogyl units per 100 ml serum within the first few hours of acute pancreatitis (Normal : 150 to 340 units/L or 80 to 180 Somogyl/100 ml) Serum amylase estimations are of *little value* in the diagnosis of chronic pancreatitis. Provocative tests with *'secretin'* or *'pancreozymin'* demonstrate low volume of secretion and reduced concentration of amylase and bicarbonate in chronic pancreatitis.

(c) LUNDH TEST : Duodenum is intubated, pancreas is stimulated by prior administration of a meal, pancreatic juice is aspirated and *tryptic activity* assessed. Pancreatic insufficiency (of the exocrine pancreas) is said to be present if the mean tryptic activity is below 6 IUL.

(d) TRIPLE TEST : It consists of 3 parts. A special double lumen tube is made to swallow and positioned into the loop of the duodenum under screening. After that—

 (i) Duodenal aspiration is done after secretin injection and again after pancreozymin injection; the aspirate is then subjected to physical and chemical examinations for bicarbonate, lipase, amylase and trypsin.

 (ii) Fresh aspirate is subjected to Pap's stain and cytological examination.

 (iii) Hypotonic duodenography after injecting an antispasmodic drug e.g. *hyoscine butylbromide* (BUSCOPAN) is performed.

(e) ERCP : This has been described earlier and is contraindicated in *acute pancreatitis* and *suspected pneudopancreatic cyst.*

OTHER TESTS FOR INTESTINAL DISORDERS

(i) The nitrogen content of the stool should be estimated as mentioned above.

(ii) Glucose tolerance test will show a flat curve.

(iii) Xylose excretion test in the urine will reveal diminished excretion as the intestine cannot absorb them properly.

(iv) Examination of stool–

(a) Passage of bulky, offensive and pale stool is due to defective absorption of fat in case of steatorrhoea.

(b) Liquid stool with pus and some amount of mucus and blood may indicate intestinal malignancy.

(c) Semiliquid and small amounts of stool mixed with mucus blood and pus may be due to bacillary dysentery.

(d) When the colour of the stool is tarry it indicates gastroduodenal haemorrhage, common blood dyscrasias or intussusception.

(e) The stool may be greenish and semiliquid in case of diarrhoea in children and sometimes in typhoid fever.

(f) The stool may be blackish if the patient has been taking iron or too much of *green vegetable* and also sometimes after taking bismuth *meat.*

(g) The stool may show cysts or vegetative forms of Entammoeba histolytica, ova or tapeworms, round worms or hookworms, as well as round worms or segments of tapeworms etc.

(h) Benzidine test reveals occult blood in gastrointestinal haemorrhage.

VOMITUS

Vomiting may occur in (i) acute gastric ulcer; (ii) peritonitis; (iii) liver diseases; (iv) acute cholecystitis; (v), acute haemorrhagic pancreatitis; (vi) fulminating pneumonias; (vii) whooping cough; (vii) increased intracranial tension; (ix) pregnancy; (x) diabetic coma; (xi) Addison's disease : (xii) following anaesthesia; (xiii) acute intestinal obstruction; (xiv) Meniere's syndrome; (xv) after consuming alcohol, emetics etc.; (xvi) digitalis toxicity; (xvii) terminal stages of uraemia; (xviii) acute myocardial infraction especially of the inferior wall. In most of these cases nausea is associated with vomiting. Huge quantity of vomitus may be seen in congenital and acquired pyloric stenosis, carcinoma of the stomach etc.

In intracranial diseases especially with raised intracranial tension *nausea is usually absent* or less conspicuous, vomiting occurs suddenly and without warning; there is no relation with food intake. This is generally known as 'cerebral' vomiting.

Haematemesis means blood vomiting: it occurs in; (1) acute gastric erosion; (2) chronic duodenal ulcer; (3) gastric ulcer; (4) carcinoma stomach; (5) cirrhosis of the liver with or without portal hypertension; (6) blood dyscrasias like haemophilia; (7) Mallory-Weiss syndrome (mucosal rupture of the lower end of the oesophagus); (8) portal hypertension syndrome resulting from various causes; (9) Rendu Osler Weber's syndrome (hereditary haemorrhagic telangiectasia). In haematemesis the blood is usually dark red in colour due to conversion of Hb into acid haematin by HCl of gastric juice.

N.B.–Remember that the *Munchausen syndrome* may present with malingering of haematemesis which is a not uncommon condition.

EXAMINATION OF URINE

(1) *Amount*

Normal excretion of urine in 24 hours is about 1500 ml.

It may be persistently increased (polyuria) in : (a) diabetes mellitus, (b) diabetes insipidus, (c) kidney diseases associated with uraemia, (d) hypercalcaemia, (e) hypokalaemia, (f) administration of diuretics, (g) after successful treatment of heart failure, (h) recovery from nephrotic syndrome etc.

The urinary output may be so small that it may fail to maintain life processes in a steady state (oliguria) in— (a) acute glomerulonephritis, (b) congestive cardiac failure, (c) acute renal failure, (d) cirrhosis with huge ascites etc. Less than 400 ml urine in 24 hours in an average adult subject is conventionally known as oliguria. Less than 100ml/24h is known as anuria.

(II) *Colour*

Normal urine has an amber or straw colour when freshly passed, and is quite transparent. Urine may be *opalescent* due to the presence of various substances in suspension e.g. pus, bacteria or phosphates, Add a few drops of 10% acetic acid;–if the opalescence disappears, it is due to *phosphates*. Filter the urine, if the opalescence persists after filtration it may be due to the presence of bacteria.

Urine may be high coloured in conditions like (a) excessive heat as in the tropics; (b) high rise of temperature in any infectious disease; (c) jaundice; (d) acute glomerulonephritis (smoky urine due to microscopic haematuria): (e) haemoglobinurias (dark red to brownish black); (f) prophyria (port wine colour due to prophobilinogen which condenses to prophyrins); (g) drug induced e.g. phenylindanediones (pink), anthracene purgative (orange), rifampicin and phenazopyridium (red), methyldopa and iron sorbitol (grey), desferrioxamine (reddish brown) and furazolidone (brown).

There may be frank blood in the urine (*haematuria*).

(i) If the haematuria is due to diseases of the bladder,

the first part of the urine is clear and the last part contains blood.

(ii) If the haematuria is due to urethral haemorrhage, the first part of the urine is mixed with blood and the last part is clear.

(iii) In case of haematuria of renal origin in the urine is uniformly mixed with blood.

Chemical examination with benzidine and the guaiac test are positive in microscopic or frank haematuria.

Common causes of haematuria

(i) Prerenal – (a) haemorrhagic diseases, (b) excessive anticoagulant therapy.

(ii) Renal–(a) acute glomerulonephritis, (b) renal tuberculosis, (c) neoplasm, (d) traumatic, (e) malignant hypertension, (f) idiopathic (essential haematuria), (g) renal stone, (h) collagen diseases etc.

(iii) Ureteric–(a) ureteric stone, (b) pyelitis.

(iv) Bladder–(a) calculus, (b) cystitis, (c) carcinoma and papilloma.

(v) Urethral–(a) calculus, (b) enlarged prostate, (c) rupture of the urethra.

(III) **Specific gravity**

The concentration of urine is expressed as its specific gravity for all practical purposes. The specific gravity depends on the type and the number of solute particles. Normal specific gravity varies from 1010 to 1035.

The specific gravity is determined by the *urinometer.* Urine is taken in a clean long cylindrical glass jar and the urinometer is made to float freely in it when it remains partially submerged. The urinometer reading at the upper level of the urine (at the bottom of the concave meniscus) is recorded and this indicates the specific gravity of the urine. Falsely low specific gravity may be recorded if the urine is tested while it is warm (shortly after it has been passed). So it should be first cooled to the room temperature. In the normal urine the specific gravity is proportional to the concentration of the sodium and the urea content of the urine. Also presence of glucose, protein, radio-opaque media etc. in the urine increases its specific gravity. Presence of 1% protein raised the specific gravity by 3 points. In a normal individual who has not taken any water for 10-12 hours and who is on a normal diet; the specific gravity of the urine should be about 1020. In chronic renal failure due to chronic nephritis, malignant hypertension or chronic pyelonephritis the specific gravity becomes *low* and *fixed* (1010) when it is known as *isosthenuria*; whereas in diabetes mellitus, acute glomerulonephritis, nephrotic syndrome, water deprivation and in any condition causing proteinuria the specific gravity of the urine becomes high.

(IV) Character of any visible deposit

Normal urine is clear and transparent. Urinary ingredients like phosphate, urates, uric acid etc. may separate out as a deposit on standing. A white deposit is formed by phosphate whereas a light yellow, brown or at times red deposits are formed by uric acid and urates. A wooly appearing cloudy deposit at the bottom of the tube may be formed by calcium and mucus only. Magnesium phosphate deposits are found in an alkaline urine whereas ammonium, sodium and potassium urates are found in acidic urine.

(V) Reaction (pH) of the urine

Normal urine is acid and the reaction is examined by dipping in it a litmus paper. An acid urine turns blue litmus red. An alkaline or neutral urine indicates either impairment of renal tubular capacity to excrete acid or ingestion of a systemic or urinary alkaliser.

(VI) *Chemical constituents*

(1) **Protein**–Proteinuria is the excretion of a sufficient amount of protein in the urine which can be detected by– (a) heat coagulation or (b) sulphosalicylic acid test or (c) commercial strips (e.g. Albustix). Quantitative estimation of protein can be done by Esbach's albuminometer. Normal daily protein excretion is up to 150 mg.

Heat coagulation test– Urine is taken in a test tube and the upper part of the column is heated to boiling;–a white cloudy precipitate appears which may be due to phosphate or protein. On addition of 10% acetic acid drop by drop, in *exces phosphate precipitate disappears but the protein precipitate persists.* A false positive result may be due to the presence of radio-opaque media in the urine or if the patient is being treated with *tolbutamide* or large doses of *penicillin.* Bradshaw's test–This indicates the presence of globulins including light chains and is negative in presence of *albumin only.* Urine is genlty layered on to few millilitres of conc. HCl when a heavy white precipitate indicates the presence of globulins.

Albustix – It is a commercial strip whose test area is impregnated with *buffered tetrabromophenol* blue. When dipped in urine the test area shows a change of colour from yellow to various shades of green depending on the amount of protein in the urine.

Causes of proteinuria :

(A) *Tubular proteinuria*–This occurs in tubulointerstitial disease like–

(i) Analgesic and lead nephropathy.

(ii) Gouty and acute uric acid nephropathy.

(iii) Hypercalcaemic and hypokalaemic nephropathy.

(iv) Acute and chronic pyelonephritis.

(v) Hereditary nephritis or Alport syndrome.

(vi) Multiple myeloma.

(B) *Overflow proteinuria*–This is essentially a form of tubular proteinuria and occurs when the filtered load of protein overwhelmes the tubular reabsorptive capacity. This is exemplified by–

(i) Bence Jones proteinuria.

(ii) Myoglobinuria.

(C) *Glomerular proteinuria*–This is caused by the loss' of normal selective filtration mechanism and is exemplified by–

(i) Acute glomerulonephritis.

(ii) Rapidly progressive glomerulonephritis.

(iii) Chronic glomerulonephritis.

(iv) Nephrotic syndrome.

(v) A symptomatic urinary abnormalities due to glomerular causes including *orthostatic proteinuria*,–a primary glomerular disease.

An abnormal protein, the Bence Jones protein consists of the light chains of immunoglobulin molecules and is diagnostic of multiple myeloma and it coagulates at $55^{0}C$ and again disappears at $85^{0}C$.

(2) **Glucose**–It can be detected by Fehling's or Benedict's reagent. *Benedict's test*–To 5 ml of Benedict's reagent 8 drops of urine is added and boiled for 2 minutes. On cooling, a coloured precipitate will appear, and this colour indicates the approximate concentration of sugar, as follows–

(i) Light green turbidity (0.1 t0 0.5% sugar).
(ii) Green precipitate (0.5 to 1.0% sugar).
(iii) Yellow precipitate (1.0 to 2.0% sugar).
(iv) Brick red precipitate (2.0% or more sugar).

More simple methods of testing urine for sugar by clinitest tablet, clinistix test strip or Diastix test strip are available now-a-days.

Sugar in the urine is found in (a) diabets mellitus (b) thyrotoxicosis, (c) acromegaly, (d) renal glycosuria, (e) lactosuria in cases of pregnant and lactating women etc.

N.B.–Benedict's test with urine may be positive, other than glycosuria in–(i) lactosuria, pentosuria, fructosuria and galactosuria; (ii) conditions where drugs are excreted as glucuronides e.g. salicylates, chloral etc. and (iii) excretion of some metabolites or homogentisic acid. However, *90 per cent of all cases of positive Benedict's test is due excretion of glucose in urine.*

(3) **Calcium**–Excess of calcium in the urine can be detected by Sulkowitch's test. This may be due to (a) hyperparathyroidism, (b) prolonged immobilisation; (c) hypervitaminosis D. (d) renal rickets, (e) malignant disease of the bone, (f) sarcoidosis and (g) idiopathic causes.

(4) **Ketone bodies**–Acetone, aceto acetic acid and belahydroxybutyric acid are ketone bodies. Their presence in the urine can be detected by (i) Rothera's test or (ii) Gerhardt's (ferric chloride) test.

Rothera's test–10 ml urine in a test tube is supersaturated with ammonium chloride. To this is added 3 drops of freshly prepared sodium nitroprusside solution. Then liquor ammon forte is added to it very gently; pouring by the side of the test tube (about 2 ml). At the junction of the two luquids a *deep purple ring* appears. Simple methods of detecting ketone bodies in the urine are by (i) Acetest tablet or by (ii) Ketostix reagent strip Ketone bodies are found in the urine in severe diabetes mellitus and often in starvation.

(5)   **Bilirubin**–Unconjugated bilirubin or haemobilirubin cannot be excreted by the kidney. If only the circulating level of conjugated bilirubin or bilirubin glucuronide (cholebilirubin) is high it is excreted in the urine. Absence of bilirubin in the urine of a jaundiced patient suggests either *haemolytic disease of congenital hyperbilirubinaemia,* while its presence suggests *obstructive or hepatocellular jaundice.*

(6)   **Urobilinogen**–Bilirubin excreted by the liver into the intestine gets converted into urobilinogen and urobilin. Some of this enters the circulation from the intestine by reabsorption. Majority of this circulating urobilinogen is reexcreted into the bile but a small amount is excreted in the urine. Presence of urobilinogen in the urine can be tested by using Erhlich's aldehyde reagent or urobilistix.

If in a jaundiced patient no urobilinogen of urobilin is found in the urine it indicates complete obstruction of the bile ducts (*obstructive jaundice*). If in patients with jaundice an excess of urobilinogen is found in the urine it indicates either *hepatocellular* or *haemolytic jaundice.* If in patients without jaundice an excess of urobilinogen and urobilin is found in the urine it indicates *hepatic cell dysfunction* and inability of the liver to excrete these substances and may be due to (i) preicteric stage of infective hepatitis; (ii) congestion of the liver in congestive heart failure (iii) cirrhosis of the liver provided haemolytic disorder can be excluded.

(VII) **Microscopical constituents**

Microscopical examination of the urine may show RBC, WBC, pus cells, epithelial cells, casts, crystals, microorganism, occasional parasites (bilharzia e.g. Schistosoma haematobium), spermatozoa and elongated prostatic threads (in chronic inflammation of the prostate).

(a)   **Casts :**

These are cylindrical structures produced by the precipitation of Tamm-Horsfall mucoproteins (THM) in the renal tubules and hence shaped by the tubules. They are of microscopic size.

(i)   *Hyaline casts* are pale, hamogeneous, transparent casts produced by the precipitation and coagulation of protein (Tamm-Horsfall protein). This is the basic cast found at times in normal individuals and in cases of proteinuria.

(ii) *Epithelial cast* is a hyaline cast covered with renal epithelial cells, found in acute glomerulonephritis.

(iii) *Granular cast* is a hyaline cast covered with degenerated renal epithelial cells and the cells show granular degeneration.

(iv) *Fatty cast* is a hyaline cast covered with epithelial cells showing fatty degeneration. Found in lipoid and diabetic nephrosis.

(v)   *Blood cast* is a hyaline cast covered with RBC; found in acute glomerulonephritis.

(vi) *Waxy cast* is a larger hyaline cast found in any case of proteinuria.

(vii) *Broad casts* are unusually wide and possibly arise in the dilated tubules which have undergone compensatory hypertrophy due to reduced functioning renal tissue. Found in chronic glomerulonephritis.

Casts are easily missed if the urine is centrifuged too long with very rapid rotation;–too long and too rapid centrifugation of the urine leads to a disruption of the fragile casts. Prolonged standing of the urine also disrupts the cells and casts–so it is best to examine a fresh sample.

In bright illumination it is difficult to see the casts; so the microscope diaphragm should be kept partially closed and the condenser should be racked down. Casts must be differentiated from the rolled up epithelial cells (so-called cylindroids) and prostatic threads.

(b) *Cells* :

(i) Pus cells in the urine are commonly found in acute and chronic, pyelonephritis cystitis and gonococcal urethritis. Pus cells or leucocytes are easily seen if the red cells are disintegrated by the addition of a few drops of glacial acetic acid. Pus cells disintegrate rapidly on standing; so they should be examined in fresh urine.

(ii) RBC–Normal uncentrifuged urine do not contain more than 3 to 5 RBC/cmm. Presence of RBC in the urine is known as haematuria. *Microscopic haematuria* is found in *infective endocarditis*.

Intact RBC in the urine indicates that there is whole blood in the urine, this is *haematuria*. But when only haemoglobin is present in the urine and no blood corpuscles, it is called *haemoglobinuria*.

If by microscopic examination no RBC is found then the suspected haemoglobinuria can be confirmed by benzidine or orthotoluidine test. A positive benzidine or orthotoluidine test indicates the presence of blood or haemoglobin in the urine. These can also be tested by dipping a Haemostix reagent strip in the urine.

Haemoglobinuria may occur in incompatible blood transfusion, (iii) autoimmune haemolytic anaemias, (iv) DIC, (v) march haemoglobinuria (exertional), (vi) haemolytic uraemic syndrome (vii) blackwater fever, (viii) snake and spider bites, (ix) Oxidant drugs in G6PD deficiency, (x) septicaemia e.g. due to Clostridium welchii, (xi) Thrombotic thrombocyto-penic purpura etc.

(c) *Bacteria and Parasites* :

(i) Bacteria may be seen by staining a smear of the centrifuged deposit of urine by Gram's method. Gram-negative bacilli are found in E. coli pyelitis.

(ii) In urine of women most often you find E. coli (escherichia coli) or S. saprophyticus (Staphylococcus). Trichomonas may be found.

(iii) Male urethritis might be caused by E. coli (most common) or N. gonorrhoeae (Neisseria) or Chlamydia etc.

(d) *Deposit* :

(i) Ca phosphate and Mg phosphate are found in alkaline urine. They are colourless deposits and are usually mistaken for pus. Phosphates dissolve on addition of dilute acetic acid but not the pus.

(ii) Ammonium, sodium and potassium urates are found in acidic urine. They are found in normal

individuals. They disappear on heating and reappear on cooling.

(iii)   Ca-oxalates are found in acid urine; these are
        envelop-like crystals.

Other investigations for the confirmation of disorders of
the genitourinary system include :–

(i)   Urine culture and antibiotic sensitivity.

(ii)   Ultrasonography of kidney and urogenital system,
       down to bladder.

(iii)   Cystoscopy and urethroscopy.

(iv)   Intravenous pyelography or excretory urography.

(v)   Micturating cystourethrography.

(vi)   Retrograde pyelography.

(vii)   Renal biopsy.

RESPIRATORY SYSTEMS

CHAPTER 4

The respiratory system is concerned mainly with the oxygenation of blood by the lungs which are contained within a bony cage, the thorax or chest. The thorax is the region between the abdomen and the neck. It contains the heart and the great vessels, the lungs, the terminal part of the trachea and the bronchi; and is traversed by structures that pass from the neck to the abdomen. The bony thorax is bounded by 12 thoracic vertebrae behind, the sternum in front and 12 pairs of costae (or ribs and costal cartilages) which extend from the vertebrae behind to the sternum in front.

The respiratory tract is composed of –

(A) Upper respiratory tract which is up to the lower border of the cricoid cartilage and consists of (1) nose and nasal septum, (2) air sinuses, (3) nasopharynx, and (4) larynx.

(B) Lower respiratory tract which includes the trachea, the bronchi, the bronchioles and the alveoli.

(A) Upper Respiratory Tract :

(1) Nose and nasal septum–Examine with the help of a torch and a nasal speculum and–

(a) Look for any deviation of the nasal septum. This may cause constant nasal obstruction and mouth breathing leading to chronic upper respiratory tract infection.

(b) Inspect the nasal mucosa for congestion polyps or bleeding areas. If it is red-boggy and oedematous,it indicates nasal allergy or acute rhinitis. Look for any obvious swelling of the nose, or any obvious nasal discharge or bleeding through the nose.

257

In case of bleeding from the nose (epistaxis) an area in the anterior part of the nasal septum just beyond the mucocutaneous junction of the nasal vestibule, called the Littles area or Kiesselback's area should be carefully examined because in the majority of epistaxis bleeding occurs from this place.

(c)   Note if there is excessive nasal discharge (rhinorrhoea) Paroxysmal rhinorrhoea(hay fever) is characterised by sneezing and excessive nasal discharge. It is the manifestation of an antigen antibody reaction; the antigen being dust, pollen grain, smoke etc. Inflammation of the nasal mucosa by Rhinoviruses is known as common cold which is characterised by stuffiness of and watering from the nose and sneezing but no fever. Vasomotor rhinitis is due to vasomotor imbalance in the blood vessels of the nasal mucosa. The triad of symptoms include nasal obstruction, bouts of sneezing, and excessive nasal discharge which is usually watery but occasionally thick and mucoid. On examination, the nasal mucosa is found to be slightly oedematous, often slightly bluish or pallid in colour and covered with excess secretions and at times a mucous polyp may be seen in the middle meatus if the vasomotor rhinitis is associated with allergic rhinitis. If sinus infection complicates the picture, mucopus will be visible in the middle meatus and postnasal space.

Search for the causes of epistaxis which are—

(I)   Physiological–vicarious menstruation, change of climate (extreme hot) etc.

(2)   Pathological–

(i)   *Local causes :* Acute rhinitis, ulcers and polyps of the nose, foreign body in the nose, head injury, local trauma, neoplasms, separation of crusts as in rhinitis sicca or atrophic rhinitis.

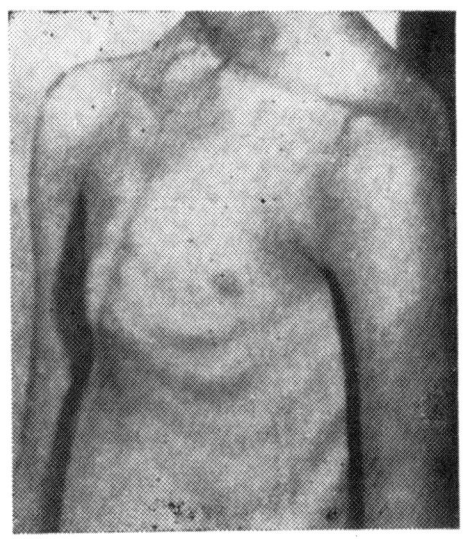

Fig. 2A : Funnel shaped chest.

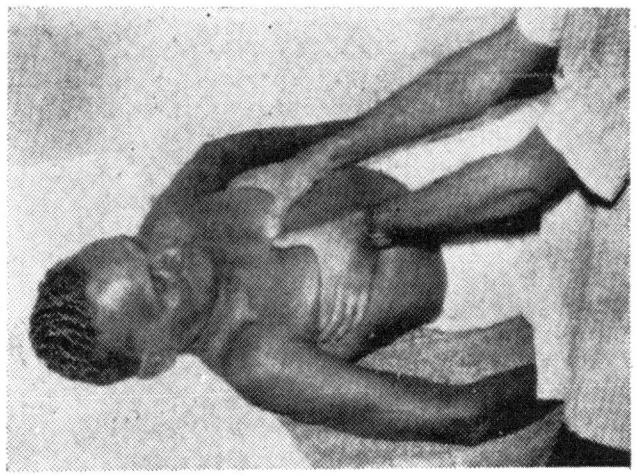

Fig. 2B ; Showing how to examine respiratory
movements of the two sides of the chest.

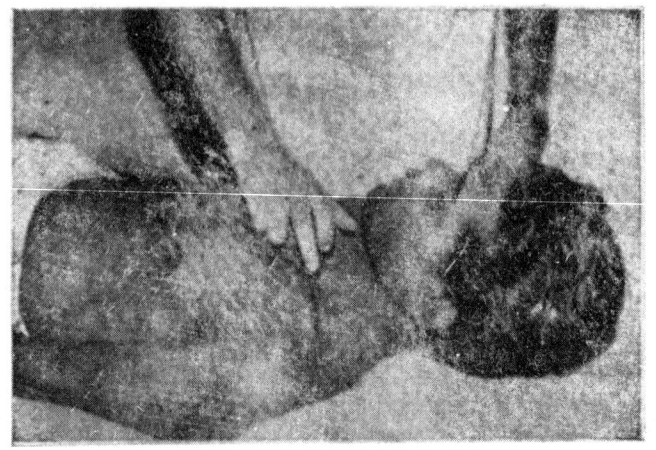

Fig. 2C : This is how clavicular percussion is done.

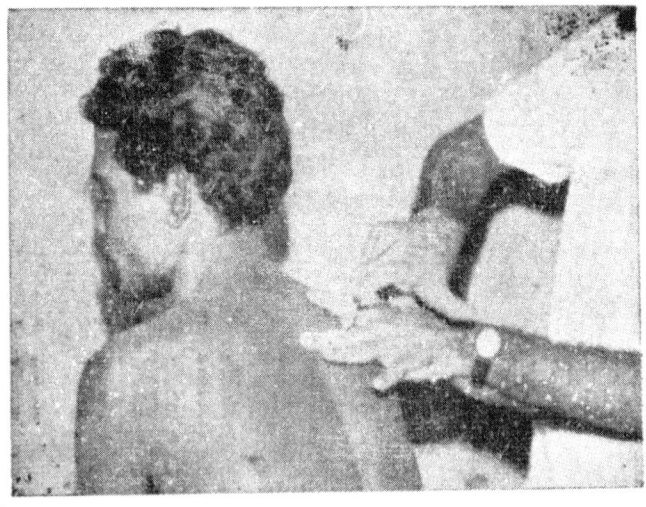

Fig. 2D : Demonstrating the percussion
of the back of the chest.

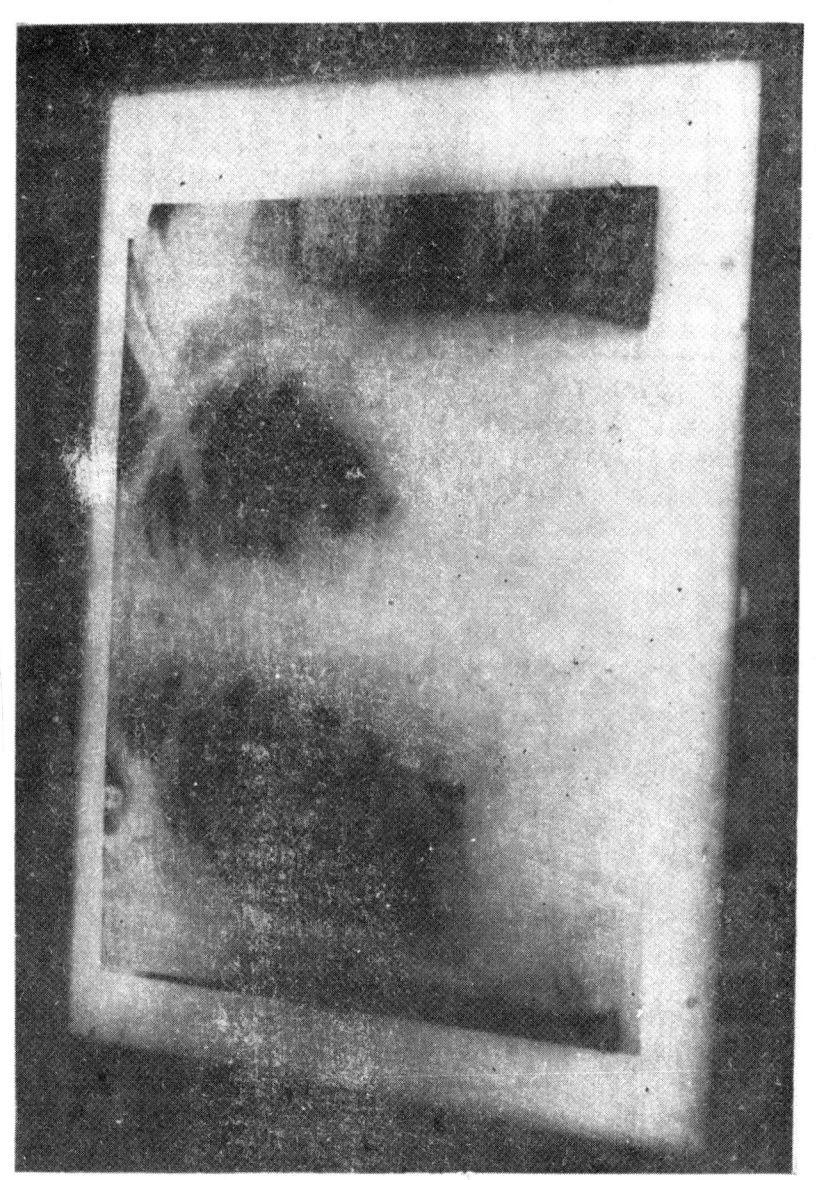

Fig. 2E : Left sided Pleural Effusion.

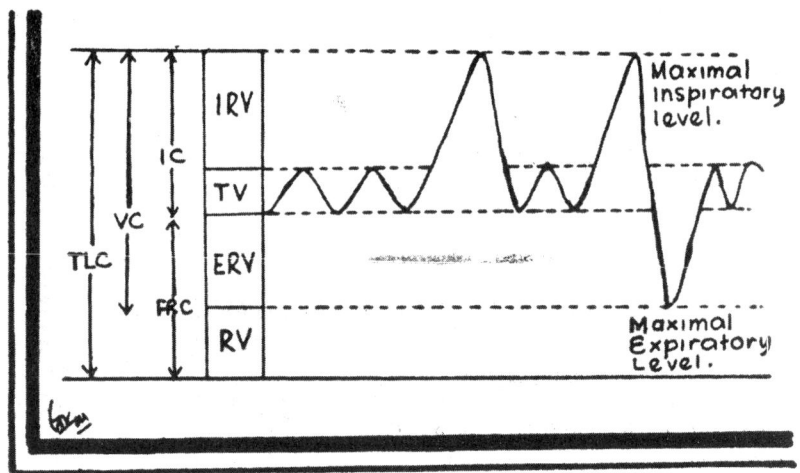

Fig. 2F : TLC : Total lung Capacity ; VC : Vital Capacity ;
IC ; Inspiratory Capacity ; FRC : Forced Residual Capacity : IRV :
Inspiratory Releive Volume ; TV : I : dal Volume ; ERV : Expiratory
Reserve Volume ; RV : Residual Volume.

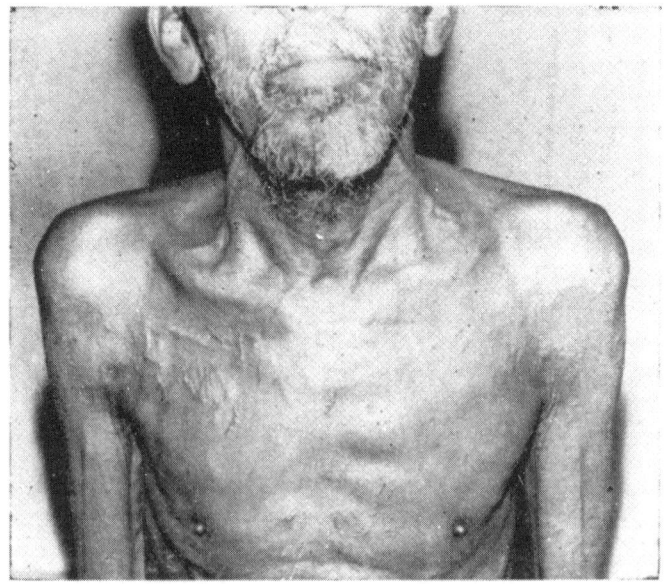

Fig. 2G : A case of superior Vena Cava obstruction
by Bronchogenic carcinoma.

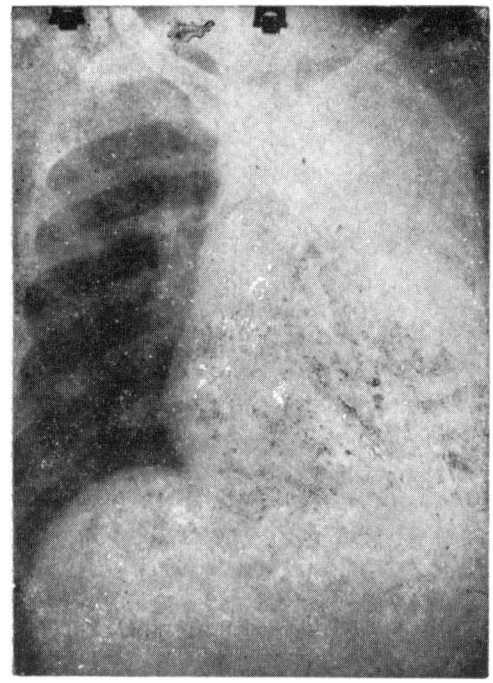

Fig. 2H : Massive pleural effusion of the left side.

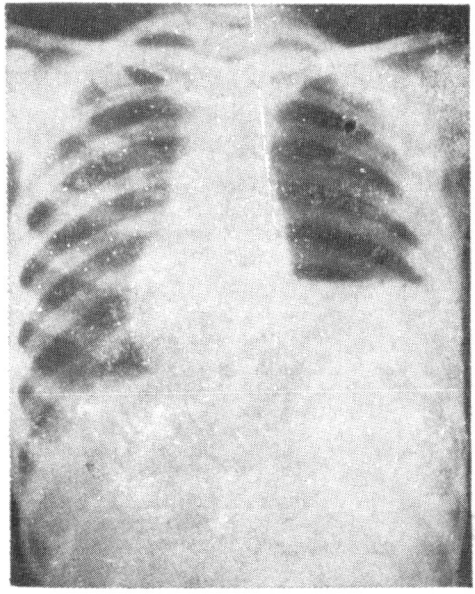

Fig. 2 I : Hydropneumothorax of the left side

(ii) *Systemic causes* : Hypertension, blood dyscrasias, lymphomas. hereditary haemorrhagic telangiectasia, prolonged anticoagulant therapy and rarely over-dose of drugs such as quinine and salicylates.

(d) Alae nasac–These usually work with the other accessory muscles of respiration when the latter are brought into play.

(II) Sinuses (frontal and maxillary air sinuses)–Gently press over the sinuses for tenderness and ask the patient to sit up and lean forward and note if he complains of any heaviness of head. Look for nasal regurgitation and palatal palsy by asking the patient to swallow water. These are found in bulbar palsy which may be due to bulbar poliomyelitis, diphtheria, brain tumours, disseminated sclerosis etc.

(III) Inspection of the tonsils and faucies should be done for diphtheritic patch, follicular tonsillitis etc.

Note whether there is any stridor or hoarseness of voice. Stridor is defined as inspiratory difficulty in breathing which may be due to foreign body in the larynx, laryngeal oedema (in angioneurotic oedema) or involvement of larynx in diphtheria and in vocal cord palsy due to involvement of the recurrent laryngeal nerve. Constant stridor since birth may be due to laryngeal webs. Stridor in infants which becomes more pronounced during crying or becomes worse during respiratory infection is due to persistence of infantile appearance of epiglottis and aryepiglottic fold in exaggerated form. About the age of three these stridors disappear. Infantile larynx is relatively smaller than that of the adult and readily develops oedema and spasm during acute inflammation. Consequently a stridor (often termed as croup) is not a rare finding in infants during any respiratory infection or exanthems. Two very important causes of stridor are acute laryngotracheo bronchitis and laryngeal diphtheria.

(IV)   *Nasopharynx* should be carefully examined for any diphtheritic patch.

Cough : Cough is a forceful reflex or voluntary expulsion of the inspired air from the respiratory tract and one of the most frequent cardiorespiratory symptoms. It is an explosive expiration that provides a means of clearing the tracheobronchial tree of secretions and foreign bodies.

Afferent and efferent paths of cough and control of cough centre–

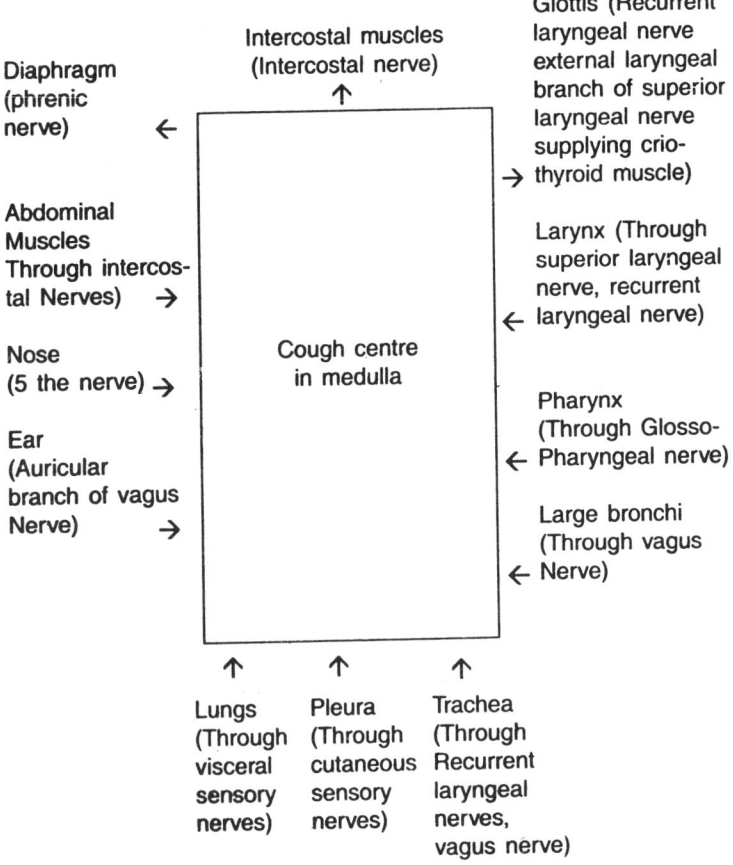

Diaphragm (phrenic nerve) ←

Abdominal Muscles Through intercostal Nerves) →

Nose (5 the nerve) →

Ear (Auricular branch of vagus Nerve) →

Intercostal muscles (Intercostal nerve) ↑

Cough centre in medulla

Glottis (Recurrent laryngeal nerve external laryngeal branch of superior laryngeal nerve supplying crio- → thyroid muscle)

Larynx (Through superior laryngeal nerve, recurrent ← laryngeal nerve)

Pharynx (Through Glosso- ← Pharyngeal nerve)

Large bronchi (Through vagus ← Nerve)

↑ ↑ ↑

Lungs (Through visceral sensory nerves)

Pleura (Through cutaneous sensory nerves)

Trachea (Through Recurrent laryngeal nerves, vagus nerve)

Cough may be :
(1) Dry–Acute tracheobronchitis, acute dry pleurisy.
(2) Wet–Resolution stage of pneumonia. Bronchopneumonia, bronchiectasis.
(3) Bovine–Recurrent laryngeal nerve palsy (e.g. due to bronchogenic carcinoma.)
(4) Hacking–Heavy smokers.
(5) Whooping–It is characterised by paroxysms of dry cough interrupted by a whoop.

The most sensitive areas stimulation of which initiates the cough mechanism are (i) bifurcation of the trachea (known as carina); (ii) upper part of the larynx, and (iii) the pharynx.

The cough centre is *depressed* (i) in deep unconsciousness, and (ii) by morphine and codeine administration.

Effects of cough : A paroxysm of violent cough may lead to–
(1) Severe vomiting.
(2) Sudden unconsciousness due to cerebral anoxia.
(3) Rupture of an emphysematous bulla resulting in spontaneous pneumothorax.
(4) Subconjunctival, retinal or bronchial haemorrhage. If cough is severe, cerebral haemorrhage may occur in susceptible individuals.
(5) Fracture rib in old age.
(6) Hernias and prolapse of the rectum or uterus.

Recurrent laryngeal nerve palsy :

Signs : (1) Bovine cough. (2) Stridor. (3) Hoarseness of voice.

Causes :
(1) Neurological–Bulbar poliomyelitis, motor neurone disease, vascular lesions of the brainstem, dephtheritic neuritis etc.

(2)   Others–Carcinoma oesophagus, carcinoma thyroid after thyroidectomy, enlarged hilar lymph node secondary to bronchogenic carcinoma, aneurysm of the arch of the aorta, right subclavian aneurysm, after operation on lungs or heart etc.

Hoarseness of voice may be the presenting symptom of–

(1)   Acute laryngitis–usually found in measles.

(2)   Inhalation of irritant gas or smoke.

(3)   Chronic laryngitis due to repeated attacks of acute laryngitis due to heavy smoking and excessive use of voice as in case of pleaders and actors.

(4)   Obstruction at the vocal cord due to foreign bodies, diphtheria tetany, angioneurotic oedema and recurrent laryngeal nerve palsy etc.

(B) *Lower Respiratory Tract*

Anatomy

Surface making of the lungs (Fig. 2-1)

(1)   Oblique fissure–It starts from the 2nd dorsal spine posteriorly and goes downwards, forwards and medially to the 6th costochondral junction.

(2)   Transverse fissure–It start from the right 4th costochondral junction and proceeds transversely up to the midaxillary line and joins the oblique fissure.

(3)   Upper border–2.5 cm above the medial third of the clavicle.

(4)   Lower border–
On midclavicular line–6th rib.
On midaxillary line–8th rib.
On scapular line–10th rib.

(5)   Lower limit of the pleura–
On midclavicular line–8th rib.
On midaxillary line–10th rib.
On scapular line–12th rib.

(6)   The hilum of the lung lies opposite the spines of the 4th, 5th and 6th thoracic vertebrae at a site between the midline and the vertebral (i.e. medial) borders of the scapulae.

When seen from behind, greater part of each lung is composed of the lower lobes, only a minor area near the apex belongs to the upper lobes. But seen from the front, the middle and the upper lobes on the right side and the upper lobe on the left side occupy most of the area.

(7)   Angle of Louis—At the junction of the manubrium stemi with the body of the sternum there is a well defined ridge called the angle of Louis. It is a very important anatomical landmark because—

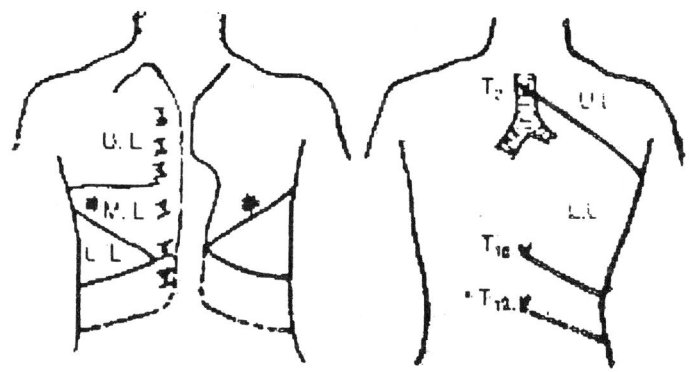

Fig. 2-1 : Surface markings of the lungs on the anterior and postenior chest walls UL–upper Lobe, KL-Middle Lobe. LL-Lower Lobe.

(a)   it is the anterior level at which the trachea divides into its two main bronchi;

(b)   behind, it corresponds with the disc between the fourth and fifth thoracic vertebrae;

(c) traced laterally, the transverse ridge that indicates the angle conducts the palpating fingers to the second costal cartilage and second rib.

The 12th rib is not always palpable and even may be absent. So the ribs and intercostal spaces should be counted from above downwards. First the sternal angle or the angle of Louis should be found out–and the rib that lies at its level laterally is the 2nd rib and the intercostal space just below this is the 2nd intercostal space. Count from this space or rib downwards.

Transverse and anteroposterior diameters of the chest are increased by the movements of inspiration. The vertebrosternal ribs move forward and upward during inspiration, thereby increasing the anteroposterior dimensions. They are also everted, around the anteroposterior axis through their ends, thereby increasing the transverse diameter. Elevation of the vertebrochondral ribs result in outward and backward movement to produce and increase in the transverse diameter only.

Muscles of respiration :
(1) Normal–External and internal intercostals, diaphragm.
(2) Accessory–Alae nasi sternomastoid, pectoralis, serratus anterior, trapezium scalenii.

Normal respiration–The rate is 18 to 20 per minute.
(1) Tidal air   – 500 ml.
(2) Supplemented air during inspiration   – 1500 ml.
(3) Supplemented air during expiration   – 1500 ml.
(4) Vital capacity – Approximately 4,800 ml in males and 3,100 ml in females.

Divisions of bronchi

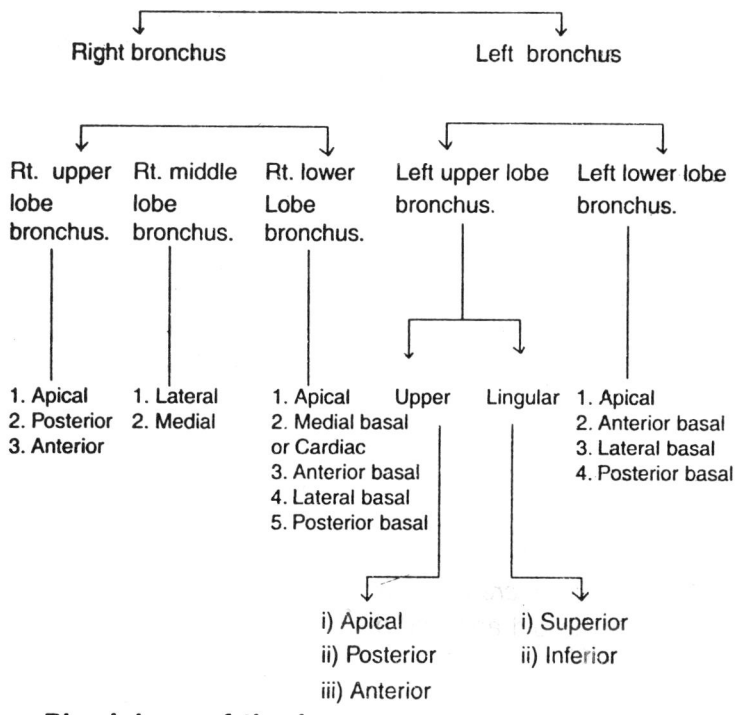

Physiology of the Lungs

(a) Primary function of the lungs is gas exchange—a process by which transfer of oxygen and carbon dioxide between environment and blood occurs. (b) Another function is regulation of hydrogenion concentration (which is also influenced by functions of the kidneys). The gas exchanges process can be considered to consist of four steps; (i) Ventilation, (ii) Gas transfer, (iii) Pulmonary blood flow, (iv) Blood gas transport.

(i) *Ventilation* : It is the mass movement of air into and out of the lungs and distribution of air within them. Rhythmic contractions of the respiratory muscles produce pulmonary ventilation by expansion of the thorax and the lungs.

By contracting, these muscles overcome both the elastic forces of the tissue as well as the resistance of the airways to the flow of air through them. The physiological dead space is not much greater than the anatomical dead space in the recumbent position, but in the erect position, physiological dead space is increased because of little blood flow to and gas exchange in the apical regions. Of the subdivisions of total volume of air in the lungs, those that need remembering are :– (a) Tidal volume – volume of air inspired or expired during breathing. (b) Vital capacity –The volume of air expelled by maximum voluntary expiration after maximum inspiration. (c) Functional residual capacity–The volume of air remaining in the lungs at the end of normal expiration. (d) Residual volume–Volume of air remaining in the lungs after maximum expiration.

The *vital capacity* is related to the size and development of the individual. Normal values have been mentioned above. It is *increased* in swimmers and divers and *decreased* in old age and diseases of respiratory apparatus e.g. poliomyelitis, pleural effusion, respiratory obstruction, pneumothorax, pulmonary fibrosis, emphysema and pulmonary oedema. It is also diminished in pregnancy and ascites.

(ii) *Gas transfer* : Oxygen and carbon dioxide exchange between alveolar air and capillary blood depends on :

(a) Distribution of ventilation and blood flow–of major functional importance in the distribution of ventilation in relation to blood flow. If the proportion of ventilation to blood flow in all the alveoli is neither uniform nor appropriate to the mixed venous and inspired gas composition, the arterial blood gas composition will not be normal.

(b) Diffusion–Total surface area of functional respiratory membranes is approximately 70 sq. metres and at any given moment the amount of blood present in the capillaries of the lung is about 100 ml. This 100 ml of blood is effectively spread over the 70 sq. metres surface area. Diffusion of gases into pulmonary capillary blood depends upon the functional alveolar surface area and the distance through which the gases diffuse. Diffusion of carbon dioxide occurs almost instantaneously and more readily than that of oxygen because of its greater solubility. If the surface area for gas exchange decrease (e.g. emphysema) or the thickness increase (e.g. increased interstitial fluid), gas exchange is impaired.

(iii) *Pulmonary blood flow* : This is primarily determined by gravity. At the apex the arterial pressure is less than the alveolar pressure and no blood flow occurs. In the middle of the lung arterial pressure is more than the alveolar pressure which is again more than the venous pressure,– the blood flow is determined by the arterial alveolar pressure difference. At the base, the arterial and venous pressures are higher than the alveolar pressure–blood flow is determined by the arterial-venous pressure difference.

Under normal conditions, distribution of blood flow is matched to distribution of ventilation. Homeostatic mechanisms exist to maintain this relation, even in the presence of considerable maldistribution of air or blood. But they may be overwhelmed by severe widespread diseases when enough functioning lung tissue does not remain.

(iv) *Blood gas transport* : A detailed account of blood gas transport is beyond the scope of this book and students should consult text-books of respiratory medicine or physiology for the same.

Examination of lower respiratory tract :
INSPECTION

Inspection of the chest should be done after proper exposure in good light and warm atmosphere. Inspection of the chest may be carried out in the sitting, standing or lying down position. It is important that the patient be sitting or lying down absolutely straight. A slant will cause a curvature of the spine and in turn lead to apparent asymmetry of the thorax. The front of the chest is inspected systematically for size, shape, symmetry, respiratory movements and obvious swelling etc. and the back is also inspected similarly. Then the chest is inspected from the sides in profile; patient being seated on a tool; particularly for evidence of any kyphosis or lordosis or for any increase in the anteroposterior diameter of the chest as in emphysema. Finally the upper part of the chest is inspected standing behind the seated patient and looking from above downwards over the shoulders of the patient.

When the patient is recumbent, the chest should be inspected first from the foot end of the bed and later from its sides in profile, keeping the eyes of the examiner at the level of the anterior wall of the chest of the patient either by sitting on a tool or by kneeling beside the patient.

Following features must be noted in all cases :

(a) Size and shape of the chest.

(b) Presence of any asymmetry e.g. any prominence of any side of chest, any localised bulging any depression of the chest wall or any localised retraction.

(c) Respiration—its rhythm, rate, type, movement of both sides of the chest along with respiration, presence of any intercostal suction or retraction along with inspiration, and whether the accessory muscles of respiration are working.

(d) Additional features e.g. sternomastoid sign, and dilated veins over the chest wall etc. should be looked for.

I. *Shape of the chest*–The normal healthy adult chest is elliptical in cross-section, the transverse diameter being greater than the anteroposterior diameter (in a ratio of 7 : 5), more or less bilaterally symmetrical. In a normal chest the subcostal or epigastric angle is about 90. In males this angle is more acute than in females.

In childhood the chest is more or less circular in cross-section.

(i) *Pigeon chest*–It is characterised by an unduly prominent sternum; triangular shape of the chest; rickety rosary i.e., bead-like enlargements of the costochondral articulations particularly of the 4th, 5th and 6th ribs; and Harrison's sulci i.e., sulci or grooves extending transversely from the sides of the xiphoid process on either sides of the chest wall producing a transverse constriction on the thorax. Harrison's sulcus is caused by the depression of the ribs at the costal attachment of the diaphragm due to pulling in of the softened ribs by diaphragmatic contractions during respiration. Pigeon chest is found in rickets and recurrent lung infections in infants.

(ii) *Funnel chest* (pectus excavatum)–This comprises of depressed lower part of the sternum, prominent costochondral junction and diminished anteroposterior diameter of the chest.

Pectus excavatum is usually asymptomatic.

Dangers of severe funnel shaped chest are–

(a) Prevents proper ventilation leading to the development of corpulmonale in later life.

(b)   Prone to develop repeated lung infections.

(c)   Obstruction of right ventricular outflow tract by depressed sternum may lead to functional pulmonary stenosis and congestive cardiac failure. Children who suffer from repeated lung infections can develop funnel shaped chest.

(iii) *Barrel shaped chest*–It has the following features.

(a)   Chest cavity is held in the position of deep inspiration. It is circular in cross-section.

(b)   Anteroposterior diameter is increased with marked kyphosis.

(c)   Supraclavicular fossae are full.

(d)   Intercostal spaces are prominent and ribs are wide apart and more horizontal.

(e)   Subcostal angle is wider than normal.

(f)   Venous girdle is present in the lower part of the chest.
      Bilateral emphysema (centriacinar or panacinar) is the cause of barrel shaped chest.

(iv) *Alar chest*–This is characterised by drooping of the shoulder and the ribs are more obliquely placed with prominent shoulder blades and the chest looks tubular. It is found normally in some thin built persons.

(v)   *Deformity due to kyphosis and scoliosis*– Kyphosis means backward bending of vertebral column with convexity posteriorly and concavity anteriorly. Causes of kyphosis are–

(a)   Carries spine–There may be gibbus formation in late stage.

(b)   Osteoarthritis.

(c)   Occupational.

(d)   Secondary to osteoporosis – e.g. after prolonged steroid therapy.

(e)   Bilateral emphysema, ankylosing, spondylitis. Scoliosis means the lateral bending of the vertebral column which may give rise to unilateral depression of the chest and is usually congenital in origin. Kyphosis and scoliosis may lead to an asymmetry of the chest wall and may diminish the size of the thoracic cavity and restrict pulmonary movements. Clinical and radiological displacements of the trachea and the apex beat may be found in cases of simple scoliosis. *Extensive unilateral fibrosis* or collapse of the lung in childhood can lead to scoliosis. Kyphos coliosis may be associated with *neurofibromatosis, poliomyelitis, Friedreich's ataxia, cerebral palsy* etc.

II.   *Unilateral fullness or bulging of the chest* Look whether there is any unilateral fullness of the chest. If present, it may be due to massive pleural effusion, empyema thoracis, pneumothorax, bronchogenic carcinoma etc.

III. *Localised fullness or bulging of the chest wall* can be detected in cases of empyema necessitates (due to accumulation of pus under the skin of the chest wall due to rib infection or empyema communicating with the chest wall), encysted pleural effusion, lung abscess, bronchogenic carcinoma, enlargement of one of the cardiac chambers, pericardial effusion, fibroma, lipoma and metastatic nodules of the chest wall, aortic aneurysm, surgical emphysema etc.

IV.   *Unilateral depression of the chest* is a presenting feature of unilateral fibrosis and collapse of the lung.

V.   Localised depression of the chest is encountered with segmental collapse of the lung, localised pulmonary fibrosis and after rib resection in thoracotomy. Localised flattening of the upper part of the 'chest wall may be due to apical tuberculosis.

VI. *Visible veins*–Superficial veins in the chest wall are visible in superior vena caval obstruction and in azygos vein obstruction. In superior vena caval obstruction there is venous engorgement with oedema of the face and upper limbs. Superficial veins are engorged in the chest with flow of blood from above downwards, towards the inferior vena cava. This is known as the superior mediastinal syndrome or reversed congestive cardiac failure and is almost always due to malignant conditions e.g. bronchogenic carcinoma, lymphomas or leukaemias.

VII. *Accessory nipples* (Polythelia) Accessory nipples may be associated with the development of systemic and pulmonary hypertension, cardiomyopathy or congenital heart diseases.

VIII. *Sinuses over the skin of the chest*–These are common in tuberculous osteomyelitis of the rib and sometimes in cases of empyema after drainage, and also in actinomycosis of lung.

IX. *Herpes zoster*–It is a cluster of vesicles on an erythematous base of viral origin, distributed over an area of skin supplied by one or more spinal nerve segment. It manifests as severe chest pain and is most commonly unilateral.

X. *Intercostal suction*–It is produced either by positive atmospheric pressure pressing the lower intercostal spaces when the intrathoracic pressure in negative due to failure of air entry through upper respiratory tract as in vocal cord palsy (always associated with stridor) or due to withdrawing of the lower posterolateral aspect of chest with each ventricular systole. The latter is due to adhesions of the parietal pericardium with the diaphragm in case of adherent pericarditis (Broadbent's sign).

XI. *Cardiac pulsation*–Apical impulse should be located carefully because displacement of the cardiac apex may reveal mediastinal shift due to underlying lung diseases as occurs in massive pleural effusion, empyema thoracis, pneumothorax and hydropneumothorax.

The apex beat is shifted to the opposite side of the lesion in the above mentioned cases whereas pulmonary fibrosis and collapse draw the apex beat to the side of lesion.

Epigastric pulsations should be looked for in a case of chronic corpulmonale as there is right ventricular hypertrophy with a low diaphragm due to emphysema.

XII. *Movements of the chest*– Look for the movements of the two sides and both upper and lower parts of the chest on quiet respiration. The movement may be restricted on both sides or on one side only.

Causes of bilateral diminution of chest movement:
(1) Bilateral emphysema.
(2) Bilateral hydrothorax.

The unilateral restriction of movement of the chest may be observed in pleural effusion pneumothorax, hydropneumothorax, fibrosed lung, collapse of the lung and bronchogenic carcinoma.

Respiratory movement–Type of respiration is next noted. In men the diaphragm moves more freely than the intercostal muscles and its downward excursion with inspiration causes free movements of the abdominal wall. Thus it is a predominantly abdominal type of respiration. This type of breathing is also seen in children. On the other hand, in women movements of the intercostal muscles are greater than the movements of the diaphragm. So the respiration is predominantly of thoracic type. Various combinations of thoracic and abdominal breathing may be seen in health. Normally during respiration the two sides of the chest should move symmetrically and simultaneously.

The rate of respiration for a normal adult is 18-20 per minute. It is higher in childhood, and at birth it is about 40 per minute. Increased rate of respiration is called *tachypnoea*. It is an important sign of pulmonary disease. The rate and depth of respiration should be observed without the patient's knowledge as consciousness of this act tends to make it irregular. Depth of respiration should also be observed. An increase in rate or *tachypnoea* and increase in depth or *hyperpnoea* is found when there is an increased demand for ventilation.

The ratio between the respiration and pulse is 1 is to 4 (18 respirations to about 72 pulse beats per minute). In pneumonia the rate of respiration is very much increased. In narcotic poisoning the respiration rate is much depressed changing the respiration to pulse ratio to about 1 is to 7. The depth of breathing or tidal volume is about 500 ml at rest. This can be measured with the help of a spirometer.

Types of abnormal breathing

(a)   Cheyne-Stokes breathing : The amplitude progressively depends to a maximum and then gradually decreases to a period of apnoea and after this short apnoea the whole cycle is repeated. It is due to diminished sensitivity of the respiratory centre to CO_2 and is most conspicuous when the patient is unconscious or is in sleep. It is rarely found except in gravely ill patients. It is found in severe cardiac failure renal failure. pneumonia, narcotic poisoning and increased intracranial pressure.

(b) Stertorous breathing : It is a noisy breathing found in comatose and dying patients. The noise is produced by the vibrations of the soft tissues of the nasopharynx, larynx, and cheeks. It is produced by the laxity of the soft palate and is found in patients who are unconscious as a result of severe brain damage, caused by trauma, haemorrhage or infraction.

(c) Kussmaul breathing (air hunger) : In this, there is an increase in both depth and rate of breathing; the hyperventilation being a conspicuous feature of metabolic acidosis. It is found in diabetic coma, uraemia cerebral tumour, and in some cases of acute alcoholism. The hyperventilation is often without dyspnoea or consciousness of laboured respiration.

(d) Asthmatic breathing or wheezy respiration : Here the expiratory phase is unduly prolonged associated with an expiratory wheeze. It is typically found in bronchial asthma.

Dyspnoea : It is a subjective state in which the effort of breathing reaches consciousness. It is defined as the undue awareness of every respiratory effort. Normally breathing is an involuntary act carried out by the voluntary muscles. Hyperpnoea is a state where the volume of ventilation or depth of respiration is increased and tachypnoea is a state where the rate of respiration is increased.

Orthopnoea or upright breathing : In this, the patient remains in a sitting posture because the dyspnoea increases greatly in recumbency.

Causes of dyspnoea : **Respiratory** : Lobar and bronchopneumonia.

Pneumothorax.

Pleural effusion.

Bronchial asthma.

Chronic bronchitis with emphysema.

Bronchogenic carcinoma.

Advanced pleural endothelioma.

Fibrosing alveolitis.

Interstitial pulmonary fibrosis.

Pulmonary embolism.

Congenital cystic lung diseases, obstructed air passage anywhere from nostrils up to the bronchioles by a foreign body or pressure by enlarged mediastinal lymph gland over the lower respiratory tract, bilateral extensive pulmonary tuberculosis and miliary tuberculosis.

Cardiovascular : Left ventricular failure.

Mitral stenosis ("critical" uncompensated).

Pulmonary hypertension.

Constrictive pericarditis.

Pericardial effusion.

Superior mediastinal syndrome.

Rapid cardiac arrhythmias.

Blood disorder : Severe anaemia.

Metabolic : Diabetic acidosis, thyrotoxicosis, high fever etc.

Neurological : Poliomyelitis.

Increased intracranial tension.

Acute ascending myelitis.

Anoxia : High altitude (pulmonary oedema).

Severe exercise or exertion.

Mechanical : Huge ascites

Psychogenic : Hysteria.

PALPATION

During palpation the patient's head must be placed in a midline and neutral position. The patient must be lying down straight. The palpation should be very gentle and systematic. At the outset it would be wise to put the hand on that part of the chest where there is any obvious swelling or where the patient is complaining of pain.

Assess the severity of the pain or tenderness at that particular site by looking at the face of the patient. This helps the examiner to avoid causing unnecessary pain to the patient.

This pain may be due to

(i)   Inflammatory conditions e.g. abscesses or boils on the chest wall.

(ii)   Injury to the chest wall e.g. fractured ribs.

(iii) Costochondritis.

(iv)   Pre-eruption stage of herpes zoster.

(v)   Secondary malignant deposit (s) on the ribs.

(vi)   Acute dry pleurisy.

(vii) Pericarditis.

(viii) Intercostal myalgia.

After this the following points should be noted carefully:

I.   *Movement :* Normally the two sides of the chest move equally. This is assessed by placing the palms laterally on the chest in such a manner that the thumbs touch each other at the midline in front of the chest with a fold of skin between the thumbs.

Note the separation of the thumbs with each inspiration. The procedure should be repeated from above downwards and also similarly in the back.

The movement of the apex of the lungs are determined by placing the palms on the shoulders in a way such that the thumbs are touching each other on their radial borders over the nape of the neck and the fingers are lying flat on the supraclavicular fossa. The patient should be in a sitting posture while the procedure performed from the back. If the patient is lying down the hands of the examiner should be placed over the two clavicles from the front. But noting the extent of lifting of the hands during deep inspiration the expansion of the apical region of the chest is assessed.

The clinicial should now measure the expansion of the chest with a tape. The expansion of the chest during inspiration is at least 2 inches in normal adult individual.

II.   *Trachea* : Extend the neck and lightly grip the trachea with the help of index and middle fingers in the suprasternal notch and decide whether it is placed centrally or deviated to one side in relation to the suprasternal notch and sternomastoid muscles. Deviation of the trachea to one or the other side of the midline is an important sign of *shifting of the superior mediastinum.* Another way of examining the position of the trachea is to push gently and carefully the index finger of the examiner's right hand directly backwards in the suprasternal notch;–normally the trachea is felt in the midline. If a tracheal deviation to any side is present the finger will slide down along the other side of the trachea.

The sternomastoid muscle becomes prominent (*sternomastoid sign*) on the side of deviation of trachea as both of these are covered with the same endotracheal fascia.

Normally the trachea remains slightly diviated to the right. In upper lobe lesions a mediastinal shift is judged by the deviation of the trachea and not by the apex beat.

In dextrocardia the trachea is central in position but the apex is on the right side; in dextroversion due to extracardiac causes, the trachea and apex beat will be shifted to the right. But the term dextrocardia is now used for any acquired or congenital causes where the heart is in the right hemithorax and the apex palpable on the right.

The trachea may be shifted in parenchymal lesions of the lungs or pleura and also in some local conditions such as enlargement of a lobe of the thyroid, mediastinal growth, aneurysm of the arch of the aorta etc.

Shifting of the trachea to the *opposite side* of the lesion occurs in pleural effusion, (massive) pneumothorax, hydropneumothorax, empyema, bronchogenic carcinoma with pleural effusion etc. Tracheal shift may be to the *same side* of the lesion in fibrosis and collapse of the lungs. In combined pleural effusion and collapse of the lung of the same side the upper part of the trachea is pulled to the same side due to collapse while the lower part of the trachea may be pushed to the opposite side due to pleural effusion. This is known as 'S' shaped trachea, found in bronchogenic carcinoma.

Tracheal tug (Oliver's sign) is the up and down movement of the trachea with each cardiac cycle found in aneurysms of the arch of the aorta as the left bronchus is then pulled down by the arch of the aorta during each cardiac systole. This sign can be elicited by raising the chin of the patient and applying a firm upward traction on the trachea with two fingers placed on the borders of the cricoid cartilage. A downward pull or tug on the trachea is felt with each heart beat.

III.   *Apex beat* : Position of the apex beat offers information about the shifting of the lower mediastinum in the diseases of respiratory system.

Palpate the apex to find out the exact site. Normally it is in the left 5th intercostal space half an inch inside the midclavicular line in adults and in the left 4th space in children.

The apex may be shifted to the left in cardiac diseases with left ventricular hypertrophy or dilatation e.g. mitral regurgitation aortic stenosis, hypertension, aortic regurgitation, cardiomyopathy etc.

Pulmonary diseases are reflected in the form of shifting of the apex to the same side of the lesion in fibrosis or collapse of a lung and scoliosis; and to the opposite side of lesion in pleural effusion pneumothorax, hydropneumothorax and empyema thoracis.

Scoliosis alone may displace the cardiac impulse or apex beat. The commoner form of scoliosis with its convexity to the right side displaces the apex beat to the left side and vice versa.

The apex beat may be palpable on the right side in dextrocardia.

IV. *Vocal fremitus* :

Definition . These are the vibrations of the sounds produced at the vocal cord, transmitted by the larynx, trachea, bronchi, bronchioles and alveoli and picked up by the palm of the clinician from the chest wall. In other words, these are palpable vibrations of the chest wall which are produced during the act of phonation.

Method : The palm of the hand is placed flat on the chest. The patient is asked to utter the word 'ninetynine' repeatedly and clearly keeping the intensity and pitch of the voice constant, at the same time the conduction of the vibrations of vocal cords, are felt over the two sides of the chest. Vocal fremitus over equivalent areas of the two sides of the chest are compared for relative intensities. Only one palm is used on both sides of the chest in order to exclude the possibility of an unequal sensitivity of the two palms.

Remember that the vocal fremitus is slightly more on the right infraclavicular regions as the right bronchus is close to the chest wall and is slightly less over the bare area of the heart which remains close to the left middle part of the chest wall.

The palm should be placed anteriorly over the

upper, middle and lower zones of the chest, laterally below the axilla and posteriorly on the interscapular and infrascapular regions.

The bare area of cardiac dullness should be skipped during palpation.

The causes of *increased* vocal fremitus are (i) consolidation of the lung, and (ii) a big superficial cavity with patent bronchus : due to the surrounding consolidation.

Diminished or *absent* vocal fremitus can be elicited on one side in (a) pleural effusion, (b) pneumothorax, (c) hydropneumothorax, (d) fibrosis of lung, (e) thickened pleura; and *bilaterally* in (a) chronic asthmatic bronchitis, (b) bronchopneumonia, (c) emphysema (d) bronchial asthma etc.

In pleural effusion the vocal fremitus is diminished or absent, though fluid is not a bad conductor of sound or vibration; and is due to a failure of conduction of the vocal fremitus by the collapsed lung itself. In fact fluid is a good conductor of sound or vibrations.

V.   *Rhonchial fremitus* : Rhonchi are the sounds produced by passage of air through the narrowed lumen of the bronchi or bronchioles in chronic bronchitis or bronchial asthma. The vibrations produced by these sounds on the chest wall may also be palpated by the palm of the hand. These are called Rhonchial fremitus–found in bronchial asthma and severe chronic bronchitis.

VI. *Friction fremitus* : Whenever the opposing surfaces of the visceral and parietal pleura are roughened by inflammation as in dry pleurisy, a friction sound or rub is produced during the phases of respiration. This is due to a friction of the two roughened surfaces of the inflammed pleura over one another. When present this sound or rub produced a vibration or sensation which can be felt by a palm placed on the chest wall. This is called the Friction fremitus or palpable pleural rub.

Palpable coarse crepitation :

Crepitations are discontinuous, bubbling or crackling sounds produced by air traversing the alveoli, bronchi, or cavities filled with liquid secretions. When the crepitations are coarse enough they may be palpable by the palm.

PERCUSSION

Method of percussion :

(1)   The middle finger of the left hand is placed firmly and flatly on the part percussed. This is the pleximeter finger.

(2)   No space should be left between the pleximeter finger and the skin.

(3)   Back of the middle phalanx of the pleximeter finger is struck by the tip of the middle finger of the right hand; the percussing finger.

(4)   Strokes should be delivered from the wrist and finger joints, not from the elbow.

(5)   The percussing finger should be bent in such a way that when the stroke is made its terminal phalanx strikes the middle phalanx of the pleximeter finger perpendicularly.

(6)   As soon as the stroke is made, the striking finger should be taken off.

(7)   The wrist joint must move loosely and the stroke should not be too heavy unless the percussion is done over a solid viscus.

(8)   The tip of the percussion finger should be away from the examiner.

Three vital principles of percussion :

(1)   Percuss from a resonant to a dull area.

(2)   The long axis of the pleximeter finger should be parallel to the edge of the organ which is to be delineated.

(3)   The pleximeter finger should be in close contact with the chest wall. Strokes should be made not more than 2 or 3 times and must be light except over viscera.

Types of percussion :

(1)   Diagnostic percussion–The main purpose of percussion is to determine the state of the underlying tissue such as the lungs or the pleura etc.

(2)   Topographical percussion–Percussion to delineate the boundaries of a particular organ.

(3)   Tidal percussion–Percussion of the lower border of the lung at the heights of deep inspiration and expiration.

Areas to be percussed :

(1)   Directly over the most prominent part of the clavicle without using a pleximeter finger and only with the percussing finger.

(2)   Along the midclavicular line, from above downwards. On the right side find out the upper border of the liver dullness and on the left side up to the upper limit of the area of cardiac dullness. Map out

the area of the cardiac dullness and then find out the upper border of the splenic dullness.

(3)   Along the midaxillary line, go on percussing up to the 8th space from the axilia. During this technique the patient's hands should be kept above his head.

(4)   Percuss over the back of the chest between the two scapulae in a bat-wing fashion till the infrascapular region is reached; then percuss from above downwards up to the 10th space. The patient should sit up and lean forward with his hands crossed on the knees.

(5)   Traube's space. It is a triangular space bounded laterally by the spleen medially by the left lobe of the liver and above by the inferior surface of the diaphragm. It is resonant because of the fundus of the stomach and is obliterated by a left sided pleural effusion, an enlarged left lobe of the liver, an enlarged spleen and a carcinoma of the fundus of the stomach.

(6)   Kronig's isthmus is the area of resonance over the shoulder bounded medially by the neck muscles and laterally by the shoulder joint. This represents the apex of the lung. Dullness of this area indicates an apical tuberculosis or a bronchogenic carcinoma of the apex or Freidlander's or staphylococcal pneumonia.

Characters of the percussion note :

(1)   *Tympanitic* : It is the variant of hyperresonant note found over a hollow viscus containing air e.g. stomach and is found in–
(i) an open pneumothorax.

(ii) over a superficial cavity with a patent bronchus.

(iii) over an emphysematous bulla.

(2) *Hyperresonant* : It is an increased resonate note where there is obliteration of the hepatic, cardiac or splentic dullness and mimics the note elicited over the lungs after a deep inspiration in normal individuals. Pathologically it is found bilaterally in emphysema and lung cysts. In the diagnosis of emphysema the increased limits or resonance with loss of hepatic and cardiac dullnesses are more important than the quality of the resonance.

(3) *Resonant* : It is the usual note produced by the air present in multiple alveoli of the normal lung parenchyma separated by numerous septa.

(4) *Impaired resonance* : The normal resonance is slightly diminished by pulmonary tuberculosis especially of the apical area, patchy fibrosis of the lung and thickened pleura. It is normally present at the upper limits of the liver and splenic dullnesses. It may be found at the bases of the lungs in pulmonary oedema or in small bilateral effusions.

(5) *Dull note* is found over consolidations, pulmonary tuberculosis, atelectasis, thickened pleura, lung abscess, bronchogenic carcinoma, pleural endothelioma etc.

(6) *Stony dullness denotes* dull percussion note with a peculiar feeling of resistance in the percussion finger and can be elicited in pleural effusion over the fluid in hydropneumothorax and empyema. This change of resonant note to dullness is due to a

superimposition of fluid or solid media between the lung tissue and the percussing finger.

Skodaic resonance. It resembles the resonance heard by percussing a wooden box. Found just above the upper level of a moderate pleural effusion.

Tidal percussion : Both lungs are percussed posteriorly along the infrascapular line downwards in full inspiration and also after full expiration. Normally there is an increase in the area of resonance by one space during full inspiration due to movement of the diaphragm and downward excursion of the normal lungs. The findings may be—

(1) A little change in resonance on inspiration and expiration in bilateral emphysema as the hypertrophied lung has restricted the diaphragmatic movement.

(2) A dullness both on inspiration and expiration in cases of basal pleurisy and basal pneumonia.

(3) The note may be dull on inspiration and resonant on expiration (paradoxical resonance,–seen in diaphragmatic palsy.)

AUSCULTATION

The following should be noted during an auscultation of the chest :

(1) Character of the breath sounds on both sides of the chest.

(2) Character of vocal resonance with comparison between the two sides.

(3) Added sounds, if present.

The diaphragm should be placed firmly over the chest.

Ask the patient to breathe regularly and deeply without making any noise. Shivering of the patient may jeopardise the utility of auscultation.

Breath sounds

These are the sounds produced by the passage of air through the respiratory tract up to the alveoli and picked up by the stethoscope placed over the chest.

Types of breath sounds

(A) **Vesicular breath sound**

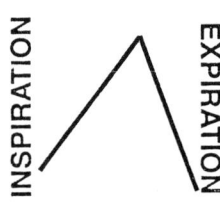

Features. (1) It is heard over the normal lung tissues (typically in infraaxillary inframammary and infrascapular areas).

(2) Intensity of the inspiration is greater than that of the expiration.

(3) Duration of the inspiration is more than that of the expiration because–

(i) Air is moving away from the chestpiece.

(ii) Intensity of the sound becoming low pitched from a high pitch as the air is moving from smaller bronchioles to bigger bronchi.

(iii) Expiration is a passive process.

(4) There is no gap between the inspiration and the expiration.

(5) It is rustling in character and low pitched.

(6) Expiration is heard only in its earlier part.

Variations :

(1) Puerile : Intensities of both inspiration and expiration are more than normal though the ratio is maintained. It is found normally in thin built children where the lung is very close to the chest wall.

(2) Jerky : Interrupted or cog wheel breathing, found in nervous or hysterical individuals. It may also be observed in early pulmonary tuberculosis.

(3) Vesicular breathing with prolonged expiration. In this type the duration of expiration is more or less equal to that of inspiration. There is no gap. The cause of the prolongation of expiration is due to a partial obstruction of the bronchial tree as in bronchial asthma acute and chronic bronchitis, emphysema and early pulmonary tuberculosis. The increased duration of expiration is explained by the fact that the whole of the expiratory phase of respiration becomes high pitched as a result of narrowing of the lumen of the bronchioles and bronchi either by spasm or inflammatory exudates.

The pitch and intensity of the breath sounds diminish if two media prevail between the patent bronchus and the chest piece of the stethoscope e.g. air and fluid in moderate pleural effusion of solid and fluid in consolidation with pleural effusion. If the medium is single, be it fluid, solid or air, the bronchial breath sound can be transmitted to the chest piece in massive pleural effusion, consolidation or massive pneumothorax.

Breath sounds may be *diminished* or *absent* in thickened pleura pleural effusion, empyema, lung abscess pneumothorax, hydropneumothorax, pulmonary tuberculosis at the apex, bronchogenic carcinoma, fibrosis or collapse of lung, over the lung bases in left ventricular failure, huge ascites and liver abscess etc. The last two disorders produce collapse of the lung bases by pushing up the diaphragm.

E.C.D (I)-19

(B) Bronchial breath sound

This is produced normally by the passage of air through the trachea and bronchial tree.

INSPIRATION

EXPIRATION

Features

(1) Typically heated over the trachea and infraclavicular and interscapular regions.

(2) Intensity of the expiratory sound is more than that of inspiration. The expiratory sound is also of high pitch.

(3) The duration of inspiration is equal to that of expiration.

(4) There is a gap between the inspiration and the expiration.

(5) It is blowing or aspirate in character and harsh in quality.

Varieties

(1) Tubular : It is a *high piched* bronchial breathing due to passage of air through the small bronchioles and conduction of the same by a solid media e.g. consolidation and is usually associated with aegophony.

(2) Cavernous : It 'is a *low pitched* bronchial breath sound heard over fibrotic lung tissues or a superficial moderately big cavity with a patent bronchus and is not associated with aegophony.

(3) Amphoric : It is a special variety of the high pitched bronchial breathing which resembles the sound produced by blowing air across the mouth of a jar. There is a tinge of metallic character e.g. tension pneumothorax and very large superficial cavities with patent bronchus.

(C) Bronchovesicular breath sound

It is a breath sound combining the characters of the vesicular and the bronchial breath sounds to some extent. It is heard when a breath sound from a superficial bronchus is transmitted through the normal lung tissue. In a healthy individual it is typically heard near the roots of the lungs at the back, at the upper part of the right lung about an inch below the clavicle and the expiratory sounds have a more bronchial character than the inspiratory sounds.

Added sounds (adventitious sounds)

These may be dry, moist, or pleural origin.

(A) Dry sounds (rhonchi)

These are prolonged, uninterrupted high pitched sounds arising in the bronchi or bronchioles due to partial obstruction of the lumen by mucosal swelling in acute and chronic bronchitis, viscid secretions in bronchiectasis, spasms in bronchial asthma or a partial infiltration of the bronchial lumen by bronchogenic carcinoma.

Rhonchi may be high pitched, produced in smaller bronchi and of squeaky quality–known as *sibilant rhonchi.* It may be low pitched, produced in larger bronchi and of snoring quality–known as *sonorous rhonchi.*

Localised rhonchi are found in bronchogenic carcinoma and generalised rhonchi are heard in chronic bronchitis and bronchial asthma.

(B) Moist sounds (crepitations)

These are discontinuous, crackling or bubbling sounds produced either in alveoli, terminal bronchioles or cavities. They are produced only in the presence of liquid secretions.

Classification–

(1) Fine crepitations–These are produced when the stickly walls of the alveoli separate by the passage of air during the last phase of inspiration and are heard in early stages of consolidation or lobar pneumonia, acute pulmonary oedema, pulmonary tuberculosis and bronchopneumonia. Fine crepitations occur only near last part of inspiration and indicate the presence of exudates in the

alveoli of a particular region. It is also heard at the bases of the lungs in left heart failure.

(2) Coarse crepitations–These are produced in the bronchi, bronchioles, alveoli or in the big superficial cavities due to the presence of exudates and are heard in both phases of respiration in bronchiectasis, bronchopneumonia, chronic bronchitis, resolution stage of lobar pneumonia, lung abscess and cystic diseases of the lungs.

Localised crepitations are heard in pneumonia, lung abscess and/or cavity, pulmonary tuberculosis and *generalised* crepitations are characteristic of pulmonary oedema, bronchiectasis and cystic diseases of the lungs. When coarse crepitations are restricted to the lung bases the possibility of bronchiectasis or fibrosing alveolitis should be kept in mind.

Post-tussive crepitations–These are the crepitations brought out by coughing and are diagnostic of superficial tubercular cavity.

Normally the crepitations are not easily heard as the secretions remain deep in the cavities and are only brought out by coughing when the secretions become superficial.

(C) Added sounds of pleural origin.

Pleural rub–It is a leathery or creaking sound produced by movements of an inflamed and roughened visceral pleural over the parietal pleura.

Features : (1) It can be heard in any phase of respiration.

(2) Rough, grating in quality.

(3) More or less localised.

(4) Disappears when the breath is held.

(5) No change in character after coughing.

(6) On pressing the chest-piece over the chest wall, the intensity increases.

(7) May have relation with the cardiac cycle in case of pleuropericardial rub.

(8) In some cases this pleural rub may be

palpable when it is called friction fremitus.

Causes : (1) Acute dry pleurisy

(2) Over an area of consolidation due to adjacent pleuritis.

(3) Over an area of pulmonary infraction due to adjacent pleuritis.

(4) Over an area of bronchiectasis or lung abscess or bronchogenic carcinoma due to adjacent pleuritis.

(5) Maliganancy of pleura e.g. pleural endothelioma.

Causes of dry pleurisy

(1) Pulmonary.

(a) Pulmonary tuberculosis.

(b) Bronchogenic carcinoma.

(c) Pulmonary infraction.

(d) Pneumonia.

(e) Bornholm disease (due to coxsackie B virus.)

(2) Inter lobar.

(a) Pulmonary tuberculosis.

(b) Lobar pneumonia.

(c) Pulmonary infraction.

(3) Diaphragmatic.

(a) Subdiaphragmatic abscess.

(b) Liver abscess.

(c) Perihepatitis.

(d) Perisplenitis.

(e) Perinephric abscess.

(f) Pyogenic peritonitis.

Signs of diaphragmatic pleurisy

(a) Pain radiates to the tip of the shoulder (4th cervical segment irritation)

(b) Abdominal pain and tenderness over the (i) epigastric and hypochondriac regions. (ii) area or a point 2" away from the midline on the right side in the subcostal plane. This is known as "Bouton diaphragmatique of Gueneau de Muss."

(c)   Hiccough.

(d)   Restricted movements of the diaphragm on screening.

Hippocratic succussion or *succussion splash* : It is the splashing sound heard when the chest of the patient is shaken vigorously by the examiner. It can be heard even with the unaided ear. Normally it can be heard over an empty stomach just after taking any liquid e.g. a glass of water. When heard over the chest it is always pathological which may be due to hydropneumothorax or herniation of the stomach into the thoracic cavity through the diaphragm. It is also heard in pyloric stenosis.

VOCAL RESONANCE

The procedure is the same as that of vocal fremitus but here we hear the resonance with the help of the chest-piece.

So this is nothing; but auscultation of the laryngeal vibrations on the chest wall.

Vocal resonance being the auscultatory equivalent of vocal fremitus the same principle is involved in the mode of production, transmission, elicitation and abnormalities of both phenomena.

How to elicit : The patient is asked to repeat the word 'ninety nine' in a constant tone and voice and symmetrical areas on both sides of the chest are auscultated alternately, starting from the upper zone, up to the lower zone, on the front, sides and back.

Types :

Normal. It generally conveys the impression of the sound being produced at the chest-piece. It is heard as an indistinct rumbling sound where the individual syllables are blurred and indistinguishable.

Bronchophony : The sound is increased and it seems to arise from the ear-piece. It is found in lobar pneumonia tubercular consolidation and above the level of the fluid in some cases of pleural effusion. Bronchophony and bronchial breathing are usually present in similar cases.

Whispering pectoriloquy : If the bronchophony becomes so intense that the acute syllables are heard distinctly the term pectoriloquy is used.

Here the sound is so much increased that it seems to be spoken right into the ear even with a whisper. It is detected in consolidation, a superficial big cavity with a patent bronchus, collapse of the lung with a patent bronchus and above the level of the fluid in pleural effusion.

Aegophony : This is nothing but the high pitched nasal intonation or bleating character of the voice characteristically found just above the level of a pleural effusion and in some cases over an area of consolidation. It resembles the bleating of a goat and is due to the interceptions of the low pitched elements of the sound and the fluid level.

Pneumothorax click

This is a sharp sound synchronous with the cardiac systole if there is air under tension inside the mediastinal pleura below the hilum.

Coin sounds (bruit d' airain : airain means brass) : When a metallic coin is placed over the affected side of the chest on the posterior wall and is percussed with a second coin a high pitched tympanitic or metallic sound can be heard by placing the chest piece of the stethoscope on the anterior wall of the chest of the affected side. It is also called brass sound, bell sound, or bell tympany. It is frequently found in pneumothorax. *Causes of pneumothorax* include rupture of subpleural emphysematous bulla or the pulmonary end of a pleural adhesion;

rupture of a subpleural tuberculous focus into the pleural space; benign spontaneous pneumothorax, following staphylococcal lung abscess, pulmonary infraction, bronchial carcinoma etc. Pneumothorax can also occur following a stab injury, fracture rib or any chest injury or may be *iatrogenic* following a lung or pleural biopsy, thoracocentesis and surgery in the lower neck.

Spontaneous pneumothorax is also associated with congenital cysts, pneumoconiosis particularly that associated with aluminium (bauxite) and cystic fibrosis. A special form of pneumothorax may be seen at the time of menstruation (*catamenial pneumothorax.*)

Pericardial and pleuropericardial rub

The former is related with systole and diastole and seems to be increased if the chest-piece is pressed against the precordium. If the patient is asked to hold respiration, the pleuropericardial rub usually disappears but the pericardial rub remains unchanged.

Causes of pericardial rub :

(1)   Viral pericarditis
(2)   Pyogenic pericarditis
(3)   Koch's pericarditis
(4)   Mycotic pericarditis
(5)   Acute myocardial infraction
(6)   Uraemia
(7)   SLE
(8)   Rheumatoid arthritis
(9)   Scleroderma
(10)   Dressler's syndrome
(11)   Traumatic pericarditis etc.

Physically signs in some common diseases of the respiratory system :

	Shifting of Mediastinum	Vocal fremitus	Percussion note	Breath sound	Vocal Resonance	Any other adventitious sound on auscultation
Emphysema Lung	No mediastinal shift	Diminished	Hyper resonant; obliteration of area of Hepatic and Cardiac dullness	Diminished in Intensity, expiration prolonged	Diminished	No adventitious sounds. At times an expiratory wheeze may be heard
Pulmonary Fibrosis	Mediastinum shifts towards the side of fibrosis	Diministed	Impaired resonance or dull	Diminished in intensity or may be bronchial	Diminished in Intensity or may be bronchophony	No other adventitious sounds heard
Pneumothorax	Mediastinum shifts to the opposite of Pneumothorax	Diminished or Absent	Hyper resonant or Tympanitic	Diminished or absent. At times amphoric. Coin bell sound	Diminished in Intensity. or absent.	No adventitious sounds heard
Pleural Effusion	Mediastinum shifts to the opposite side of effusion	Diminished or absent	Dull or Stony Dull	Diminished or absent. At times may be bronchial over collapsed lung in massive pleural effusion.	Diminished in Intensity Aegophony heard just above the fluid level	No other adventitious sounds heard
Collapse of lung	Mediastinum shifts towards the side of collapse	Diminished	Dull on percussion	Absent or Bronchial breath sounds.	Diminished in Intensity or bronchophony	No other adventitious sounds heard
Cavitation	No Mediastinal shift.	Increased usually.	Hyper resonant (when filled with air); Dull (when filled with fluid)	Amphoric or Cavernous breath sound (if communicating with a patent bronchus	Bronchophony but a times Whispering pectoriloquy	Crepitations after cough Creptiations are better heard at times.
Consolidation of Lung.	No mediastinal shift	Increased	Dull on Percussion	Bronchial breath sounds	Bronchophony at times whispering pectoriloquy	In the early stages and at the time of resolution. Fine crepitations at the end of inspirations

METHOD OF ASPIRATION :

(1)   Position of the patient--Prop up the patient near the edge of the bed and ask him to keep the hands over his head.

(2)   The area is sterilised with iodine and spirit.

(3)   Site of puncture—The 5th or 6th intercostal space in the mid-axillary line or the 8th intercostal space below the inferior angle of the scapula is the usual site if there is a huge amount of fluid and in case the amount of fluid in the pleural cavity is small or in an encysted pleural effusion the site selected should be the area of maximum dullness. In these cases, to localise the exact position of the fluid it is better to have an X-ray of the chest (both P A and lateral views).

(4)   For local anaesthesia at the site of puncture infiltrate 2% novocaine.

(5)   The aspiration needle connected with a three-way tube is then introduced into the pleural cavity. At first there will be a resistance due to the skin and muscles but it falls as soon as the needle enters the pleural cavity. The puncture should be done through an intercostal space, just above a rib margin.

(6)   Now connect the three-way tube with a 50 cc syringe and aspirate the fluid.

(7)   There are two opinions regarding the volume of the fluid to be aspirated. Some advocate that pleural fluid should be aspirated in several sittings, not more than 300–500 ml at a time. The other group observes that the fluid should be aspirated as much as possible and only to be stopped when the patient shows some complications like severe bouts of cough.

For diagnostic purposes at least 40 ml fluid must be aspirated for cytological, biochemical and physical studies.

(8)   Withdraw the aspiration needle and seal the wound with tincture benzoin when the required amount of fluid is obtained. If the patient is restless or anxious it is better to give a sedative half an hour before the aspiration.

INDICATIONS OF ASPIRATION :

(1)   Diagnostic : To know the physical, cytological and biochemical characters of the fluid for the detection of the cause of the pleural effusion.

(2)   Therapeutic : To relieve the patient from respiratory distress in the following conditions :

(i)   If fluid is up to the clavicular level;

(ii)   If fluid persists even 15 days after the previous aspiration;

(iii) When there is rapid collection of fluid in the pleural cavity.

DANGERS OF ASPIRATION :

During aspiration of pleural fluid there is a chance of introducing infection giving rise to empyema thoracis and also air giving rise to hydropneumothrorax. If the fluid is rapidly aspirated there may be cardiorespiratory embarrassment or noncardiogenic acute pulmonary oedema.

INVESTIGATION OF THE PLEURAL FLUID :

The fluid is collected in separate sterile test tubes and is to be examined for physical, cytological and biochemical characters.

(A)   **PHYSICAL CHARACTER :**

(1)   *Appearance*

(a)   The fluid may be turbid or frankly purulent in

empyema thoracis. The pus is due to streptococcal or staphylococcal infections. Greenish pus may be obtained in infections due to pneumococcus or Pseudomona pyocyaneous.

(b)   In tuberculous effusion the fluid is amber or straw coloured.

(c)   Clear serous fluid in hydrothorax is due to congestive cardiac failure, nephrotic syndrome, severe anaemia etc.

(d)   Haemorrhagic pleural fluid is commonly found in malignant pleural effusion. Haemorrhagic fluid may also be due to tuberculous effusion, following pulmonary infraction, haemorrhagic diseases, in viral infections or trauma and in congestive cardiac failure.

(e)   Milky white turbid chylous fluid may be due to filarial or malignant obstruction of the thoracic duct, eosinophilic lung, lymphomas, lymphangiomyomatosis etc.

(2)   *Specific gravity*
In empyema or tuberculous effusion the specific gravity is more than 10, 6. In hydrothorax it is less than 1012.

(3)   *Spontaneous coagulation*
In empyema thoracis and rarely in tuberculous effusion the fluid may clot if left in a test tube, due to its high protien content.

(4)   Odour
In empyema caused by E. coli the fluid may be offensive fishy odour.

(B)   **CHEMICAL EXAMINATION :**
In empyema and tuberculous effusion the total protein content is more than 3 gm%. In hydrothorax the protein

content is less than 3 gm%. Sugar is grossly reduced in empyema and in tuberculous effusion. In hydrothorax there will be no alteration of the sugar content of the fluid.

(C) **CYTOLOGICAL EXAMINATION**

In transudates due to hydrothorax of any cause only a few endothelial cells are present per cmm of fluid. In empyema the cell count is more than 1000/ cmm and the majority of the cells are polymorphs. In tuberculous effusion the cell count is more than 1000/cmm and there is preponderance of lymphocytes. Plenty of RBC in the fluid indicates haemorrhagic effusion. Eosinophils may be found in the pleural fluid of those cases where repeated aspiration has been done or in chylous pleural effusion. In malignant effusion the malignant cells may be demonstrated by special staining.

(D) **BACTERIOLOGICAL STUDY :**

(1) In empyema a smear prepared from the centrifuged deposit should be stained by Gram's method for microscopical examination to identify the type of organism. This should be confirmed by culture and animal inoculation.

(2) In suspected tuberculous effusion the prepared smear from the centrifuged deposit is to be stained with Ziehl Neelsen's method for demonstration of acid fast bacilli. Culture and guineapig inoculation are to be done for confirmation of the diagnosis.

(3) Milky white fluid is to be examined for microfilaria by staining a smeared slide by Leishman's technique or by a cover slip preparation of the centrifuged deposit. The colour of this may become clear on adding ether.

Pleural effusion may be post pneumonic; tuberculous; malignant (following bronchogenic carcinoma or pleural mesothelioma); or following lymphomas or penetrating wounds of the chest and myxoedema. In these cases the pleural fluid is exudative in nature. *Transudative pleural effusion* (hydrothorax) may occur following cardiac failure, nephrotic syndrome, hepatic failure (cirrhosis of liver, gross hypoproteinaemia. Meigs syndrome etc. *Haemorrhagic pleural effusion* is caused by penetrating wounds of the chest, neoplastic implant on pleura, primary mesothelioma of pleura and occasionally due to tuberculosis. Amoebic liver abscess may burst into the pleural cavity producing an anchovy sauce coloured fluid. Rarely coxsackie virus, psittacosis or infectious mononucleosis and very rarely a fungal infection such as coccidioidomycosis or blastomycosis also causes pleural effusion.

Differences between transudates and exudates

TESTS	TRANSUDATE	EXUDATE
colour	Usually colourless but may vary from, slight yellowish tint to milky or reddish tinge.	Usually variously coloured according to the cause
Appearance	Usually clear	Usually turbid
Coagulation	Does not coagulate	Coagulates often on standing.
Specific gravity	< 1015	>1020
pH	<7.8	>7.8
Protein	< 3gm%	>3gm%
Fluid to serum protein ratio	<0.5	>0.5
LDH	Low (>200 I.U.)	High (>200 I.U.)
Fluid to serum LDH ratio	< 0.6	> 0.6
RBC	Usually<10000/mm^3	May be>10000/mm^3
WBC	Usually<1000/mm^3	Usually>1000 mm^3

TESTS	TRANSUDATE	EXUDATE
Differential leucocyte count	Usually>50% lymphocytes Polymorphs usually absent	> 50% in Koch's and malignancy Polymorphs>50% in acute inflammation
Sugar	Same as in blood	Slightly or markably diminished
Amylase	–	>500 units/cc usually in pancreatitis, rarely in infection or neoplasm
Complements	–	C^3 and C^4 components are diminished in rheumatoid arthritis and SLE

SPUTUM AND ITS EXAMINATION

The term sputum is used in a broad sense and includes any material that is spitted out. The material may come from any portion of the respiratory tract. However, here we are concerned with the expectoration that comes from the larynx and below that.

(A) *MACROSCOPICAL*

In the process of examination, it is easy to pour the sputum into a petridish and place this against a black back ground and inspect through a hand lens. Some amount of sputum should also be taken in a test tube and allowed to settle and the following points are to be noted.

(i)   *Amount*

To obtain precise information about the amount, it is better to collect the sputum in a graduated container for 24 hours.

Small amounts of sputum are expectorated in many lung diseases but large quantities (10-20 oz) are found only in bronchiectasis, pulmonary abscess or when an empyema ruptures into a bronchus. An increase in amount following a change of posture is characteristic of bronchiectasis.

(ii)   *Character*

(a)   Serous : It is described by the patient as thin and watery and sometimes forthy. Usually it is pinkish in colour due to the presence of RBC. The commonest cause is acute pulmonary oedema and rarely alveolar cell carcinoma. A ruptured hydatid cyst will cause expectoration of a clear salty fluid. It may be pinkish in colour due to the presence of RBC.

(b)   Mucoid : It is clear, tough jelly-like and sticky and the amount is small. It is characteristic of early bronchitis. The amount becomes copious in a later stage of bronchitis when it becomes mucopurulent (indicating active bacterial infection of the respiratory tract) and in bronchial asthma.

(c)   Mucopurulent : This is one of the commonest types of sputum. At the time of collection of such sputum, a lump of dense mucopus will be seen sinking down in the clearer media to the bottom of the test tube and becoming flat. This is usually seen in cases of pulmonary tuberculosis with cavity formation. If watery fluid is present in addition on standing the sputum will separate in three layers. The uppermost layer is thin forthy mucus. The middle layer is serous and may look greenish. The lowermost layer is brownish in colour consisting of mucopus, anaerobic bacteria, Charcot-Leyden crystals, putrefactive products and foul smelling organic acids, RBC, tissue debris and yellow bodies called Dittrich's plug and sometimes elastic tissues if erosion has developed. This is characteristic of bronchiectasis.

(d) Purulent : In a pure form it is present only in cases of lung abscess, empyema and an extrinsic abscess rupturing into a bronchus.

(e) Expectoration resembling anchovy sauce. This is seen when an amoebic liver abscess bursts into the lung and the material is expectorated through a communicating bronchus.

(f) Haemorrhagic : Small amounts of blood mixed with sputum giving rise to a rusty appearance is seen in pneumonia. The pink, frothy sputum is the result of acute pulmonary congestion while red streaked sputum is frequently seen in pulmonary tuberculosis. Blood mixed with mucus, giving rise to prune-juice appearance is sometimes found in pulmonary neoplasms.

(g) In laryngeal diptheria pieces of membrane may be coughed out.

(h) Food particles may be found in the sputum in cases of tracheo-oesophageal fistula.

(iii) *Colour*
A serous sputum is colourless while a mucoid sputum looks grey. A purulent sputum is usually yellowish or greenish but may be only white. Black

discolouration due to presence of soot particles is found in coal miners, cigarette smokers etc. Rusty to golden yellow discolouration is characteristic of pneumococcal pneumonia. Blood streaked sputum may be seen in chronic bronchitis, pulmonary tuberculosis and sometimes in bronchial carcinoma while blood stained sputum is common in bronchial carcinoma, lung abscess, bronchiectasis etc. Pinkish colour occurs in acute pulmonary congestion. Anchovy sauce expectoration is the result of bursting of an amoebic liver abscess into the lungs.

(iv) *Odour*

'Nasty' odour is usually referred to that of purulent sputum. When the odour is extremely unpleasant and described by the patient as that of rotten egg or of sewer, it suggests the presence of bronchiectasis, more rarely of pulmonary suppuration following spirillum infection or of gangrene of the lung. Because of effective antibiotics this form of sputum is now rarely seen.

(B) *MICROSCOPICAL*

Microscopical elements in the sputum may have different origins. It may come from any portion of (i) respiratory tract and lungs, (ii) from blood, or (iii) It may be foreign bodies.

(i) *From the respiratory tract and lungs :*

(a) Epithelial cells are commonly seen in chronic bronchitis which may contain iron pigment following corpulmonale.

(b) Casts of smaller bronchi and their ramifications are found in fibrinous bronchitis. These casts may be mistaken for diphtheritic membranes, when culture of the latter will be diagnostic.

(c) Elastic fibres due to destruction of lung tissue may be obtained in bronchiectasis, gangrene of the lung, lung abscess, tuberculosis etc.

(d) Calcareous materials are sometimes obtained in pulmonary tuberculosis of long duration.

(e) Groups of malignant cells in the form of cell nests or sarcomatous tissue may rarely be seen in alveolar carcinoma.

(ii) *From blood* : RBC are found in the stage of red hepatisation while WBC are found in the stage of grey hepatisation in case of lobar pneumonia. Eosinophils are found frequently in asthma. Pus cells may be found in any acute infection of lung. Charcot-Leyden crystals and crystals of uric acid are occasionally found in asthma.

(iii) *Foreign bodies :* Asbestos bodies which are golden yellow and dumb-bell shaped are met with in cases of asbestos pneumoconiosis. Hooklets and scolices are found in hydatid cysts of lung. Fungus of actinomycosis are rarely seen. Structure of liver cells, crystals of lecithin and tyrosin are very rarely seen in amoebic liver abscess bursting into the lungs.

(C) BACTERIOLOGICAL

For a proper bacteriological examination the sputum should be collected in the morning in a sterile container after mouth wash with only warm water and then it should be examined immediately by making a smear and staining. Culture followed by animal inoculation should be done if necessary. Smear should be stained by both Gram's and Zeihl-Neelsen's methods and examined under the microscope with the oil immersion lens. In suspected cases of Koch's infection, repeated examination is necessary if the first examination proves negative.

However, it is essential to remember that the sputum may normally contain many nonpathogenic bacteria. Certain variety of streptococcus, pneumococcus, diphtheroid bacilli and H. Influenzae may be discovered in the sputum even though there had been no respiratory disease.

SPECIAL DIAGNOSTIC PROCEDURES

I. RADIOLOGY

It is needless to mention the importance of X-ray examination of the chest which includes the following :

(A) Posteroanterior and lateral views of skiagram of chest

The posteroanterior film is taken with the film against the front of the chest and the X-ray tube placed six and a half feet behind the patient. A lateral view is essential for localisation of the lesion in terms of lobe, zone, particularly the midzone, and proximity of lesion to the anterior or posterior wall of the chest. A systematic plan of examination of the film is advised so that all the possible information that can be had from the film are ensured. The following points should be examined :

(i) Bony skeleton–scoliosis bony erosions, tumours and fractures.

(ii) Position of the trachea–This is seen as a dark line (due to air inside) in front of the upper dorsal vertebrae.

(iii) Position of the diaphragam–This is important because it may be pulled up by a collapse or fibrosis of the lower lobe of lung. The angles between the ribs and the diaphragm on both sides laterally (costophrenic anlges) and the angles beetwen the heart and the diaphragm (cardiophrenic angles) should be looked carefully to note whether they are clear, opaque or obliterated. Normally the costophrenic and cardiophrenic angles should be clear.

(iv) Heart shadow and other mediastinal contens– This will help to detect right and left ventricular hypertrophics (in the lateral view) and also other cardiovascular disorders.

(v) Lung fields–Excessive translucency indicates emphysematous change. More than 60% of the parenchymatous lesions can be diagnose by means of P A and lateral views of the film.

For radiological diagnosis, the lung fields are examined in reference to three zones :

(i) Upper zone–It extends from the apex down to the

level of the 2nd costochondral junction.

(ii)   Mid-zone—It extends from the lower limit of the upper zone to the lower borders of the 4th costal cartilages.

(iii)   Lower zone—It corresponds with the part of lungs below the lower limit of mid-zone. In posteroanterior view of the skiagram of chest sometimes a transverse line may be seen in the 3rd and 4th intercostal spaces on the right side which is the transverse fissure separating the right upper and middle lobes of the lung. The oblique fissure which separates the upper and lower lobes on both sides is not visualised in the P A skiagram of the chest.

(B) *Fluoroscopy*

It is not much helpful in the diagnosis of lung diseases as compared to its diagnostic importance in cardiovascular diseases and diaphragmatic paralysis. The latter will show paradoxical movements of the diaphragm, that is the diaphragm descending when it should ascend (during expiration) and ascending when it should descend (during inspiration).

(C) *Bronchography*

In this procedure a radio-opaque iodised oil is introduced via the trachea into the bronchial tree and then X-ray pictures are taken in PA and lateral views to visualise the particular bronchi or the whole of the bronchial tree. The oil may be introduced either,

(a) by a needle through the crico-thyroid membrane into the trachea, or,

(b) by a nasal catheter in the trachea through one of the nostrils, or,

(c) through a bronchoscope.

This is helpful in the diagnosis of bronchiectasis and to select preoperatively the particular lobe to be operated.

(D) *Tomography*

Tomography is a particular method of X-ray in which structures at a particular plane and depth are kept in focus and anything out of the plane is kept out of focus so that they do not superimpose on the X-ray picture. In fact, it is nothing but an X-ray picture at a particular plane and depth. Its main use is to detect narrowing of the bronchus in cases of bronchogenic carcinoma and to detect a cavitation of the lung in an apparently opaque shadow.

II. BRONCHOSCOPY

This is done for direct inspection of the main bronchi and their branches and taking a biopsy especially to confirm the diagnosis of a bronchogenic carcinoma. It is also helpful in visualising and removing any foreign body from inside the bronchial lumen.

III. THORACOSCOPY

By this procedure the pleura is inspected after induction of an artificial pneumothorax.

IV. MEDIASTINOSCOPY

This is a recent procedure by which the structures in the mediastinum are directly inspected. The instrument is inserted behind the sternum and biopsy of the mediastinal structures e.g. lymph glands can be obtained.

V. LUNG BIOPSY

Drill biopsy of the lung is performed for histopathological

confirmation of the diagnosis of diffuse lung diseases e.g. diffuse interstitial fibrosis.

VI. LUNG FUNCTION TESTS

Detailed discussion of the different lung function tests is beyond the scope of this book; but a few simple clinical tests are briefly described. The lung function tests enable us to make a physiological and functional rather than a pathological diagnosis. They are useful *diagnostically* for objective assessment of the patients and their disabilities and *prognostically* to assess the progress of the disease and the effect of the treatment.

Spirometry– It is one of the most commonly used laboratory methods for evaluation of the patient. This includes measurement of vital capacity.

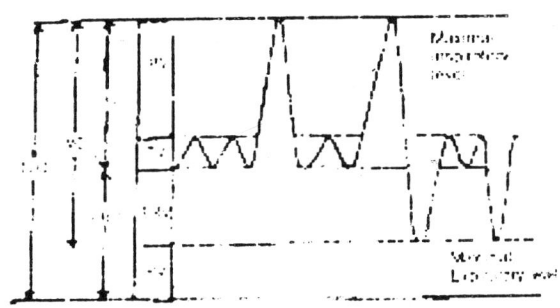

Fig. 2-2 The lung volumes TLC–Total ling capacity. VC–Vital capacity TV–Tidal volume IRV–Inspiratory reserve volume ERV –Expiratory reserve volume. RV–Residual volume.

Vital capacity is defined as the largest volume of air which the patient can exhale voluntarily beginning with the fully inflated lungs. The result is expressed in litres. Weakness, pain on deep breathing, lack of co-operation on the part of the patient etc. may result in an underestimation of the vital capacity (normal 3 to 5 litres).

Reduction of vital capacity in the absence of obstruction is indicative of a *restrictive* ventilatory defect e.g. deformities of thoracic cage, pleural thickening, pleural effusion and lung fibrosis.

Spirometer tracings recorded during forced expirations (expiratory spirogram) are the most convenient indirect method of confirming the presence and assessing the severity of an obstructive ventilatory defect.

In normal subjects about 75 per cent of the vital capacity is expelled in the first second of forced expiration and the rest in about three seconds. So a normal forced expirogram is very steep in its initial portion, then smoothly curved and finally reaches a plateau in 3 to 6 seconds.

Forced expiratory volume in the first second (FEV) is 70 to 75 per cent of the vital capacity in normal individuals under sixty. When there is an obstruction to the outflow of the air from the lungs as in asthma, bronchitis, emphysema or intraluminal obstruction owing to mucus or oedema, this curve is flattened. By recording the FEV_1 a numerical value can be given to the degree of flattening of this curve. It is expressed as the ratio of FEV_1 FVC. In patients suffering from *obstructive* airway disease the percentage is below 70. In the presence of *restrictive* ventilatory defects the FEV_1 will remain 75 to 80 percent of the vital capacity or more depending on the age of the patient; provided the airways are not obstructed.

The test should be repeated after the use of aerosol bronchodilators for prognostic evaluation. Airway obstruction is said to be reversible if the FEV_1 improves. In cases of bronchial spasm due to bronchitis and bronchial asthma the obstruction is partial; it is not reversible in emphysema.

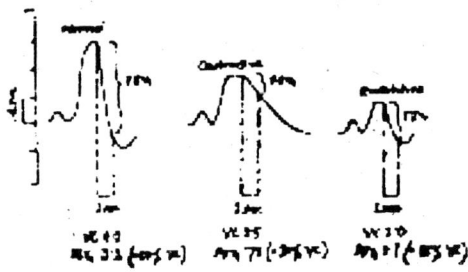

Fig. 2-3 : *Graphical representation of obstructive and restrictive defects of ventilation*

Alternatively, with the help of Wright's peak flowmeter, peak expiratory flow rate (PEFR) can be measured. The peak expiratory flow rate is reduced in airways obstruction. It is to be remembered that 150 ml of air fills the conducting airway which constitute the 'anatomical dead space' and take no part in gas exchange.

Defects of ventilatory capacity can be obstructive and or *non obstructive*. Obstructive defect of ventilatory capacity may be due to chronic bronchitis and bronchial asthma where variable airways obstruction occur due to bronchial secretion, oedema of bronchial mucosa and bronchospasm. Nonobstructive defect of ventilatory capacity may be due to (i) restrictive lung disorders and (ii) hypodynamic ventilatory defects.

A restrictive lung disorder is due to reduced lung compliance as in (a) diffuse infiltration of lung, (b) fibrosis of lung, (c) pulmonary oedema or stiffness or pleura of chest wall as in, (d) pleural thickening or, (e) kyphoscoliosis respectively or may be due to diminished ventilable pulmonary volume as in, (f) pulmonary resection, (g) malignant tumour, (h) pneumothorax and, (i) pleural effusion.

Hypodynamic ventilatory defect may be due to (a) failure of central respiratory drive as occurs after depressant drugs, anaesthetics, cerebrovascular accidents or, (b) due to neuromuscular failure as in poliomyelitis, polyneuritis or after muscle relaxant drugs.

Lung function tests, thus include

(i) Tests for ventilatory capacity.

(ii) Tests for regional lung function.

(iii) Arterial blood analysis.

(i) *Tests for ventilatory capacity* : This includes the followings :

(a) *Forced expiratory time* (FET) : It is the best physical sign for diffuse intrathoracic airways obstruction – requiring no special instruments and can be readily performed at the bedside. FET is the time taken to deliver the vital capacity. In normal subjects this is accomplished in 3.4 seconds. Prolongation of FET beyond 6 second indicates airways obstruction and that FEV_1 FVC is less than 60%.

(b) *Forced expiratory volume* (FEV) *and forced vital capacity* (FVC) *:* In diseases causing diffuse airways obstruction e.g. asthma, bronchitis, emphysema etc. the inequality of the disease process in different airways causes them to close irregularly and progressively as expiration is continued. Result is that in severe cases less than 40% of the FVC is expelled in the first second and the rest of the air takes still much longer, or in other words FEV/FVC $\leq$ 40%. This is called obstructive type of ventilatory defect. In interstitial lung diseases, ankylosing spondylitis etc. both FEV and FVC are nearly equally reduced. So FEV/FVC% will either remain normal or may even increase because of increase elastic recoil. This is restrictive type of ventilatory defect.

(c)   *Peak expiratory flow rate* (PEFR) : It can be measured by the Wright peak flowmeter and the reading is obtained in litres/min. PEFR is diminished in obstructive airways diseases and as such, it is a good indicator of the severity of obstruction.

(d)   *Maximum breathing capacity* (MBC) or *maximum voluntary ventilation* (MVV) : It is measured by instructing the patient to breathe as deeply and as repidly as he can for about 15 secs. The volume breathed may be recorded by a spirometer or collected in a bag. The result is expressed in litres min. It is rarely used now-a-days.

(ii)   *Tests for regional lung function :* These include fluoroscopy bronchospirometry and radioisotope techniques. By fluoroscopy the proportion of ventilation received by each individual   lobe and regional differences of pressure in the lungs can be ascertained from the intensity of 'lighting up' of the lungs and also from the movements of the ribs, mediastinum and diaphragm.

Bronchospirometry involves differential bronchial catheterization and collection of air separately from each lung. It is rarely used.

In radioisotope technique and isotopically labelled gas is administered and its concentration in different regions or 'cores' of lung is determined by external counting. Xenon[33] is an insoluble gas which is very suitable. Scanning of the radioactivity of the lungs after-IV administration of macroaggregated 1[31] or, Tc[99] labelled albumin is also widely used.

(iii) *Arterial blood analysis* : The pH, PaCo and PaO_2 are determined by special apparatus for arterial blood gas analysis and with these data, the type of respiratory failure (vide infra), the state of acid base balance, the therapy to be instituted and the response to therapy can all be ascertained.

Overall function of the lung is to maintain the physiological limits of blood gases needed for normal tissue metabolism by oxygenation of deoxygenated blood and elimination of CO_2. In respiratory failure carbondioxide is inadequately eliminated and so its level in the blood rises. Normal arterial oxygen saturation is above 97% and arterial carbon dioxide tension (PCO) is normally 37-43 mm of Hg and the pH of blood is 7-38 to 7-42. The partial pressure of oxygen in arterial blood (PO_2) is normally about 100 mm of Hg.

When PCO rises above 49 mm of Hg it indicates *respiratory failure* due to alveolar hypoventilation. Its level falls in hyperventilation and is less affected by diffusion impairment or right to left shunting of blood because of the relatively high diffusibility of Co. Routine PCO_2 estimation in arterial blood is not always possible. An easier method has been introduced by Campbell and Howell, where

the patient breathes and rebreathes into a bag until the gas mixture in the bag is in almost same gas-
eous equilibrium with the alveolar air and hence
indirectly with the arterial blood. Final analysis of
the gas mixture in the bag is then carried out using
simple instruments and apparatus.

VII. **PLEURAL BIOPSY**

This is one of the indispensible diagnostic techniques for confirmation of tuberculosis and malignancy of pleura.

VIII. **SKIN TESTS**

In the diagnosis of the chest diseases skin tests
can prove valuable Allergic asthma is associated
with immediate skin reaction to allergen e.g.
pollens etc. This is type I immune reaction or
immediate hypersensitivity reaction. Cell mediated (delayed) hypersensitivity or type IV immune
reaction is seen in Mantoux test used to detect the
tuberculous infection (either past or recent). For
sarcoidosis, an intradermal Kveim test is done
which is relatively specific for this disease.

COR PULMONALE

Cor pulmonale is defined as enlargement of right
heart secondary to malfunctioning of the lungs.
The enlargement may be due to both hypertrophy
and dilatation and malfunctioning of the lungs may
be due to causes other than intrinsic lung diseases. The most obvious mechanism is obstruction of the pulmonary vessels. It may be due either
to vasoconstriction from hypoxia or to distortion,
compression or obliteration of the vessels by the

underlying disease process. Hypoxaemia may impair myocardial contractility and reduced left ventricular performance may contribute to the consequent cardiopulmonary derangements. Cor pulmonale may be either *acute* or *chronic*. In acute cor pulmonale the right heart dilates because of acute pulmonary embolism. Chronic cor pulmonale may be caused by–(i) intrinsic diseases of the lungs of airways, (ii) malfunctioning of the chest belows, or (iii) insufficient drive from the respiratory centre. Of all these causes chronic obstructive lung diseases (chronic bronchitis and emphysema) are the commonest. But cor pulmonale resulting from chronic obstructive lung diseases may remain undiagnosed till there is an episode of overt right heart failure. Diagnosis may be confirmed by arterial blood gas analysis (showing arterial hypoxaemia, hypercapnia and acidosis); roentgenographic and electrocardiographic evidences of enlargement of right ventricle; and if necessary, by catheterization of right side of the heart. Recently echocardiography has proved valuable in detecting pulmonary hypertension based on the movements of the pulmonary valve.

RESPIRATORY FAILURE

Respiratory failure is a clinical condition characterized by abnormality of blood gases present at rest and caused by a disorder of respiration or of its control mechanisms.

There are two types of respiratory failures in both of which the arterial O_2 tension is diminished, but may be distinguished by arterial CO tension.

In type I the $PaCO_2$ is normal or low associated with a low PaO_2

In type II there is elevated $PaCO_2$ associated with a low PaO_2

Type I respiratory failure is due to a defect in gas transfer caused by uneven distribution of inspired air and pulmonary blood flow. It is found in (i) Pulmonary oedema, (ii) Pulmonary fibrosis or infiltration, (iii) Pulmonary thrombo embolism and (iv) transiently in severe asthma and acute bronchial infection.

Type II respiratory failure is caused by deficient total alveolar ventilation. It is found in (i) chronic obstructive lung diseases like chronic bronchitis, emphysema and asthma, (ii) depression of respiratory centre caused by narcotic group of drugs or anaesthesia or vascular disorders, (iii) neuromuscular failure in conditions like poliomyelitis, polyneuritis, myasthenia gravis, chest injury etc. and (iv) end stage of type I respiratory failure.

PART-II

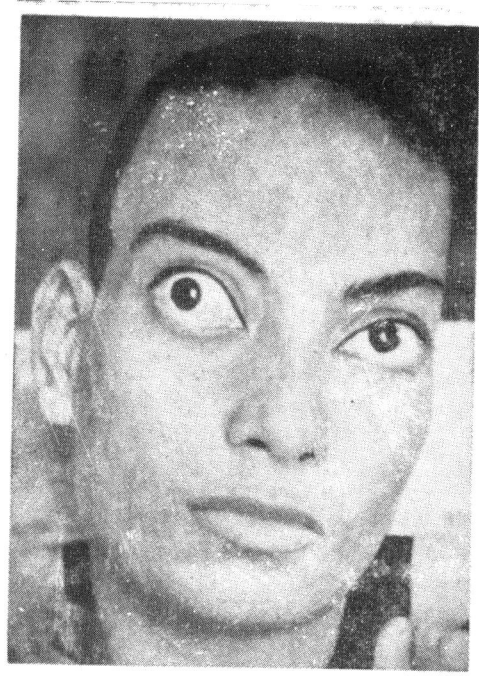

Fig. 1A : This Patient had Grave's Disease
Note the exophthalmos and Dalrymple's Sign.

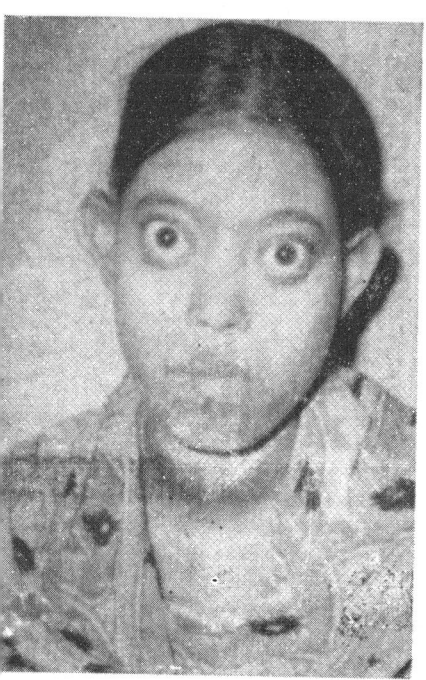

ig. 1B : Another patient with Grave's
Disease.

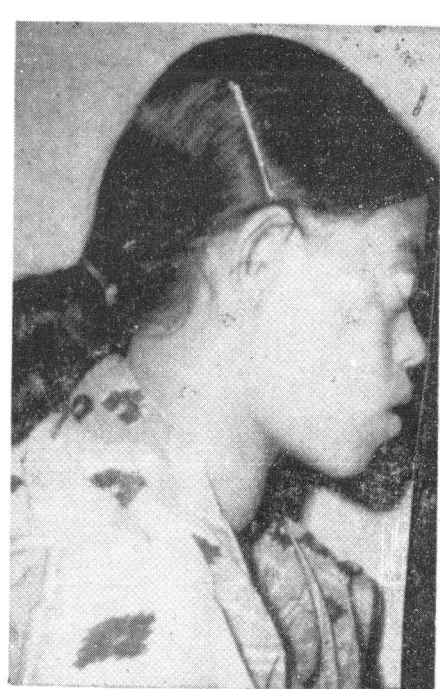

Fig. 1C : Same patient as in Fig. 1B,
Note the protrcsion of the eye balls.

ENDOCRINE AND METABOLIC DISORDERS

CHAPTER 1

The endocrine organs are considered a system since they are closely interrelated. The effects secondary to their dysfunction usually have predominant clinical signs reflected in different organ systems other than the gland itself which is actually diseased.

The manifestation of endocrine diseases are either due to increased or decreased functions of the glands resulting in over production or diminished production respectively of their hormones resulting in the various clinical syndromes e.g. Cushing syndrome or Sheehan syndrome.

It must be remembered that like the diseases of the bones and joints many of the endocrine disorders can be diagnosed chiefly by inspection and can be confirmed subsequently by other clinical methods and relevant biochemical procedures.

THE THYROID GLAND

The examination of the thyroid gland proper has already been discussed and also vide infra. The important symptoms in *hyperfunction* of the thyroid gland are increased appetite, loss of weight, gradual weakness, excessive sweating insomnia, nervousness, palpitation, heat intolerance, diarrhoea. Personal history regarding any psychological trauma should be carefully noted as this might have precipitated the thyrotoxicosis.

In *hypofunction* of the thyroid gland information must be obtained as regards the mental condition, psychosis (myxoedema psychosis or madness), aches and pains, or paraesthesia of the fingers; subjective symptoms of anginal pain or breathlessness; constipation; recent change in voice and history of menorrhagia in the female. Also specifically ask about cold intolerance increasing lethargy and fatigue etc.

Clinical examination :

(1) 'Facies' gives valuable information. In hyperthyroidism the bright glittering eyes, the fixed stare and exophthalmos and retraction of the upper eyelids are the classical features. In hypothyroidism a defective mentality, puffiness of the face, swelling of the lower eyelids, malar flush, dry, rough and scaly skin and delayed dentition in young patients are usually found.

(2) Closely look for evidences of hyperfunction—excitability, trembling, sweating, nervousness, predominantly proximal and to some extent generalised muscular wasting etc.

Narrow palpebral fissures, dull look, thick lips, potruded tongue, abdominal distension and umbilical hernia etc. are to be looked for in hypothyroid state in a child which may be confused with *mongolism* which is clinically characterised by a rounded samll head, hypertelorism, small palpebral fissures, inner canthus directed downwards, mental retardation, nystagmus, low set ears, single transverse crease in the palm (simian crease) etc.

N.B.–Myasthenia gravis may be associated with both hyper and hypothyroid states (autoimmune aetiology).

(3) Next examine for the toxic manifestations in hyperfunction of the gland.

(a)   *Pulse rate* especially the 'sleeping pulse rate' is a better guide. The rate may have a wide range between 90 and 160 per minute without a rise of temperature and this may be because of atrial fibrillation which will be confirmed by the irregularly irregular pulse, pulse deficit more than 10/min and varying intensities of the first heart sound.

(b)   *Tremor* :

  (i)   Ask the patient to stretch out the arms with the fingers wide apart. Now look at the fingers which will exhibit fine tremor.

 (ii)   The patient is asked to put out of the tongue when a fine tremor may be visible.
Trembling of big muscles such as those overlying the shoulder joint may be present.

(c)   *Eye signs* :

  (i)   Exophthalmos (protrusion of the eyeball)–Ask the patient to look straight. Visualisation of the lower sclera for more than 2mm confirms exophthalmos and is an early sign of thyrotoxicosis. Lid retraction which is of spastic type is one of the commonest eye signs in thyrotoxicosis. Lid retraction is said to exist when the patient looks forward and a portion of sclera between the upper eyelid and the cornea becomes visible. Normally this remains covered by the upper eyelid in the forward position of gaze. The staring look and widening of the palpebral fissures thus produced is known as *Dalrympl's sign.*

Bilateral exophthalmos may also be found in retroorbital tumours, cavernous sinus thrombosis, carotidocavernous fistula, empyema of the accessory nasal sinuses, symmetrical orbital tumours as in lymphoma, oxycephaly and leontiasis osseum. *Unilateral* exophthalmos may be caused by orbital cellutitis, granuloma, cavernous sinus thrombosis, orbital periostitis, meningocele, encephalocele, neoplasms, orbital haemorrhage or emphysema etc. Exophthalmos may occurs as a part of the classical triad of *Hand. Schuller Christian* disease in which diabetes inspidus and skull defects are the other two components.

(ii) .Failure of accommodation (*Moebius's sign*). The patient cannot converge the eyes for near vision. Also there may be ophthalmoplegia producing limitations of eyeball movements in one or more directions. Diplopia which is common in thyrotoxicosis, occurs when the patient attempts to look in the direction of limited movement.

(iii) Lagging behind of the upper eyelids when the patient is asked to look downward exposing the sclera between the upper eyelid and the cornea– is known as *Von Graefe's sign* (lid lag).

(iv) Infrequent blinking is the *Stellwag's sign.*

(v) Absence of wrinkling of the forehead on looking upwards with the face directed downward, due to impairment or absence of contraction of the frontal belly of the occipitofrontalis is *Joffroy's signs.*

(vi) Periorbital oedema.

(vii) Inequal dilatation of the pupils.

(viii) Diplopia, weakness of superior and lateral rectus muscles producing exophthalmic opthalmoplegia.

(ix) Chemosis of the conjunctiva and exposure keratitis might occur and this might later on lead to panophthalmitis.

(4) Local examination–The patient is asked to swallow (which he will find easier if given a glass of water) and note whether the swelling moves upward on swallowing. The thyroid gland should be examined from the front and also from behind.

Examination from the front–The neck is well exposed and slightly extended (Kocher's method) and the following points are noted while palpating the gland :

(a) Shape–Localised, nodular or diffuse collar like.

(b) Size big or small.

(c) Surface–smooth or not.

(d) Consistency–Hard shotty feeling in Riedel's thyroiditis or Hashimoto's disease but hard and fixed to the underlying structures usually in carcinoma of the thyroid gland.

(e) Movement of the gland with deglutition. Note whether it is possible to get the lower limit or not. In *retrosternal goitre*, the lower limit cannot be outlined and dilatation of the subcutaneous veins may be visible over the upper anterior part of the thorax due to obstruction of the great veins at the thoracic inlet. This can also be demonstrated by asking the patient to raise the arm and keep in that position for a few seconds when congestion of the face, cyanosis, and discomfort become evident. This is the *Pemberton's sign.* The thyroid gland is pushed sideways to make the gland more prominent.

(f) Deviations of the trachea are to be noted because an enlarged lobe of the thyroid gland may push the trachea to the opposit side.

(g) The carotid pulsation is to be examined as it is often exaggerated in thyrotoxicosis or may be impalpable when thyroid carcinoma spreads to the carotid sheath.

(h) Evidences of venous engorgement as in secondary nodular goitre with congestive cardiac failure should be searched for.

(i)   Feel for a thrill of the thyroid gland. In Graves' disase either a systolic thrill or rarely a continuous thrill may be palpable.

(j)   Neck glands should be examined routinely as they may be involved by metastasis from a carcinoma of the thyroid.

Examination from behind–The neck is slightly flexed and the thyroid gland is palpated from behind as before.

Percussion of the manubrium sterni is of importance since the note is dull in retrosternal goitre which can be confirmed by a lateral X-ray of the neck.

On auscultation, a systolic bruit may be audible in a hyperfunctioning thyroid. This should be distinguished from carotid souffles and venous hum.

Measurement : The circumference of the neck at the most prominent part of the swelling is to be measured at fortnightly intervals to assess any alteration in the size of the gland.

'Goitre' is present in most cases of hyperthyroidism but it may be accompanied with signs of *hypothyroidism* in Hashimoto's disease, in a carcinoma of the thyroid or in prolonged treatment with antithyroid drugs in case of thyrotoxicosis.

(5) *Examination of the hand*–It is warm and moist in hyperthyroidism. Cold and dry in hypothyroidism. Clubbing may be present in myxoedema as also a Carpal tunnel syndrome (entrapment neuropathy due to compression of the median nerve). Clubbing may also be found in Graves' disease associated with a dermopathy in the form of localized of pretibial myxoedema.

Fine tremor may be present in hyperfunction of the gland. Dilated veins may be visible in thyrotoxicosis.

Pulse rate is to be carefully noted because sinus

tachycardia in thyrotoxicosis and sinus bradycardia in myxoedema are commonly encountered.

Atrial fibrillation may be found in an otherwise covert thyrotoxicosis and also quite commonly in elderly individuals without other obvious clinical manifestations of hyperthyroidism. Waterhammer pulse is frequently found due to hyperkinetic circulatory state in hyperthyroidism. Arterial wall may be thickened in myxoedema due to associated hypercholesterolaemia. Inequality of pulsations in radial and dorsalis pedis arteries may be present in myxoedema due to associated atherosclerosis. Hypotension is usually encountered in myxoedema whereas a high pulse pressure is found in thyrotoxicosis.

(6) Examination of the *lymph nodes* is essential to find out any enlargement (due to proliferation of reticuloendothelial cells) found in hyperthyroidism in about 10% of cases or metastasis from a thyroid carcinoma.

(7) Examination of the *cardiovascular system* may reveal hyperdynamic apex, loud first heart sound with a systolic scratch due to an abnormal vigour of the heart beat inside the pericarcium, systolic murmur, accentuated pulmonary second sound, atrial fibrillation and congestive cardiac failure in hyperthyroidism. The scratchy sound heard in midsystole in the left second intercostal space during expiration is the *Means Larman* scratch and is possible due to rubbing together of the normal pleural and pericardial surfaces by the hyperdynamic heart.

Diffuse or impalpable apex with an increased area of cardiac dullness, muffled heart sounds, evidences of pericardial effusion or congestive cardiac failure due to cardiomyopathy may be present in myxoedema.

(8) Gastrointestinal system–Hepatosplenomegaly and increased peristaltic sounds are frequently encountered in

hyperthyroidism whereas a distended abdomen with minimum peristaltic sounds, palpable faecolith, ascites and
abdominal angina with hepatic enlargement are the classic
features of myxoedema. The typical "frog-belly" of cretinism
is commonly associated with an umbilical hernia.

(9) Genitourinary system–Glycosuria with creatinuria
are commonly found in hyperthyroidism and traces of
albumin may be detected in the urine in hypothyroidism.

(10) (a) Nonpitting oedema is commonly found in
myxoedema but a pitting one may be present when
complicated with congestive cardiac failure. Oedema may
also be present in hyperthyroidism when congestive cardiac failure occurs.

(b)   Thyroid acropachy–Clubbing of the fingers and
       toes associated with characteristic changes in
       bones unlike that of pulmonary hypertrophic
       osteoarthopathy and some skin disorders are
       collectively called thyroid acropachy.

(11) A rapid loss of weight in hyperthyroidism and a
gradual increase in weight in myxoedema are the characteristic features of the two diseases.

(12) Thyrotoxic myopathy–Weakness and wasting of the
proximal (i.e. shoulder and hipgirdle) group of muscles are
common. The weakness is most felt in climbing upstairs.
This myopathy resolves completely with treatment.

In hypothyroidism the changes in the skeletal muscle
consist of increased volume, stiffness and slowness of
contraction and relaxation. Action myospasm, percussion
myoedema and commonly slowness of tendon reflexes are
classical findings. Hypothyroidism may be associated with
pseudomyotonia, polyneuropathy and cerebellar ataxia in
addition to the above.

(13) Dermopathy : Pretibial myxoedema–Localised thick-

ening of the skin over the dorsum of the foot and legs, found in patients of active or past thyrotoxicosis. The skin is hyperpigmented, pruritic and has a peaud orange appearance.

INVESTIGATIONS

(i) Basal Metabolic Rate–The   rate is high in hyperthyroidism and low in hypothyroidism. The test lacks specificity. In anxiety states, cardiac failure, pyrexia, blood dyscrasias, lymphoma, phaeochromocytoma etc. the rate becomes high. In severe malnutrition and nephrotic syndrome the rate becomes low. Despite these drawbacks, the BMR is the only way of assessing the effects of thyroid hormones on the body as a whole. In normal subjects BMR remains within 15% of those expected from the tables. A higher or lower value respectively indicates hyper or hypothyroidism when other disease states are excluded.

(ii) Estimation of cholesterol– A high value is suggestive of hypothyroidism especially the primary one, but low cholesterol concentration has little value in the diagnosis of thyrotoxicosis.

(Normal value is 150 to 250 mg. per 100 cc of blood). A value greater than 300 mg% is a fairly constant finding in hypothyroidism.

(iii) Protein bound iodine–Normal value is 3 to 8 microgram%. It is also elevated, besides thyrotoxicosis, in pregnancy, in patients taking oestrogen containing contraceptive pills or iodides in form of cough mixtures or in patients who have been investigated recently with administration of contrast media. Low values are found in patients with nephrotic syndrome or those who are being treated with steroids and in some patients with Cushing syndrome and acromegaly. For a lack of specificity this test has been replaced by a measurement of serum T_4 concentration.

Butanol extractable iodine (BEI) is approximately 0.5 mg/ 100 ml less than PBI.

(iv) Radioactive idoine uptake (RAIU)–The patient is given the isotope (I_{131} or preferably I_{123}) in water to drink and estimation of the radioactive iodine in the thyroid is measured generally after 24 hours. Normal uptake is 5 to 30% and so RAIU is of value in detecting hyperthyroidism but not of hypothyroidism. High uptakes of radio iodine also occur in iodine deficiency states. In iodine excess states, the value may be low.

(v) Serum T_4 concentration–Measured by competitive protein binding method. Recently, it is measured by radioimmunoassay. Normal value is 4 to 11 Ug per 100 ml.

(vi) Serum T_3 estimation–Done by radioimmunoassay.

(vii) T_3 resin uptake test.

(viii) Free thyroxine index–The free thyroxine index is derived by multiplying the serum total thyroxine by the thyroxine resin uptake (normal range of free thyroxine index– 4.5 to 11.5).

(ix) Thyroid scan–Radioactive iodine isotope (1131) or technetium (Tc 99 m) are used. It helps in the detection of a 'hot' nodule (i.e. secreting excess hormone) or 'cold' nodule (i.e. not secreting hormone).

(x) Effective thyroxine ratio (ETR)–Measurement of serum T_4 and binding capacity of the thyroid hormone binding proteins in a single manouevre. This is a reliable test of thyroid function.

(xi) T_3 suppression test is particularly useful to note whether the high radioiodine uptake is due to hyperthyroidism or due to iodine deficiency. Tri-iodothyronine when given for 10 days at a rate of 100 ug T_3/day in divided doses,–suppresses or reduces the radio iodine uptake in normal subjects and in iodine deficiency states (where it suppresses the increased TSH secretion due to iodine deficiency) but do not reduce radio iodine uptake in hyperthyroidism where the thyroidal overactivity is due to circulating long acting thyroid stimulator (LATS).

(xii) Serum TSH levels in response to TRH stimulation—Serum TSH is low in thyrotoxicosis. 20 miuntes after IV injection of TRH, the TSH level is measured, little or no response is found in thyrotoxicosis but very high response is found in hypothyroidism due to primary thyroidal failure. The TSH secreting mechanism is impaired in intrinsic pituitary disease.

(xiii) Thyroidal antibodies. (1) *Thyroglobulin antibodies:* Precipitation and immunofluorescence tests are done to detect circulating antibodies against thyroglobulin. The test is positive in Hashimoto's disease and Grave's disease. (2) *Microsomal antibody*–detected by complement fixation test and immunofluorescence. (3) *Long acting thyroid stimulator* (LATS). It is an immunoglobulin (IgG) found in excess in the serum of patients with Grave's disease. This antibody is formed against the components of plasma membrane of the thyroid cells. (4) In Grave's disease the serum also contains the immunoglobulins–TSH binding inhibitory immunoglobin (TBII) and thyroid (cyclic AMP) stimulating immunoglobulin (TSI).

(xiv) Relaxation Time of Tendon Reflexes : The time course of muscular relaxation after the induction of a stretch reflex is characteristically altered by thyroid deficiency. This causes a delay in the relaxation phase,–but not due to any change in the conduction of nerve impulses. Several mechanical devices can record the duration of the contraction and relaxation phases of the ankle jerk. Usually the 'time to half relaxation' is measured. This is prolonged in hypothyroidism and shortened in hyperthyroidism. It is a simple procedure causing no discomfort to the patient, and if diseases like primary muscular disorders can be excluded, is a very useful procedure in thyroid disorders.

THE PITUITARY GLAND

The pituitary gland is situated in the sella turcica and is connected to the hypothalamus by the infundibular stalk. It has two lobes. (i) The anterior lobe or adenohypophysis, and (ii) the posterior lobe or neurohypophysis (Pars nervosa).

The anterior lobe of the pituitary gland secretes–

(i) Growth hormone (GH) or somatotropin.

(ii) Adrenocorticotrophic hormone (ACTH)

(iii) Thyroid stimulating hormone (TSH)

(iv) Gonadotrophic hormones–Follicle stimulating hormone (FSH) and luteinising hormone (LH), in the male which is known as interstitial cell stimulating hormone (ICSH).

(v) Prolactin and,

(vi) Melanocyte stimulating hormone (MSH)

The neurohypophysis secretes–

(i) Antidiuretic hormone (ADH or vasopressin), and (ii) Oxytocin.

N.B.–The anterior lobe develops as an upwardly displaced group of cells from the primitive buccal endothelium while the neurohypophysis developes as a downward projection of neuroectoderm from the base of the brain. The anterior lobe is predominantly supplied by the portal venous blood coming from the capillaries of the hypothalamus and this has two significance–(i) the hypothalamic regulatory peptides are carried to the anterior pituitary via this portal venous system, and (ii) the adenohypophysis being perfused predominantly at the pressure of a venous system is susceptible undergo infarction in hypovolaemic shock e.g. in post partum hae-morrhage especially because the pituitary is enlarged in pregnancy.

THE ROLE OF THE HYPOTHALAMUS

Hormones of the anterior pituitary are controlled by the specific factors released from the hypothalamus through the portal vessels of the infundibular stalk which is con-nected with the median eminence, supraoptic and paraventricular nuclei. Pituitary hormones with specific target glands like TSH, ACTH and LH or FSH receive only releasing factors like TRH, CRF, LH or FSHRH but those pituitary hormones which have no specific target glands are controlled both by releasing and inhibitory factors for example GHRF and GHIH or MSRH and MSHIF or, PLRF(?) or PLIF. Growth hormone inhibitory factor is also known as *somatostatin* or SRIF (somatotrophin release inhibiting factor) and some of its other actions are – (i) decreasing the TSH response to TRH; (ii) inhibition of insulin and glucagon secretion : (iii) inhibition of secretion of gastrin and vasoactive intestinal peptide etc. SRIF is present in the D cells of pancreas and other parts of gut and brain; (iv) SRIF or somatostatin has profound effects on splanchnic and portal vascular beds and on IV admin-istration has shown to decrease the urinary volume, effec-tive renal plasma flow and GRF (BMJ, 1701, 297, 1986) and has recently been advocated in the management of patients with GI bleeding.

Axons of the ganglion cells of the supraoptic and paraventricular nuclei comprise the hypothalamico-hypophyseal system. These axons carry the secretory granules from the above nuclei to the neurohypophysis and vasopressin and oxytocin are released from the granules into the blood stream. ADH secretion is controlled by (i) the osmoreceptors in the supraoptic nuclei, (ii) volume receptors of the left atrium. and (iii) baroreceptors of the carotid and aortic bodies. Oxytocin release is primarily stimulated by suckling or stimulation of the female genital tract.

Increased secretion of GH before puberty causes *gigantism* and *acromegaly* after puberty.)

Excessive secretion of ACTH may present as *Cushing disease*.

Premature secretion of gonadotrophins may cause *precocious puberty.*

Failure of function of the pituitary gland may be progressive and usually follows the following order : *gonadotrophins decline first* to be followed by GH, ACTH *and last the* TSH. It is *Simmond disease*–where the gonadal, adrenocortial and thyroid failure present a composite picture. But if this total failure of the anterior pituitary occurs after a severe post partum haemorrhage it is called *Sheehan syndrome* (vide supra).

Deficient secretion of the ADH causes *diabetes insipidus.*

Prepubertal panhypopituitarism (e.g. due to craniopharyngioma) usually causes dwarfism due to failure of the growth hormone. Later on due to gonadotrophic deficiency puberty fails to appear, causing a combination of dwarfism and *sexual infantilism* called pituitary infantilism.

Rerely the prepubertal pituitary and hypothalamic dysfunctions lead to deficient or inappropriate skeletal growth, obesity, hypogonadism (and may be, diabetes insipidus) which is called *Frohlich syndrome* or *dystrophia adiposogenitalis.*

In a patient suffering from hypo or hyperfunction of the pituitary gland proper elicitation of the history is most essential to come to a diagnosis. A patient below 25 years who abnormally rapidly grows in height (maintaining the proportion of growth) is possibly suffering from *pituitary gigantism*. A patient above 25 requiring gradual larger sizes of hats, gloves, boots and complaining of headache, palpitation and somnolence is probably suffering from *acromegaly.*

A child abnormally rapidly gaining weight with deposition of fats around the hips and with evidences of hypogonadism is possibly suffering from *Frohlich syndrome* whereas immature general, skeletal, and sexual developments without obesity is the characteristic feature of *pituitary infantilism.*

History of amenorrhoea in a woman after the birth of a child, failure of lactation, loss of axillary and pubic hair indicate that she is probably suffering from *Sheehan syndrome.*

Clinical Examination :

(i) Facies is the most characteristic in hyperpituitarism. Prominent supraorbital ridges, thickening of the nose with wide nostrils, thickening and enlargement of the lips and the tongue, presence of prognathism (lower incisors in front of the upper with a prominent mandible) are the classic features of *acromegaly.* Mooning of the face is the characteristic of Cushing disease.

(ii) Hands and feet are to be examined as these are often enlarged and thickened; fingers and toes are square shaped in acromegaly.

(iii) Length of the limbs (including the height of the patient).

(iv) Measurement of the circumference of the head are to be noted at frequent intervals as bony growth chiefly affects this part in hyperfunction of the pituitary gland.

(v) The spine is routinely examined for any evidence of kyphosis.

(vi) Examination of the skin reveals a warm, moist,

thickened and coarse skin with fibromata mollusca and increased pigmentation and body hair in acromegaly and purple striae with acne in *Cushing syndrome*. Absence of pubic and axillary hair, scanty hair on eyebrows and scalp are observed in *hypofunction of the pituitary. Soft, shiny and elastic* skin is the feature which *differentiates* it from *myxoedema*.

(vii) Buffalo hump like obesity is the characteristic of Cushing syndrome but the distribution of fat chiefly around the buttock and hip is encountered in hypofunction of the pituitary gland. The confidence of the patient is to be established first by explaining about the disease process prior to the examination of the secondary sex characters.

(viii) Routine examination of the cranial nerves and ophthalmoscopy, perimetry and scotometry should be done in patients with pituitary tumours.

Visual defects very depending upon the position of the prtuitary tumour in relation to the optic chiasma. Colour vision for red may be impaired; visual field defects range from an upper temporal quadrantic defect to bitemporal or homonymous hemianopia. Unilateral blindness with optic atrophy and enlargement of the blind spot in scotometry may be detected. In every case of visual field defect an X-ray of the skull should be taken. *Retinitis pigmentosa* may be found in the congenital familial disorder of Laurence-Moon-Biedl syndrome which is characterised by obesity. hypogonadism, dwarfism, mental deficiency and polydactyly.

(ix) As overgrowth of bone, cartilage, soft tissue and viscera are the effects of increased secretion of growth hormone, palpation of the abdomen may reveal hepatosplenomegaly; cardiac enlargement may also be detected by palpation and radiography.

(x) Features of diabetes mellitus, hypertension, hyperthyroidism, alteration of sex functions and excess lactation, if any, are to be noted while examining a case of acromegaly. Similarly any lack of pigmentation and features of diabetes insipidus are to be looked for in hypofunction of the pituitary gland.

(xi) *Measurements* : Measurement from the crown to symphysis pubis and from symphysis pubis to the sole by a tape is to be done routinely in patients suffering from pituitary disorders.

(a) The distance from the crown to symphysis pubis is more than the distance from symphysis pubis to the sole in pituitary dwarfism.

(b) Relation of the span to the height is to be determined. This span exceeds the height and the measurement from symphysis pubis to the sole is greater than the distance from the crown to the symphysis pubis in gigantism. Span and height become equal in Klinefelters syndrome. Arms and legs are stunted but the body length is essentially normal in achondroplasia.

Investigation for Dysfunctions of the Pituitary Gland

Deficient or excessive secretions of the anterior or posterior pituitary may occur as isolated or combined defects, i.e. one or more of the hormones secreted may be simultaneously deficient or excessive. As such, the presentation depends on the numbers and extent of hormone deficiencies. In the evaluation of the patient, the history and physical examination usually proves helpful with regard to aetiology. As regards laboratory evaluation, it must be remembered that although the basal hormone levels provide much information, the *pulsatile* nature of the anterior pituitary hormone secretion makes interpretation and evaluation difficult, particularly between normal and low blood levels. Hence various provocative tests are used. Investigations for each individual hormone dysfunction will be considered separately.

(A) Prolactin :

(i) **Deficiency** : The basal morning levels normally vary between 1 and 20 ng/ml in men and 1 and 25 ng/ml in women. in large pituitary lesions, prolactin values may be low and a deficient response to provocative test e.g. TRH or chlorpromazine may be seen. But testing for prolactin deficiency is rarely needed.

(ii) **Hypersecretion** : Prolactin levels over 100–150 ng/ml usually indicate a pituitary tumour. TRH by stimulating the lactotrophs and chlorpromazine by inhibiting the PIF activity, stimulate the release of prolactin. TRH 400 Ug IV and chlorpromazine 25–50 mg IM increase prolactin secretion to more than double the normal basal value. But then high basal levels are of greater diagnostic value than provocative tests. When elevated prolactin value has been demonstrated radiological studies prove most useful.

N.B.–Prolactinomas are the commonest pituitary tumours and may be a micro(<10 mm) or a macroadenoma (>10 mm).

(B) Growth hormone :

(i) **Deficiency** : The provocative tests include–(i) A fasting patient is asked to climb several flights of stairs and if the growth hormone level in blood after that is over 6 ng/ml, the result can be considered normal; (ii) Insulin test– 0.1 to 0.2 unit/kg soluble insulin is given IV as a bolus via a saline drip to a fasting patient. Growth hormone rises to a peak at 30 to 60 minutes and the value must be greater than 6–8 ng/ml. When the insulin test is contraindicated, levodopa can be used orally. All tests should be performed on a fasting patient as glucose normally suppresses growth hormone.

(ii) **Hypersecretion** : Patients with acromegaly have raised BMR. Impaired glucose tolerance is seen in about half the cases.Growth hormone levels are abnormally elevated and if measured during the glucose tolerance test, they are not suppressed and occasionally may be para-doxically elevated contrary to that in a normal person when the level goes down to below 5 ng/ml. Also there is an abnormal release of growth hormone following TRH. The serum phosphate level may be elevated.

An enlarged sella turcica is seen in the vast majority of patients on radiological study.

(C) **LH and FSH :** Determination of the basal levels will provide valuable information. LHRH test (100–150 ug) IV given and serum LH determined at 20 to 30 mins) is usually not necessary. Clomiphene citrate (that blocks the feed-back of gonadal steroids on hypothalamus) may be admin-istered to find out whether increase in LH and FSH values occur, thus testing the hypothalamic pituitary axis.

Also, urinary gonadotrophins may be measured by bioassay or radio immunoassy.

(D) **TSH** (Thyrotropin) : The levels of the thyroid hor-mones and TSH are determined. The former is low in hypothalamic, pituitary as well as primary hypothyroidism. the latter is low in hypothalamic and pituitary diseases but elevated in primary hypothyroidism. However, the low and normal TSH levels cannot be differentiated usually by radioimmunoassy. TSH response 20 to 30 min after 400-500 µg of TRH, IV—which normally doubles--can also be determined. Unfortunately, hypothalamic and pituitary dis-eases cannot be differentiated always and euthyroid and hyperthyroid patients do not respond to TRH.

(E) **ACTH** :

(i) **Deficiency** : Basal morning plasma cortisol and 24 hour urine 17 hydroxysteroid excretion are diminished.

Insulin tolernace test may be performed as

hypoglycaemia stimulates ACTH release. Normally cortisol rises by 5-7 µg% above the base line. However, some patients are too sensitive to insulin to bear the stress.

These patients may be tested with *metyrapone* which blocks 11-β hydroxylation step in cortisol synthesis pathway. Normally, ACTH, 11-β deoxy cortisol and urinary 17-hydroxysteroids levels rise. If the adrenals are normal, failure to respond to metyrapone can be taken as diagnostic of ACTH deficiency.

(ii) *Hypersecretion* : The diurnal variations of the plasma ACTH and cortisol levels are lost. ACTH release is impaired after insulin induced hypoglycaemia. *Dexamethasone suppression test*–The principle is that in ACTH hypersecretion, glucocorticoids in physiological doses fail to suppress ACTH secretion, although much higher doses suppress it. Thus, when 0.5 mg dexamethasone is given 6 hourly (2 mg/day) most patients usually show no suppression. When 2 mg 6 hourly is given, *plasma cortisol level falls below 5 µg% and urinary 17 hydroxysteroids excretion falls below 3 mg per gram creatinine.* ACTH suppression is rarely possible if there are large pituitary adenomas, and even then only by very high doses of dexamethasone.

(F) *ADH* : investigations for deficiency or hyperfunction of this hormone include–

(i) Measurement of ADH level in blood and urine by bioassay or radioimmunoassay.

(ii) *Plasma osmolality* (normal range is 280 to 300 mosm/kg) is elevated in ADH deficiency and vice versa.

(iii) *Water deprivation test* : Water deprivation stimulates ADH secretion so that urine specific gravity goes above 1020 and osmolality goes above 700 mosm/kg after 12 to 18 hours. Plasma osmolality alters very little. The values do not exceed 1014 and 300 mosm/kg respectively in diabetes insipidus. Water loss continues, dehydration develops and rapid loss of weight occurs. The test should not be continued if 3% or more of body weight is lost.

(iv) *Hypertonic saline infusion*–5% saline is given IV– this normally results in the release of ADH, increase in plasma osmolality and a fall in urine volume. It is contraindicated in those who cannot tolerate a saline load, e.g. a patient with heart disease.

(v) *Administration of nicotine*–Either by smoking cigarettes (1 to 3) or intravenously causes antidiuretic effect. This is compared with that produced by graded IV doses of vasopressin. The effect is less in diabetes insipidus.

(vi) *Response to vasopressin injection* can help differentiating nephrogenic diabetes insipidus from other varieties as also true diabetes insipidus from primary polydipsia.

(vii) *Dehydration test* : This test is due to find out the concentrating capacity of the kidneys. Fluid is with held for a period till the osmolality of the three urine samples for 3 consecutive hours becomes constant.Then 5 units of injection vasopressin given subcutaneously. Urine osmolality is measured 1 hour after the injection.

In diabetes insipidus the urine osmolality will rise by more than 9 percent after vasopressin injection. In normal persons the urine osmolality rises but less than 9 percent.

X–ray as a diagnostic aid :

(i) Typical suprasellar calcification may confirm a hypopituitarism due to a craniopharyngioma.

(ii) X-ray of the skull may reveal irregularity and widening of the sella turcica in acromegaly. In addition, prognathism and tufting of terminal phalanges may also be detected.

(iii) Wedging of the vertebrae and pathological fractures of the ribs of evidences of osteoporosis may be seen on X-ray examination in Cushing's disease.

THE ADRENAL GLANDS

They are two in number, situated on the upper pole of each kidney. Each gland is composed of two parts, the outer cortex and the inner medulla. *Adrenal cortex secretes* (i) mineralocorticoids ie, aldosterone and deoxycorticosterone, (ii) glucocorticoids i.e. cortisol cortisone and corticosterone and (iii) sex steroids i.e., androgen and to a lesser extent oestrogen and progesterone.

Zona glomerulosa, the outer zone, mainly synthesizes aldosterone, whereas the inner zone–fasciculata-reticularis synthesizes cortisol and androgens.

Adrenal medulla secretes (i) Adrenaline (epinephrine), and (ii) noradrenaline (norepinephrine).

Hypofunction of the adrenal cortex causes Addison's disease while hyperfunction of the adrenal cortex causes Cushing syndrome.

Hypersecretion of aldosterone causes *aldosteronism* which may be either *primary* hyperaldosteronism associated with an adenoma called *Conn's syndrome,* or *secondary* hyperaldosteronism as occurs in cirrhosis of liver, nephrotic syndrome or congestive cardiac failure.

A tumour of the adrenal medulla (phaeochromocytoma) secretes excessive noradrenaline and adrenaline and lead to hypertension which may be paroxysmal or sustained along with episodes of pallor, sweating, palpitations, headache, epigastric pain and apprehension.

Hypersecretion of androgenic hormones in the female causes virilization with increased muscular development, hirsutism and enlargement of clitoris. Hypersecretion of androgenic hormone in pre-adolescent boys causes *precocious puberty* but if occurs in adult male might pass unnoticed. A rare condition–*adrenogenital syndrome*–is caused by partial or complete deficiency of certain enzymes which are essential for the biosynthesis of cortisol. This is characterised by virilirzation in the female and precocious puberty in the male.

A good history takes the observer a long way towards a correct diagnosis of suprarenal disorders and points to be noted are–

(i) If the child has become repidly obese with precocious development of hair in the axilla and in the pubic region, think of hyperfunction of the adrenal cortex.

(ii) Appearence of masculine character in a female indicates hyperfunction of the cortext.

(iii) A patient complaining of generalised weakness. backache, mooning of the face, hirsutism and easy bruising may indicate hyperfunction of the cortex (Cushing syndrome).

(iv) If a young patient complains of palpitation, excessive sweating apprehension and pain in the abdomen, he is probably suffering from a tumour of the adrenal medulla *(Phaeochromocytoma).*

(v) Gastrointestinal disturbances like vomiting, diarrhoea, asthenia, fainting attacks and dark brown pigmentation of the skin and mucous membrane may be the presenting features of *Addison's disease.*

(vi) A 'critical general survey' is essential to come to a proper diagnosis. Emaciation, weight loss and evidences of dehydration may be obvious in Addison's disease whereas obesity (buffalo-hump-like) may be seen in Cushing syndrome and a recorded chart weight indicates the prognosis of the case and response to therapy.

(vii) Systolic blood pressure may fall to 60 mm Hg or even lower in hypofunction of the gland contrasted to systolic hypertension of Cushing syndrome and paroxysmal or sustained hypertension of a medullary tumour.

(viii) Hirsutism may be the feature of congenital adrenal

hyperplasia or Cushing syndrome while either pseudohermaphroditism or virilism may be seen in an adrenal cortical tumour. Increased pulse rate due to sympathetic effect may occasionally be found in phaeochromocytoma.

(ix) A lump in the abdomen and paroxysmal hypertension may favour the diagnosis of phaeochromocytoma (lump in the abdomen and hypertension may occur in coditions like polycystic kidney, hydronephrosis, hypernephroma and pregnancy). The rounded facies of *Cushing syndrome* with acne vulgaris may be recognised at first sight. Brownish black pigmentation in gum and buccal mucous membrane, the axillae, areolae of nipple, creases of palm and around genitalia is frequently found in *Addison's disease*. Purple striae in Cushing syndrome develop around the hips, anterior axillary fold, abdomen and flanks.

Features of diabetes mellitus and evidences of either active or quiescent tuberculosis are to be carefully noted in Cushing syndrome and Addison's disease respectively. Before labelling the case as hypo or hyperfunction of the adrenal gland certain biochemical investigations are to be undertaken.

Biochemical investigations :

(1) Estimation of serum sodium and potassium. These are low in Addison's disease due to electrolyte imbalance (Normal value : serum sodium 136–145 mEq/litre; serum potassium 3.5 to 5 mEq/litre.)

(2) (a) Increased urinary excretion of 17-ketosteroid and 17-hydroxycorticosteroids are respectively found in adrenal virilising syndrome and Cushing syndrome.

(b) Low urinary corticosteroid is found in Addison's disease.

(c) Estimation of vanilylmandelic acid (VMA), cate-cholamines and metanephrine in 24 hours urine. Normal upper limits for these are 7 mg, 100 mg and 1 mg respectively in 24 hours urine. In phaeochromocytoma VMA may be as high as 300 mg. But analysis for urinary metanephrine and normetanephrine appears to be the most useful biochemical screening test at present becaue of convenience and diagnostic accuracy.

(3) Estimation of basal metabolic rate–high in Cushing syndrome.

(4) Glucose tolerance test (GTT)–Diabetic type of glu-cose tolerance curve and glycosuria are found in Cushing syndrome.Hypoglycaemia is commonly found in Addison's disease and the patients are unusually insulin sensitive.

(5) *ACTH test* :

Under maximal stimulation with ACTH the cortisol secretion rises 10 times to 300 mg/day. Injection Tetracosactrin (an ACTH preparation) is given IM in a daily dose of 1 mg for three consecutive days in the morning.

Measurement of plasma *fluorogenic corticosteroid* level at 30 minutes, 60 minutes and 5 hours after the injection is done. In normal persons the value will exceed 690 n mole/litre after 5 hours. In Addison's disease the value will not rise more than 700 n mole/litre after 5-12 hours even after the third intramuscular injection. Maximal stimulation can be obtained with prolonged ACTH infusion. A synthetic variety of ACTH, *cosyntropin* is given in 500 to 1000 ml normal saline at the rate of 2 units per hour for 24 hours. Normally, 17 hydroxysteroid excretion rate increases to 25 mg/ day and plasma cortisol level rises to more than 40 µg/ 100ml. In secondary adrenal insufficiency the values respectively are 3-20 mg/day and 10-40 µg/ 100 ml. In primary adrenal insufficiency there is still smaller.

responses. This test can alternatively be performed by infusing 25 units of cosyntropin over an 8 hour period for 2 or 3 consecutive days.

(6) Suppression Tests – (i) Overnight dexamethasone suppression test is most reliable. Plasma-cortisol level is measured at 8 am after oral administration of 1 mg dexamethasone previous midnight. Normally, the level should be less than 5 µg/100 ml. (ii) Another definitive test of adrenal suppressibility is to give 0.5 mg dexamethasone every 6 hours for 2 days, and urine is collected for a 24 hour period. Normally, urine 17-hydroxysteroids fall to less than 3mg/day on second day and plasma cortisol falls to less than 5 µg /100 ml.

Tests for pituitary adrenal responsiveness by insulin hypoglycaemia or by metyrapone has been already described.

(7) Eosinophil count and its ralation with steroid therapy– Eosinophil count may be high in hypofunction of the adrenal cortex. Eosinophil count of a patient suffering from Addison's disease is done at 2 am and IV infusion of 25 units of ACTH in 500 ml of glucose saline is started and peripheral blood count of eosinophil is repeated after 8 hours. Normally, the count falls by 75 to 100 per cent. But in Addison's disease, the change ranges from a rise of 70% to a fall of 50%.

(8) Effect of injection of histamine–In suspected cases of phaeochromocytoma an injection of histamine elevates the blood pressure. This test is usually not done as it is a dangerous one.

(9) Phentolamine methanesulphonate (Rogitine) test– Injection of 4 mg of Rogitine causes lowering of systolic blood pressure and a fall of about 50 mm of Hg has a

diagnostic significance in phaeochromocytoma. Rogitine is given IV as a bolus.

Radiological investigations : Radiological evidences of the fracture of ribs and wedging of vertebrae may be seen in Cushing syndrome; X-ray may reveal evidences of tuberculosis of the lung and calcification above the upper pole of the kidneys in Addison's disease. Perirenal air insufflation and aortography are helpful for the localisation of the vascular tumour like phaeochromocytoma. Metastatic lesions may be found in X-ray in case of neuroblastoma.

The history and the above investigation will confirm the diagnosis and will differentiate the endocrine disorders from other diseases, for example–Addison's disease can be differentiated from pernicious anaemia, chronic arsenic poisoning and carcinoma of the stomach.

THE PARATHYROID GLANDS

The parathyroids are four small glands attached along the posterior borders of the lobes of the thyroid glands. They are arranged in pairs. two on each side, *Parathormone* (PTH) is the chief secretion of the parathyroid glands. *Calcitonin*, mainly secreted by the parafollicular 'C' cells of the thyroid is also secreted by the parathyroid gland.

The parathyroid glands control the concentrations of (i) calcium and (ii) inorganic phosphorus in the blood. The parathormone mobilizes calcium from the *bones* and increases calcium absorption from the *intestine* producing hypercalcaemia–thereby increasing the excretion of calcium in the urine.Parathormone also reduces *the renal tubular reabsorption of phosphate* and increases the phosphate excretion. Thus in hyperparathyroidism the concentration of serum calcium is raised and serum phosphorus level is lowered. As there is an increased excretion of calcium in the urine in *hyperparathyroidism renal* calculi is frequently formed. Calcium is deposited in and around the renal tubular epithelium giving rise to nephrocalcinosis, a form of tubulointerstitial disease.

In *hypoparathyroidism* there is a lowered concentration of calcium and a raised concentration of phosphate in the plasma.

Hyperparathyroidism may be (i) *primary* due to a parathyroid adenoma; (ii) *secondary* with a hypertrophy of the parathyroid glands as found in chronic renal failure or (iii) *tertiary* when due to a long stimulus one of the hyperplastic glands start functioning autonomously.

Pseudohypoparathyroidism is a rare condition where the patient's own parathyroid gland appears to be normal but probably due to an apparent failure of the tissues to respond to parathormone (receptor insensitivity), The clinical features of preudohypo parathyroidism are short stubby hands with short metacarpals, rounded face, frontal bossing, mental retardation, ectopic deposition of calcium and cataracts. *Biochemical features* include hypocalcaemia and hyperphosphataemia. High concentration of calcitonin may be found in the circulation.

Pseudo-pseudohypoparathyroidism probably is an incomplete form of pseudohypoparathyroidism where there is absence of biochemical features like hypocalcaemia or hyperphosphataemia but presence of other features of the hands, facies and ectopic calcification etc.

HISTORY : Amplification of the patient's description of his complaints aids in the diagnosis of disorders of the parathyroid gland.

A patient presenting with the features of extreme muscular weakness, aches and pains in the bones, repeated long bone fractures, polyuria and acute pain in the abdomen (renal colic or acute haemorrhagic pancreatitis) is probably suffering from an overactivity of the parathyroid glands.

A patient complaining of severe cramps in the muscles of the limbs, fatigue, weakness and lack of concentration following an operation in the neck (possibly for toxic goitre) may be sufficient to diagnose *tetany due to damage of the parathyroid glands.* There may be history of hoarseness, stridor (laryngismus stridulus) or convulsions. Certain clinical and biochemical tests are essential before labelling the case as hypo or hyperparathyroidism.

EXAMINATION : The hypotonicity of the muscles and the peculiar waddling gait in hyperfunction of the gland may draw the attention of the clinician.

Risus sardonicus (i.e. spasms of facial and masseter muscles) the dry and rough skin, falling off of scalp hair, malformed teeth and brittle nails may be the common manifestations of hypoparathyroidism.

Examination of the eye may reveal a cataract or "calcium deposits" in the conjunctiva or at the margin of the cornea– this can be detected by slit lamp examination–in hypo or hyperfunction of the gland respectively. Ophthalmoscopic examination should be done routinely to detect papilloedema that may be due to increased intracranial tension resulting from hypoparathyroidism.

Examination of the skeletal system may reveal tender swellings over the bones, tenderness of the hands, swelling in the jaw, kyphosis, bowing of the femur, evidences of pathological fractures associated with a tumour in the neck in *hyperparathyroidism.* Painful spasms of the hands with the fingers tightly apposed, flexion of the wrist, hyperextension of the terminal phalanges, thumb adducted and flexed across the palm (the classical "accoucheur hand") and inversion of the foot may be seen in hypoparathyroidism.

Demonstration of increased neuromuscular irritability like spasm of the muscles following tapping of the 7th cranial nerve in the parotid gland (Chvostek's sign); carpopedal spasm following inflation of the sphygmomanometer cuff to a little above the systolic blood pressure (*Trousseau's sign*) and twitching of the muscles following electrical stimulation (*Erb's sign*) must be carried out if there is at all any suspicion of hypofunction of the parathyroid gland.

Other manifestations of hyperirritability of nerves in hypoparathyroidism are–(i) *Hoffmans sign*–Tetanic muscular spasms produced by electrical or mechanical stimulation of a sensory nerve–the ulnar nerve being usually used. (ii) *Kasida's thermic sign of tetany*–Hyperaesthesias and spasms develop after application of hot and cold irritants. (iii) *Pool's Arm and Leg signs*–(a) Tension on the brachial plexus by forceful abduction of an arm causes spasms of the muscles of the hand and arm; (b) Tension of the sciatic nerve by forceful flexion of the thigh on the trunk with the leg extended leads to spasms of leg and foot muscles (iv) *Schlesinger's Leg sign*–Painful spasms of the extremity occurs within seconds to minutes when the hip joint is flexed and the leg extended. (v) *Schultze's tongue dimpling sign* is the dimpling occurring at the points of mechanical stimulus caused by tapping the protruded tongue with a percussion hammer.

Biochemical investigation

(a) Estimation of serum calcium and phosphorus.

Increased serum *calcium* and low serum *phosphorus,* and a low serum *calcium* and high serum *phosphorus* are the characteristics of hyperparathyroidism and hypoparathyroidism respectively (Normal values; Calcium 8.5 to 10.5 mg per 100 ml, Phosphorus 3 to 4.5 mg per 100 ml).

(b) Estimation of serum *alkaline phosphatase* : In hyperparathyroidism it is high—may be even 150 K. A units (Normal 3–13 K A units).

(c) Hydrocortisone suppression test for hypercalcaemia. The patient is given hydrocortisone 40 mg 8 hourly for 10 days. Serum calcium level is estimated before and after giving hydrocortisone. If the hypercalcaemia is due to hyperparathyroidism there will be no *significant change* in the serum calcium level after hydrocortisone for 10 days. If the hypercalcaemia is due to any other causes it always falls significantly usually reaching an almost normal level.

(d) Radioimmunoassay of the parathyroid hormones are done for diagnosis and to localise the tumours when blood is taken from the neck veins with percutaneous catheter.

Radiological study : The important findings are— (i) Subperiosteal erosions of the phalanges (ii) Loss of lamina dura around the teeth and (iii) Nephrocalcinosis in a straight X-ray in hyperparathyroidism. Besides these, it occasionally shows (iv) Pathological fractures (v) Renal stone and (vi) Gastric or duodenal ulcer in a barium meal X-ray of the stomach and duodenum in hyperfunction of the gland.

DIABETES MELLITUS

Diabetes mellitus is a clinical syndrome characterised by hyperglycaemia with or without glycosuria due to a deficiency or diminished effectiveness of insulin. It affects the metabolism of carbohydrate, protein fat, water, and electrolytes and in the long run may terminate in some grave complications.

Many clinical types of diabetes are encountered. At one extreme is the obese elderly person accidentally discovered to have glycosuria insulin independent type of diabetes which starts in adult life (commonly after 40 years) and

usually controlled by dietary restriction alone. This is the type 2 or non-insulin dependent diabetes mellitus (NIDDM) or Maturity Onset Diabetes. At the other extreme is the young adult or child who after a few days or weeks of polyuria, thirst and rapid loss of weight is likely to develop severe keto-acidosis and unless treated with insulin promptly, may rapidly progress of coma (Juvenile Onest Diabetes or Type I or insulin dependent diabetes). There is another group of patient known to have maturity onset diabetes in young (MODY).

Diabetes mellitus is thus classified as :

(A) Primary–*Type I or IDDM* which may be–

Type IA – transient pancreatic isletcell antibodies (PICA), no autoimmune features.

Type IB–persistent PICA, other auto-immune features.

Type II or NIDDM : In contrast to type I, these have no HLA associations and may be (i) obese, (ii) non-obese or (iii) MODY.

(B) Impaired glucose tolerance : In this the venous plasma glucose concentration 2 hr after 75 gm glucose lies between 8 and 11 mmol/L.

(C) Gestational diabetes mellitus is first recognised during pregnancy but remits afterwards.

(D) Previous abnormality (latent diabetes) : Glucose tolerance is abnormal during stressful situations e.g. CVA, AMI, infections etc.

(E) Potential diabetes : Potential diabetics are those who may eventually develop overt syndrome e.g.–(i) the identical non-diabetic twin of a diabetic, (ii) individual whose both parents are diabetic, (iii) individual with one diabetic parent, the other parent having a diabetic parent, sibling, offspring or a sibling with a diabetic child, (iv) woman giving birth to a live or still born child weighting

4.5 kg or more at birth, or to a still born child with islet cell hyperplasia not related to rhesus incompatibility. (v) individuals with HLA indentical to those of diabetic sibling, and (vi) individuals with circulating PICA.

(F) Diabetes mellitus associated with–(i) hormonal changes e.g. Cushing syndrome, (ii) drug induced (iii) pancreatic diseases, (iv) genetic and chromosomal syndromes, (v) insulin receptor abnormalities, (vi) others eg hyperlipoproteinamia, types III, IV, V, type I glycogenosis, chronic renal failure, hepatic cirrhosis etc.

Aetiologically diabetes can be classified into different types e.g. –

(A) *Primary or Idiopathic diabetes* : Majority of the patients are included in this group. Aetiology is exactly not known but certain factors are thought to be responsible for both insulin dependent and insulin independent diabetes.

(i) Genetic factors : Responsible for mainly the type II and possibly for type I. Dominant inheritance is found in maturity onset diabetes or insulin independent group.

(ii) HLA system : Association with HLAB 8 or B 15 is common in younger patients i.e. type I.

(iii) Viral infections : Mumps and Coxsackie B4 virus infection are thought to be responsible. Staphylococcal infections in older patient may unmask the latent diabetes.

(iv) Autoimmunity : Another hypothesis for insulin dependent diabetes as it may be associated with other autoimmune diseases like Hashimoto's thyroiditis, hyperthyroidism, Addison's disease etc.

(v) Obesity Frequently associated with diabetes.

(vi) Diets : Excessive eating may be a predisposing factor mainly type II.

(B) *Secondary diabetes* : A definite pathological process is mainly type II responsible for this group.

(i) Pancreatic diabetes : Carcinoma, chronic pancreatitis, removal of pancreas during surgery, haemochromatosis, cystic fibrosis, pancreatic calcification etc. lead to destruction of the islet cells.

(ii) Endocrine diabetes due to presence of circulating insulin antagonist hormones in blood :

    (a) Growth hormone e.g. in acromegaly.

    (b) Adrenocortical hormones e.g. in Cushing syndrome.

    (c) Adrenaline e.g. phaeochromocytoma.

    (d) Thyroid hormone e.g. hyperthyroidism.

    (e) Associated with other apudomas.

(iii) Iatrogenic diabetes : Corticosteroids, thiazide dieuretics oral contraceptives, frusemide, diazoxide etc. may precipitate diabetes in genetically susceptible individuals.

(iv) Genetic and chromosomal syndromes e.g. DIDMOAD (diabetes insipidus, diabetes mellitus, optic atrophy, and deafness–and autosomal recessive disorder), Friedreich's ataxia, muscular dystrophy, Down's syndrome, Turner's syndrome. Refsum's syndrome etc.

(v) Insulin receptor abnormalities,–Type A is a primary defect of the receptor and type B is due to autoantibody to the receptors.

(vi) Miscellaneous group–see (F) above.

Clinical observation

Many patients are first detected to have glycosuria during a routine examination. No symptom or abnormal physical signs may be present.Some patients are first seen complaining of the symptoms directly attributable to the diabetic state. Symptoms of hyperglycaemia – polyuria, nocturia, and temporary visual disturbances; symptoms of water and electrolyte loss–thirst and dry mouth due to dehydration, weakness and wasting of the muscles due to increased neoglucogenesis, loss of subcutaneous fat due to increased lipolysis pruritus vulvae etc. are frequently complained of by elderly obese diabetics and their external genitalia are susceptible to infection by monilia.

In the fulminating case the most characteristic features are those of dehydration—dry mouth, furred tongue, soft eyes, inelastic skin, marked loss of body weight, low blood pressure, rapid pulse, and breathing is deep and sighing if there is acidosis.

An excess loss of potassium following diabetic ketosis may give rise to extreme muscular weakness, abdominal distension, constipation, vomiting, depression and impairment of intellectual activity. Clinical examination may reveal abdominal distension associated with reduced bowel sound, depressed tendon reflex, presence of extrasystoles or other cardiac arrhythmias. ECG may reveal a low voltage curve, flattened T waves and prominent U wave following the T wave.

Diabetic ketoacidosis and diabetes with acute infections are to be considered as acute emergencies.

The physical signs will depend much 'on the mode of presentation'. Evidences of causative disease like acromegaly, Cushing syndrome, phaeochromocytoma, chronic pancreatitis, haemochromatosis are to be sought for.

Follow up examinations are necessary for the recognition of known complications affecting different systems :
I. Neurological complications :

(a) *Sensory* : Acute peripheral neuritis due to metabolic disturbance (sorbitol pathway) and chronic peripheral neuritis due to diabetic angiopathy of vasa nervorum, loss of joint and vibration sensations etc. Peripheral neuritis is symmetrical distal in distribution and usually of subacute type.

(b) *Neuromuscullar* : Loss of tendon reflexes, diabetic amyotrophy characterised by wasting and pain in the proximal muscles (thighs), weakness, paralysis, extraocular muscle palsies etc. Diabetic amyotrophy is usually asymmetrical.

(c) *Cranial nerves* : Second, third and fourth and sixth cranial nerves may be involved.

(d) *Autonomic* :

(i) Gastrointestinal disturbances like nocturnal diarrhaea, delayed gastric emptying etc.

(ii) Genitourinary complaints like atonic bladder, impotency, retrograde ejaculation etc.

(iii) Ulcers of skin, diminished or absent sweating and oedema of the lower limbs.

(iv) Pupillary changes.

(v) Vascular abnormalities like orthostatic hypotension.

(vi) Joint changes e.g. Charcot's joint or neuropathic joint.

II. Cardiovascular complications : (i) Ischaemic heart disease ranging from angina of effort to acute myocardial infarction, (ii) diabetic diffuse small vessel disease causing cardiomyopathy and (iii) vascular gangrene mainly dry gangrene occur due to atherosclerotic process. *The recent ideas* about diabetic foot ulcer, are, however, (i) they are primarily due to abnormal pressure distribution resulting from diabetic neuropathy, (ii) Secondarily aggravated by bony distortion of feet, (iii) predominantly due to sensory deficits precluding pain recognition, (iv) diminished vascularity helps in maintaining and (v) infections to which a diabetic is susceptible for other reasons too. Diabetes mellitus with acute myocardial infarction or ischaemic heart disease and cerebrovascular accident are frequently encountered in clinical practice. Thus if a patient complains of paralysis, one should enquire about symptoms of diabetes and routine examination of urine and blood should be done.

III. Respiratory complications : Pulmonary tuberculosis, pneumonia, bronchopneumonia, lung abscesses etc. are found more frequently amongst diabetics.

IV. Urogenital complications : Balanitis cystitis, pyelonephritis, K W (Kimmelstiel Wilson) syndrome (characterised by diabetes, hypertension, anasarca, proteinuria and hypoproteinaemia); renal arteriosclerosis, papillitis necroticans, acute renal failure etc.

V. Skin complications :

(a) Infections– Staphylococcal infections like, boil, carbuncle, furuncle pruritus, pyoderma, candidiasis, dermatophytosis etc.

(b) Diabetic pruritus–especially pruritus vulvae.

(c) Diabetic dermopathy–hyperpigmented and retracted scars seen in young persons, over the shin bones.

(d) Necrobiosis lipoidica diabeticorum (NLD)– patchy lesion, well circumscribed, central part yellowish in colour. Commonly seen over the lower extremities or over the forearmes.

(e) Progressive lipodystrophy and insulin lipodystrophy.

(f) Xanthoma diabeticorum.

(g) Carotenosis – Yellowish discolouration of the skin and palms sometimes seen in diabetic patients.

VI. Eye complications :

(a) Transient myopia, sometimes hypermetropia.

(b) Cataract–(i) Earliar occurrence of senile cataract– common (ii) True or juvenile diabetic cataract–not common.

(c) Diabetic ophthalmoplegia–3rd nerve (common) and 6th nerve palsies. These though due to infarction of the nerve trunk, are reversible.

(d) Vitreous humour–Two types of degenerative changes

are seen—(i) Asteroid hyalitis—these are small white innumerable vitreous opacities consisting of calcium containing acidic lipids. (ii) Synchisis scintillans—Shiny opacities containing cholesterol which settle to the bottom when head is moved.

(e) Optic atrophy :

(f) Retinal changes— These may be *simple* or *background or may progress to proliferative retinopathy.*

(a) *Diabetic maculopathy* or *simple retinopathy*— This includes the following sequential changes—

(i) Increased capillary permeability, (ii) Capillary closure and dilatation, (iii) Microaneurysms, (iv) Arteriovenous communications. (v) Dilated veins, (vi) Dot and blot haemorrhages, (vii) Cotton wool spots or soft exudates, and (viii) Hard exudates.

(b) Proliferative retinopathy— This includes—

(i) Neovascularisation. (ii) Bleeding from new vessels, (iii) Retinitis proliferans i.e. scarring following the haemorrhage, (iv) Vitreous haemorrhages and opacities and (v) Retinal detachment leading finally to blindness.

VII. Gastrointestinal complications : Emphysematous cholecystitis and cholelithiasis, superior mesenteric artery occlusion giving rise to abdominal angina, intestinal pseudoobstruction because of autonomic neuropathy causing disordered gutmotility, blind loop syndrome and malabsorption.

VIII. Obstetric complications : Birth of a large size baby (more than 10 lbs), Still birth, toxaemia of pregnancy and hydramnios.

IX. Coma : Which may be due to

(i) Diabetic ketoacidosis.

(ii) Hyperglycaemic nonketotic diabetic coma.

(iii) Lactic acidosis, which may be caused by the biguanide group of antidiabetic drugs.

(iv) Hypoglycaemic coma, which may be caused by oral-antidiabetics or insulin.

(v) Coma due to other associated diseases like cerebrovascular accidents, uraemia, hepatic failure etc.

Diagnosis of Diabetes Mellitus and Complications

Diabetes is suspected from the history of the patient, symptoms attributable to diabetes or complications of the disease and finally confirmed by certain biochemical ivestigations. Sometimes a routine blood or urine test performed for some other purpose betrays the diagnosis to the clinician.

(a) Examination of urine : (i) Determination of *specific gravity* (range may be 1035 to 1045 in diabetes mellitus)

(ii) Detection of *sugar* by Benedict's test. The details of this test have been outlined elsewhere.

Alternatives are : (a) Clinistix : Paper stick impregnated with an enzyme preparation which turns purple when dipped in urine containing glucose. No other urinary constituent gives such reaction. (b) Clinitest tablets : Semi-quantitative method of testing urine for reducing sub-stances including glucose.

(iii) **Albumin** : (a) Boiling test : The details of the test have already been described elsewhere. (b) Albustix tablet : Proteinuria may also be detected by albustix tablet.

(iv) **Acetone** : (a) Rothera's test–described earlier. (b) Ferric chloride test–A possitive ferric chloride reaction is obtained only if acetoacetic acid is present in consider-able amount. (c) Acetest tablet–It provides a simple method of testing urine for acetone. One tablet is placed on a white surface and a drop of urine is gently placed on the tablet. If acetone is present, a mauve colour develops.

(v) Microscopic examination of urine for pus cells, casts and RBC (may be suggestive of pyelonephritis or necrotising papillitis).

(B) Blood :

(i) **Routine blood examination** for haemoglobin percentage, total count and differential count and sedimentation rate. E.S.R. is raised when there is superadded infection; anaema may be due to renal failure.

(ii) **Biochemical study** : (a) In patients with symptoms a fasting venous plasma glucose concentration > 8 mmol/L is *diagnostic.* If it is < 6 mmol/L the diagnosis is *excluded.* When the fasting level is between 6 and 8 mmol/L the patient is given a 75 gm oral glucose load and if the venous plasma glucose concentration at 2 hr is > 11 mmol/L the test is diagnostic of diabetes; while a value between 8 and 11 mmol/L is *diagnostic of impaired glucose tolerance.* (b) In patients without symptoms the criteria include an additional abnormal level after the 75 gm glucose load e.g. a 1 hr value of 11 mmol/L or higher and in no case *the diagnosis of diabetes is made on the basis of a single abnormal glucose value in an asymptomatic patient.*

According to the WHO Expert Committee on Diabetes (1980), a 75 gm glucose load should be used, and the concentration of glucose in venous whole blood estimated by a specific enzyme assay should be as follows :

Glucose concentration in mg%

	Normal	Diabetic
Fasting	< 100 (5.5 mmol/1)	> 120 (7.0 mmol/1)
2 hours after glucose	<120 (7.0 mmol/1)	>180 (10.0 mmol/1)

(c) Intravenous glucose tolerance test : If the patient is unable to take glucose by mouth or if there is vomiting, intravenous glucose tolerance test is done.

(d) Estimation of plasma protein : Diminished in KW syndrome. Simultaneous examination of the urine may reveal massive albuminuria.

(e) Blood cholesterol : Raised in diabetes mellitus in some cases.

(f) Estimation of plasma non-esterified fatty acid (NEFA). Plasma NEFA level may be high with normal plasma concentration of glucose and insulin in case of maturity onset diabetes.

(g) Estimation of blood urea and NPN : These are elevated with the onset of renal failure (Normal value : 20 to 40 mg%).

(C) Test for diagnosis of primary causative diseases like acromegaly, Cushing syndrome are to be undertaken if the history is suggestive.

(D) Routine ophthalmoscopic examination particularly for microaneurysm at the venous end of the capillary.

(E) Routine chest X-ray for associated pulmonary tuberculosis and electrocardiogram to detect any cardiac involvement are done.

Recognition of prediabetes (Vide supra)

(a)   Obesity, heredofamilial history (chance of diabetes is 85% in offspring if both father and mother are diabetic).

(b)   History of recurrent spontaneous abortion, still birth, or birth of a big baby.

(c)   Hyperglycaemia during the stress of pregnancy, severe infection or injury.

(d)   Appearence of cataract in a very young age.

(i) Glucose tolerance test–Normal.

(ii) Cortisone loaded glucose tolerance test : Higher blood sugar curve than in an ordinary glucose tolerance test. The administration of cortisone often causes glycosuria.

Thus the test is helpful for detecting pre-diabetic states.

Causes of glycosuria :

A. Associated with hyperglycaemia
    (a) Idiopathic – diabetes mellitus
    (b) Affection of islets of Langerhans
        (i) Pancreatitis   (ii) Carcinoma of pancreas
        (iii) Surgical removal   (iv) Cystic fibrosis
        (v) Haemochromatosis
    (c) Endocrine-causes
        (i) Acromegaly   (ii) Hyperthyroidism
        (iii) Cushing syndrome (iv) Phaeochromocytoma
        (v) Tumour of alpha cell
    (d) Intracranial causes
        (i) Brain tumours   (ii) Injury to brain
        (iii) Damage of hypothalamus
        (iv) Emotional stress
        (v) Cerebral haemorrhage
    (e) Metabolic causes
        (i) Starvation   (ii) Obesity
        (iii) After burns of fractures
        (iv) Infections
    (f) Renal causes
        (i) Uraemia
    (g) Drugs
        (i) Corticosteroids and **ACTH** administration
        (ii) Diuretics like chlorothiazides, hydrochlorothia-
            zides etc.
        (iii) Contraceptive pill, (iv) Diazoxide.
    (h) Miscellaneous
        (i) After myocardial infarction
        (ii) Alimentary glycosuria
B. Not associated with hyperglycaemia
        (i) Renal glycosuria   (ii) Fanconi syndrome
        (iii) Heavy metals like mercury, lead poisoning

(iv) Drugs like– morphine, chloroform etc.
C. Others
    (i) Pregnancy   (ii) Rheumatoid arthritis
    (iii) Associated with malignancies
    (iv) Poisoning with organophosphorus compounds.

Appendix to Chapter 1

(1) *Kallman's syndrome*– This is a congenital disease of the hypothalamus characterised by LH and/or FSH deficiency with anaemia and midline defects e.g. cleft lip, cleft palate, ectopia vesicae etc. This is the commonest form of hypogonadotropic hypogonadism in isolated form in both sexes, is a familial condition and may be associated with renal agenesis. An incomplete form of Kallman's syndrome is the "fertile eunuch syndrome."

(2) *Prader wili syndrome* is a condition of hypothalamic obesity characterised by voracious appetite, gross obesity, mental retardation, hypogonadism, diabetes mellitus and small hands and feet.

(3) *Causes of hyperprolactinaemic* (many of which may result in galactorrhoea)–

(A) Physiological : Neonatal period; puberty is girls; coitus and orgasm; nipple stimulation; pregnancy and suckling; sleep; and stress.

(B) Drugs : Dopamine receptor blockers (e.g. phenothiazines; haloperidol; metoclopramide sulpiride etc); CNS dopamine depleting agents (e.g. reserpine, methyl dopa); miscellaneous e.g. oestrogens, TRH etc.

(C) Hypothalamic or pituitary stalk lesions : Craniopharyngiomas, gliomas, pinealomas, sarcoidosis, tuberculosis, eosinophilic granuloma, sectioning of the stalk traumatic or otherwise.

(D) Pituitary tumours : Prolactin cell, mixed prolactin cell/ growth hormone; acidophil stem cell; mixed prolactin cell/ corticotrophin cell.

(E) Others : Idiopathic or functional hypothyroidism; chronic renal failure; ectopic e.g. secreted by a bronchogenic carcinoma or a hypernephroma.

(4) *MEN (Multiple Endocrine Neoplasia) Syndromes :* These may be of three types (I. IIA and IIB) familial and inherited usually as autosomal dominant. In type I the adenomas predominantly are those of parathyroid, pituitary and pancreas, but adrenocortical and thyroid adenomas may occur. Type IIA comprises medullary carcinoma of thyroid, phaeochromocytomas that are usually bilateral and rarely parathyroid adenomas or hyperplasia. Type IIB (sometimes called III) consists of medullary carcinoma of thyroid often associated with a Marfanoid appearance, proximal myopathy, thickened lips, lingual and corneal and eyelid neuromas, ganglioneuromatosis of bowel, skin pigmentation– all these rarely may be associated with parathyroid or adrenal medullary diseases.

CHAPTER 2

THE HAEMOPOIETIC AND LYMPHATIC SYSTEMS

Students quite commonly come across patients presenting with haematological disorders. In these cases, look for the signs of haematological diseases as outlined. It should be emphasised at the outset that very often only a clinical examination is not sufficient to establish a diagnosis. A peripheral blood examination is always required, and often the examination of bone-marrow may be necessary.

Symptoms and signs of (i) anaemia and (ii) haemorrhage should be looked for at the beginning. Through these have been described already in previous chapters, the salient points are summarised here.

(i) *Anaemia :*

    (a) Pallor of the skin, mucous membrane of lips, tongue, buccal cavity, lower palpebral conjuctive, nail beds.

    (b) Dyspnoea, palpitations, angina, right heart failure.

    (c) Claudication and ankle oedema.

    (d) Lassitude, inability to concentrate, dizziness, tinnitus throbbing in the head.

    (e) Anorexia nausea, constipation or diarrhoea.

    (f) In severe anaemia. low grade pyrexia may occur mainly due to elevated basal metabolic rate.

(ii) *Haemorrhage :*

    (a) Occult blood in the stool, melaena.

    (b) Purpura–petechiae and ecchymoses.

    (c) Epistaxis.

    (d) Haemoptysis.

(e) Haematuria and menorrhagia.

(f) Haemarthrosis.

(g) Bleeding from minor cuts and wounds in the skin and mucous membrane for a prolonged period.

Haemorrhage will very often lead to post-haemorrhagic anaemia and this contributes to the signs and symptoms of anaemia already present.

(iii) *Lymph nodes* : All the principal groups of lymph nodes in the body are examined starting from those of the head. Look for enlargement of the principal lymph nodes, and if any group or groups are found enlarged, they should be examined in detail and the following points are to be noted : (a) The groups affected and whether there is generalised lymphadenopathy (vide index for causes). (b) The size of the enlarged lymph nodes. (c) The consistency and whether there is any fluctuation, as may be present due to caseous necrosis in tuberculous lymphadenitis. (d) The attachments of the nodes–whether discrete or confluent or attached to the sorrounding structures. (e) Tenderness, which is most commonly due to acute pyogenic infections. (f) Any skin abnormality in the vicinity and draining areas of the node.

(iv) *Liver and spleen* : Being parts of the haemopoietic and lymphoreticular systems, these two organs are commonly enlarged in haematological disorders. Not uncommonly they are found to be massively enlarged.

Palpate the liver and the spleen as outlined in the chapter on the gastrointestinal system. Sometimes even an enlarged liver may be difficult to feel. In such cases percussion will give valuable information regarding the degree of enlargement. The extent of enlargement should be measured in centimeters or in terms of fingers from the point of cross-section of the midclavicular line with the costal margin to the furthest extent of the organs. N.B.–Spleen is impalpable in sickle cell disease as it undergoes atrophy due to repeated infarctions and contributes to hyposplenism.

(v) *The mouth* : If the students neglect this part of examination, they might miss important findings. The lips, gums, tongue, buccal mucosa, palate, fauces and tonsils are all examined step by step as has been discussed in the examination of the gastrointestinal system. Ulcers, necrotic areas and thrush and other fungal infections of the mucous membranes are seen in immune-depressed states, and acute leukaemias and lymphomas especially during the long periods of marrow hypoplasia and neutropenia consequent upon deliberate attempts at maximum cell kill.

(vi) *The skin* : Look for pallor, icterus and purpura (Petechiae and ecchymoses), search for areas of infiltration that may be present in leukaemias and lymphomas. Look for fungal and other infections of the skin commonly present in patients with immune-deficiency. Look for any ulceration over the legs, particularly over the malleoli, that may be present in hereditary haemolytic anaemias. Scratch marks may be found on the skin since pruritus is common in myeloproliferative disorders, Hodgkin's disease and polycythaemia. Elasticity of the skin should be routinely looked for so as not to miss the rare Ehlers-Danlos syndrome and pseudoxanthoma elasticum (PXE), the connective tissue diseases that may be present with abnormal skin elasticity, bleeding and bruising.

(vii) *Sternal tenderness* : Look for sternal tenderness that may be present in acute leukaemias, thallasaemia, multiple myeloma, metastases etc. or may have resulted from too vigorous aspiration of the sternal marrow during diagnostic puncture. Ask for pain and tenderness in other bones, e.g. pelvic bones, vertebrae and long bones. These may be present in malabsorption states causing osteomalacia, or may be associated with sickle cell disease e.g. due to infarction and also in local and disseminated malignancies.

(viii) *Ophthalmoscopic examination* : A drop or two of a mydriatic solution (e.g. Drosyn) is instilled into the eyes and when the pupils are sufficiently dilated, examine the fundus oculi with an ophthalmoscope. Retinal haemorrhages may be found in severe anaemia, thrombocytopenic purpura, leukaemia etc. These may be punctate, splinter or flame shaped. Retinal haemorrhages, exudates, papillaedema and very rarely permanent optic atrophy may follow sudden massive haemorrhage, e.g. from the gastrointestinal tract. Optic atrophy may result from cyanocobalamin deficiency. Polycythaemia may cause venous engorgement and leukaemias may produce retinal exudates and also papilloedema, if meningeal involvement occurs.

Examination of blood and Bone-Marrow

Blood : Blood is usually collected by puncturing a vein

in the antecubital fossa (avoiding venous stasis as far as possible) into tubes or vials using either citrate or heparin or EDTA as anticoagulant. The following are the tests that are usually performed:

(i)   A thin smear is carefully prepared, stained by any of Romanowsky's method (usually Leishman's stain as used) and then examined under the oil immersion lens of the microscope. All the three formed elements of blood are examined. The erythrocytes are examined for their size, shape, haemoglobin concentration, immature forms (normoblasts), and arrangement of the cell (for excess rouleaux formation). Abnormalities in size is called anisocytosis, and abnormalities of shape is known as poikilocytosis.

With leucocytes, a differential count is done, and abnormal cell and immature forms are particularly looked for.

The morphology and approximate numbers of platelets are determined.

Also look for parasites e.g. malaria, LD bodies, microfilaria, Bartonella bacilliformis (in oraya fever) etc.

(ii) The haemoglobin level is determined. Sahli's haemoglobinometer is usually employed. A more improved method uses spectrophotometry after converting haemoglobin into cyanmethaemoglobin.

(iii) Volume of packed red cells (VPRC or PCV) is determined by the help of Wintrobe's haematocrit.

(iv) Total counts of red cells, leucocytes and platelets are determined commonly by using haemocytometer in well equipped centres, this is done by using electronic devices as with the former method chances of error are more. Reticulocyte count is also performed after supravital staining.

(v)   LE cells may be seen in specially prepared peripheral blood and is seen in (i) SLE (most commonly), (ii) chronic hepatitis (iii) occasionally in patients getting hydrallazine, (iv) some cases of penicillin sensitivity. (v) some cases of acquired haemolytic anaemia, (vi) aparently idiopathic thrombocytopenic purpura etc. The LE cell is to be differentiated from a somewhat similar Tart cell found in LE cell preparations of blood containing abnormally excessive globulin.

Bone-Marrow : Bone-marrow is obtained either by (i) aspiration, using a syringe and a specially designed needle or by (ii) trephine biopsy. Aspirates may be obtained either by sternal puncture or iliac crest puncture. The manubrium or body of the sternum is punctured, a little distance from the midline. Trephine biopsy is always taken from the iliac crest.

A slide is prepared, suitably, stained by Romanowsky's method and examined, or the marrow is examined histologically after fixation in formalin.

Examination includes–(i) assessment of cellularity of the marrow, (ii) the type and activity of erythropoiesis, (iii) the number and types of developing white cells, (iv) the number and type of megakaryocytes, (v) the myeloid erythroid ratio normally 3-4 : 1), (vi) the presence of foreign or tumour cells. (vii) the presence of parasites or organisms, and (viii) the iron content of the marrow by special staining e.g. Prussian blue stain that stains the iron granules blue. Marrow aspiration helps in (i) the diagnosis of megaloblastic anaemias, leukaemias, multiple myeloma, secondary carcinoma of bones, lipoid storage diseases, kala-azar, aplastic anaemias, agranulocytosis, idiopathic thrombocytopenic purpura, sideroblastic anaemia, hypersplenism, hypochromic anaemia due to iron deficiency (ii) excluding leukaemia and megaloblastic anaemia, and (iii) sometimes in assessing the response to treatment in acute leukaemias and (iv) assessing the prognosis in aplastic anaemia and agranulocytosis.

The Leukaemias

The leukaemias are a group of disorders characterised by widespread malignant proliferation of leucocytes and their precursors throughout the tissues of the body with a variable circulating component. Classification : The leukaemias are broadly classified into two groups, acute and chronic. The distinctions between the two groups are clinical as well as haematological.

Clinically, the patient with acute leukaemias almost invariably pursue a rapidly fatal course without effective treatment; whereas the chronic leukaemia patient may survive for years.

Haematologically, in acute leukaemias most primitive blast cells are characteristic findings in blood or bone-marrow; whereas in chronic leukaemias differentiation to mature types of cells is seen and blasts are few and far between.

Subleukaemic leukaemia : This variety presents with normal or low leucocyte counts with abnormal cells in the blood.

Aleukaemic leukaemia : In this variety the leucocyte count in the blood is usually subnormal with no abnormal cells. Hence the diagnosis depends on examination of the bone marrow.

Preleukaermia : This belongs to the heterogeneous group including also the myelodysplastic syndromes and refractory anaemia with excess blasts (RAEB) which have in common the anaemia not responding to conventional therapy, neutropenia, thrombocytopenia, monocytosis and splenomegaly. All these conditions subsequently develop clinicohaematological acute leukaemias, the chane of which is very high if chromosomal abnormalities remain associated.

Classification of acute leukaemias : The acute leukaemias have been classified into acute lymphoblastic leukaemia (ALL) and acute nonlymphoblastic or acute myelogenous leukaemia (AML).

The French-American-British (FAB) Co-operative Group has subdivided ALL on the basis of lymphoblast morphology into three groups–L_1, L_2 and L_3. The L_1 variety is commonly seen in children and consists of small, homogeneous blast cells with little cytoplasm and inconspicuous nucleoli. The L_2 is more frequent in adults and consists of large haterogeneous blasts with abundant cytoplasm and nucleoli.

The L_3 is the rare Burkitt' type with large blasts containing vacuolated blue cytoplasm.

ALL can also be classified on the basis of cell types– T cell type, B cell type, receptor silent type and undifferentiated type.

AML according to FAB classification is subdivided into six types–M_1 to M_6. M_1 is myeloblastic without maturation; M_2 is myeloblasitc with maturation; M_3 hypergranular promyelocytic; M_4 myelomonocytic; M_5 is monocytic either poorly differentiated with monoblasts or well differentiated with more mature monocytes; and M_6 is erythroleukaemia.

The chronic leukaemias are broadly classified into— (i) chronic myeloid leukaemia and (ii) chronic lymphatic leukaemia.

Eosinophilic leukaemia : It is a rare variant of chronic myeloid leukaemia. Some suggest that it is allied to polyarteritis nodosa and while chromosomal analysis is usually normal, the disease is usually progressive and the course can be partially influenced by steroid therapy.

Hairy cell and prolymphocytic leukaemias are variants of chronic lymphatic leukaemia. Hairy cell leukaemia is also known as leukaemic reticuloendotheliosis. It usually affects elderly males, often associated with massive splenomegaly without lymphadenopathy and while lymphocytosis may be slight, they have characteristic cytoplasmic villi or 'haris'. These cell are possibly of B-cell lineage.

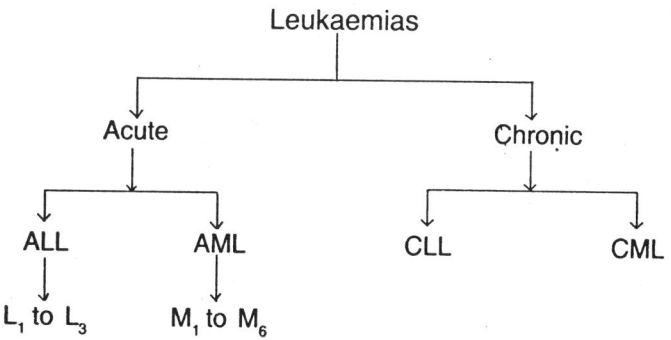

Features of acute leukaemia : It may occur at any age, and in adults is at least as frequent as in children. In children the highest incidence is during the first six years. From the clinical features the morphological types cannot be distinguished although gum hypertrophy and ulcerative lesions of the rectum and the vagina are more common in the monoblastic type, and the lymphoblastic variety is predominant in young children.

The presenting manifestations, in order of decreasing frequency, are anaemia, fever and malaise, haemorrhagic manifestations, infections of the mouth and pharynx, bone and joint pains, upper respiratory tract infection, superficial lymph node enlargement, diarrhoea and vomiting, mediastinal pressure, central nervous system involvement and skin rashes.

A typical blood picture shows normochromic anaemia, thrombocytopenia, variable leucocyte count–usually less than 100×10^9 per litre–and the majority of them are typical or atypical blast cells.

With specific therapy, on an average children survive for two years and adults for less than 12 months.

Immediate-causes of death are haemorrhage (especially cerebral), infections, anaemia, and exhaustion.

Chronic myeloid leukaemia – Usually occurring between 30 and 60 years it is usually insidious in onset. Manifestations in order of reducing frequency are those of anaemia, splenomegaly, raised metabolic rate, haemorrhage (especially bruising), acute abdominal pain, bone and joint pains, menstrual disturbances, neurological symptoms, priapism secondary gout, skin disorders and disturbances of vision or hearing. A few patients are diagnosed accidentally during routine blood examinations.

A typical blood picture shows moderate anaemia, grossly elevated leucocyte count with a complete granulocyte spectrum (with 20–50% myelocytes) and normal or raised platelet count. In the bone-marrow aspirate in 80–90% cases, the Philadelphia (Ph[1]) chromosome can be demonstrated.

Biochemically there is a high serum vitamin B_{12} concentration, while leukocyte alkaline phosphatase (LAP) is low (which is also classically seen in paroxymal nocturnal haemoglobinuria).

Average survival time is 3 years.

Most frequent termination of the chronic phase is blast cell transformation when the disease becomes refractory to treatment.

Chronic lymphocytic leukaemia – Usually occurs between 45 and 75 years. Males are affected twice as frequently as females. The onset is insidious. In order of reducing frequency, the clinical manifestations are superficial lymph node enlargement, anaemia, haemorrhage, raised metabolic rate, splenomegaly, gastrointestinal cutaneous and nervous system involvement and bone or joint pains.

A typical blood picture shows variable degree of normochromic normocytic anaemia, leucocytosis which is usually less than that of CML with raised lymphocyte count (90–95%) and normal or reduced platelet counts.

Average life expectancy is 3 to 4 years; but there is considerable individual variation. Death usually results from anaemia, haemorrhage and infections.

The Lymphomas

Lymphomas are diseases of the lymphatic system characterised clinically by progressive tumour like enlargement of lymphatic tissue with eventual fatality; and histologically by multiplication of one or more of the elements normally present in lymph nodes to the extent of destruction of nodal architecture.

The lymphomas are broadly classified into two groups—Hodgkin's lymphoma and non-Hodgkin lymphoma. The cell of origin of Hodgkin's disease is most possible the *dendritic interdigitacing cells* found in the interfollicular regions of the lymphnodes which belong to the monocyte-histiocyte series, while the non-Hodgkin lymphomas develop either from a monoclonal B cell series or do not possess any distinctive cell surface markers and very few are derivatives of tissue histiocytes.

Hodgkin's lymphoma is subdivided histologically into four groups—lymphocyte predominant, nodular sclerosis, mixed cellularity type and lymphocyte depleted type.

Non-Hodgkin lymphomas are either nodular or diffuse type. Each of these may again be well differentiated lymphocytic, poorly differentiated lymphocytic, mixed histiocytic laymphocytic, histiocytic or lymphoblastic.

The non-Hodgkin lymphomas are monoclonal proliferations of B-cells, T cells or histiocytes or which the B cell tumours are most frequent and true histiocytic lymphomas are rare (**BMJ**, 577, 293, 1986).

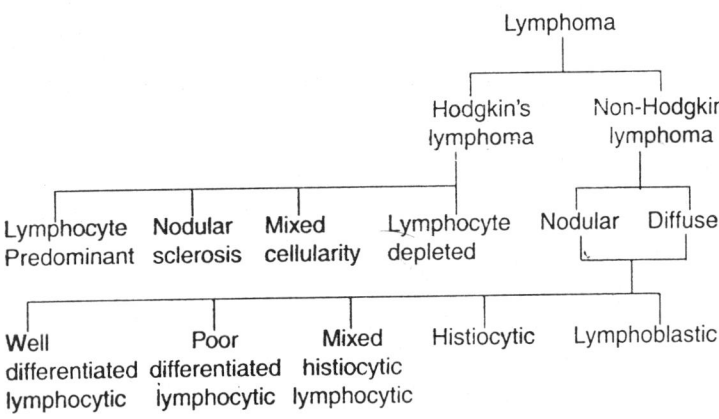

Burkitt's tumour is a variant of lymphocytic lymphoma occurring almost exclusively in children between 2 and 14 years of age. It is found mostly in low lying tropical areas of Africa. There are evidences that the Epstein-Barr virus is aetiologically associated with Burkitt's lymphoma and nasopharyngeal carcinoma.

Hodgkin's disease–Usually occurs between 20–40 years of age, males being 2-3 times more commonly affected than females. In over half the cases, superficial lymph node enlargement is the presenting features. Other features include malaise, sweating, weight loss, anorexia pruritus, pyrexia which may be Pel-Ebstein type, mediastinal pressure, abdominal pain, nervous system involvement, skin manifestation (usually herpes zoster), bone pain, splenomegaly and anaemia. One-sixth of the patients complain of alcohol induced pain. Characteristic histological picture of lymph node biopsy shows Reed-Sternberg giant cells with loss of nodal architecture and pleomorphic appearance of the cells.

Survival time, though varies widely, is 2-3 years on an average.

Clinical Staging of Lymphomas

Stage I is a single lymph node region (or an extralymphatic site or organ) involvement.

Stage II is 2 or more lymph node-regions (or one extralymphatic organ or site+one or more lymph node region) on the same side of diaphragm.

Stage III is involvement on both sides of the diaphragm splenic or localised extralymphatic organ or site involvement. In subgroup III_1 upper abdominal lymphatic structures are involved in III_2 lower abdominal nodes are involved.

Stage IV is disseminated or diffuse involvement of one or more extralymphatic tissues of organs $\pm$ associated lymph node involvement. All these different stages may be either B when associated with pyrexia (101^0F) and / or night sweats and / or unexplained weight loss > 10% in the last 6 months or A when none of these are present.

The Bleeding Disorders

Bleeding disorders may be caused by one or more of the following three factors :

(i)   Decrease in platelet count or normal but ina-equately functioning platelets or both.

(ii) Defect in or damage to the blood vessels.

(iii) Defect in the machanism of blood clotting.

In all these conditions there is an abnormal propensity for bleeding. Haemorrhages in the skin and mucous membrane that are less than 2 mm in diameter are known as petechiae. Diffuse, flat haemorrhages larger than this are known as ecchymoses. If there is a definite swelling the lesion is called haematoma.

Any condition in which there is bleeding into the skin is known as *purpura*. Purpura may be either *localised* or *generalised*.

Localised purpura may be–senile purpura, orthostatic purpura, mechanical purpura, adrenocorticosteroid induced purpura, purpura due to Ehlers-Danlos syndrome etc.

Generalised purpura may be due either to platelet abnormalities or vascular damage.

(I) **Platelet abnormalities** : Platelet abnormalities may be thrombocytopenia, thrombocytopathia or thrombocythaemia.

(i)   Thrombocytopenia is a decrease in the number of platelets in the circulating blood; the bleeding does not become troublesome so long as the platelet count remains above 30,000/cmm. Thrombocytopenia may result from–(a) increased destruction of platelets, (b) increased consumption of platelets, or, (c) failure of platelet production.

(a)   Increased destruction of platelets : The commonest disease of this group is the autoimmune idiopathic thrombocytopenic purpura. It occurs in children between 2 and 6 years of age in the form of an acute self-limiting disease. In older children and young adults, it occurs as a more chronic condition, particularly more frequently in females. The acute type usually occurs about 3 weeks after an infectious fever e.g. chicken pox, measles, rubella or infectious mononucleosis. There is an *autoantibody* of IgG type against platelets in ITP and the spleen sequesters and destroys, and sensitised platelets. The blood picture is usually normal apart from thrombocytopenia unless post-haemorrgagic anaemia complicates the disease. In the bone-marrow an excess of young megakaryocytes are found.

Platelet destruction also occurs immunologically in systemic lupus erythematosus, or may be induced by drugs e.g. hydrallazine, procainamide etc. Non-immunological platelet destruction occurs in hypersplenism.

(b)   Increased consumption of platelets occurs in disseminated intravascular coagulation and thrombotic microangiopathy.

(c)   Failure of platelet production occurs in bone marrow aplasia, acute leukaemias, myelofibrosis. multiple myeloma etc.

All the thrombocytopenic condition cause haemorrhages into the skin and mucous membrane, epistaxis haematuria, menorrhagia, and bleeding from the gastrointestinal tract. Intracranial haemorrhages may occur, but in rare is ITP.

(ii)   Thrombocytopathia–Defective platelet function in presence of a normal count (e.g. Glanzmann's thrombasthenia, Bernard-Soulier syndrome and Wiskott-Aldrich syndrome) characterises this condition.

(iii)   Thrombocythaemia–Very high platelet count associated with a bleeding tendency is found in this condition and may be essential or associated with polycythaemia vera and may cause leuco erythroblastic anaemia.

(II)   *Defect in or damage to the blood vessels :* This includes :

(a)   Henoch-Schonlein purpura.

(b)   Scurvy.

(c)   Infective conditions eg, haemorrhagic small pox, scarlet fever.

(d)   Drug induced purpuras, e.g. quinine, aspirin, phenacetin, sulfonamides etc.

(e)   Macroglobulinaemia etc.

(III)   *Defects in the mechanism of blood clotting :* This includes–

(i)   Hereditary disorders e.g.–

(a)   Haemophilia A or classical haemophilia–Affects males, transmitted by healthy women as it is an X-linked recessive disorder. There is a deficiency of factor VIII. The bleeding tendency usually appears in infancy and uncontrolled wound bleeding is the characteristic symptom.

(b)   Christmas disease or haemophilia B–Caused by factor IX deficiency, the inheritance is same as above.

(c)   Von Willebrand disease–It is characterised by a double defect of abnormal platelet adhesion and a low factor VIII procoagulant activity. The *Von Willebrand factor, a plasma glycoprotein* (required for normal platelet adhesion to the vascular subendothelium) remains complexed with antihaemophilic factor in circulation. In Von Willebrand disease this factor is absent or abnormally low or functionally defective. One of the most common of the inherited bleeding diseases, its inheritance is *autosomal codominance* or *recessive* and affects both sexes. The bleeding sites are skin, mucous membranes and surgical wounds contrasted to haemophilia or Christmas disease where the muscles, joints and surgical wounds are the bleeding sites.

In all the above 3 disorders the *prothrombin times are normal; partial thromboplastin times are prolonged; while the bleeding time is prolonged and ristocetin induced platelet aggregation is impaired only in Von Willebrand disease.*

(ii) Acquired disorders : Found in

  (a) Vitamin K deficiency.

  (b) Liver diseases.

  (c) Anticoagulant drug administration.

  (d) Disseminated intravascular coagulation.

  (e) Massive transfusion of stored blood.

Hess' Capillary Fragility Test or Tourniquet Test : This is an important part of the examination of a patient with bleeding tendencies. It is performed by placing the sphygmomanometer cuff around the upper arm and raising the pressure in the cuff to about 100 mm Hg for 5-7 minutes. If the systolic pressure is less than 100 mm Hg, the pressure in the cuff is raised to halfway between the systolic and diastolic pressures. The cuff is then deflated and 2-3 minutes later the number of petechiae in area of 3 to 5 cm diameter half an inch below the antecubital fossa is counted. Usually this is 10 or less in most normal subjects though up to 20 may be present. More than 20 is abnormal. In severe thrombocytopenia the count may be even 100; test may be negative in mild to moderate thrombocytopenia.

Blood & Blood Product Transfusion

Indications :

(i) Sudden reduction of the blood volume following a haemorrhage.

(ii) Severe anaemia that cannot be relieved by specific therapy e.g. aplastic anaemia, acute leukaemia etc.

(iii) Haemolytic disease of the new born where exchange transfusion becomes necessary.

(iv) Packed red cells, given when there is a danger of circulatory overload.

(v) Platelet transfusions in severe thrombocytopenia due to a failure of platelet production.

(vi) Fresh frozen plasma in Christmas disease.

(vii) Cryoprecipitated antihaemophilia factor in haemophilia.

(viii) Serum albumin in the treatment of haemoconcentration an shock as occurs after extensive burns, Intestinal obstruction, acute pancreatitis etc.

(ix) Granulocytes may be transfused in those with critical neutropenia ($<0.5 \times 10^9$/L) but it is still not very clear whether they significantly reduce the mortality of neutropenic patients. Transfusion of large numbers of irradiated granulocytes (derived from a cell separator) from a patient with CML may help, albeit transiently in infected patients with neutropenia.

Complications : Properly supervised transfusion usually does not result in any adverse effects. Complications occur in 2 to 50 percent of transfusions.

The immediate complications are : (i) Febrile reactions. (ii) Allergic reactions, (iii) Circulatory overload. (iv) Haemolytic reactions. (v) Infections due to contamination of the blood. (vi) Biochemical upsets after massive transfusion due to citrate intoxication. (vii) Air embolism (viii) Thrombocytopenia in rapidly repeated large transfusions leading to bleeding tendencies.

The late complications are : (i) Transmission of diseases e.g. syphilis, malaria, brucellosis, virus B and non A non B hepatitis, AIDS etc. (ii) Immunological sensitisation, (iii) Transfusional haemosiderosis. (iv) Thrombophlebitis.

AQUIRED IMMUNO DEFICIENCY SYNDROME (AIDS)

I. *Definition* by centers for Disease Control (CDC) in USA : "Presence of a reliable diagnosed disease that is at least moderately indicative of an underlying defect in cell mediated immunity."

II. *Virus* which causes at last AIDS are Human Immunodeficiency Virus-I (HIV-1), HIV-2 and HIV-0 (both mostly in Africa). HIV-1 is to be known to have 9 subtypes worldwide (A-H and O). In Thailand mostly subtype E, in Europe especially B. HIV is a retrovirus carrying a special enzyme called reverse transcriptase (RT), which changes the viral RNA into DNA to include it into the genom of the infected cell. In that stage the own immuno system hardly recognizes the virus. HIV has a so-called CD-4 tropism, that means all cells with a

CD-4 surface marker are targets of HIV (T4-lymphocytes, monocytes, macrophages etc.) CD 26 surface antigen might be a second receptor which is important for HIV.

This all leads to a destruction and a decreasing of the number of helper T cells, which is the first serological aspect of the beginning disease. The quotient of CD4/CD8 (helper T cells suppressor T cells//T_H /T_s) is normally ~2; < 1.2 the risk of opportunistic infections is enormously increasing. An other direct effect is reported in the CNS : a subacute enzephalitis caused by HIV leads to a destruction of myelin and atrophy of the brain. In Europe and USA the main group of people which have to face this disease, are homo/bisexual men and i.v. drug users, in Central Africa men and women are both equally infected (mostly caused by prostitution).

III.   *Ways of infection* :

   (a) <u>Sexual intercourse</u> : High risk in promiscuity and "unsafe sex" especially homosexual men and heterosexuals of both gender (in the last group the number is extremely increasing).

   (b) <u>Parenteral</u> : Blood transfusion, other blood products and i.v. drug users without cleaning and especially sharing of equipment. The risk of infection through an accidentally trauma during the work in medical centers etc. is very low, but be careful anyhow, you could get more easily hepatitis B or C.

   (c) <u>Vertical transmission</u> : The embryo gets the virus from it's infected mother or the new-born during birth. The risk of transmission during pregnancy or birth is about 20% world wide (Europe less, Africa more).

IV. *Epidemic aspects* :

(a) Some descriptions about sporadic outbreaks of a disease that might be AIDS in the 1970th

(b) In early 1980th in homosexual guy communities especially in California, USA.

(c) Spread out rapidly in the following ten years mainly in haterosexual adults, but also children in USA, Europe and Africa.

(d) Worldwide about 15 Mio infected people, in 2000 apporximatey 30 to 40 Mio (highest rise in incidence in Asia and Africa).

(e) In India apporximately 2-4 Mio infected people (WHO estimation end of 1996).

(f) India more detailed :

○ Most complete longitudinal seroprevalence studies in the South, among patient with sexual transmitted diseases (STD); 1% 1986-89, 8.5% 1991-92

○ Madurai : 6.5% among STD patients 1991

○ In Mumbai /Maharashtra 2.5% among antenatal clinic attenders 1994

○ Jaipur/Rajasthan prevalence among STD patients 3.3% and 0.8 among antenatal attenders

○ In Central, North and East India an epidemic not yet take off, except Manipur (injecting drug users).

These are only spotlights, exact figures are hardly available, but it is possible to immagine the necessity of general knowledge and information about pathogenesis and prevention to come along with this disease.

V.   *Clinical features* :

(a) Careful history should be taken. For HIV testing you have to get an approval of the patients. Give advice, attendance and attention to the patient.

(b) Detection of Virus :

Antibody tests : 1. ELISA (Enzyme Linked Immunosorbent Assay)

2. Western Blot (Electrophoresis of viral antigens)

Virus particles : 1. Isolation of HIV (6 weeks)

2. p24 antigen (control parameter during disease)

3. HIV-RNA (important for the diagnosis in new-born of seropositive mothers)

The three above are not for the routine diagnosis.

Quantification : Virusequivalent/ml plasma; with this parameter you are able to tell something about :

Prognosis (high virusload has got an unfavourable prognosis; amount should be <10.000 virusequivalent/ml)

Control of therapy/progress (an antiviral therapy should decrease the virus amount about factor 3)

For the most significant investigation at first carry out two ELISA test, if there is at least one positive undertake the Western Blot. Is the Western Blot positive too, the patient is HIV positive in a high perceniage?

(c) Checklist for further clinical check up :

1. History of sexual transmitted diseases (Syphilis, Gonococcal infection, Lymphogranuloma venerum (LGV), etc.

2. Skin and mouth : Look for dry skin, folliculitis, oral candidiasis, gingivitis, Herpes simplex and zoster infection Karposi's sarcoma.

3. Gastrointestinal system : Pain, diarrohea (e.g.

Cryptosporidium), dysphagia (Cytomegalie-virus (CMV) esophagitis), perianal disease (Herpes simplex).

4. Respiratory system : Cough, dysponea (Pneumocystis carinii pneumonia (PCP).

5. Neurological status : Visual condition (CMV retinitis). headache (toxoplasmic cerebral abscess), peripheral neuropathy, concentration, mood.

6. (a) T_H cell count (normal = 500 cells/mm^3)
   (b) Microbiological detection of opportunistic germs, sexual transmitted diseases and Tbc
   (c) Hepatitis serology
   (d) Total blood count
   (e) Blood electrolytes
   (f) Urine tests
   (g) X-ray of the chest.

7. Prove the state of vaccination. Be careful with life vaccines, BCG is contraindicated.

VI. *Clinical classification* (Centers for Disease Control/CDC) of HIV infection : 4 groups

Group I - Acute HIV disease :

6 days to 6 weeks after infection occuring as a picture like mononucleosis with fever, lymphadenopathy, splenomegali angina, sometimes meningoencephalitis and exanthema. Rule out mononucleosis with Paul-Bunell test and blood count. Is there no HIV antibody result 6 month after possible infection, the possibility of an infection is nearly ruled out.

Group II - Asymptomatic infection (latent period) :

A) No clinical signs, but the person is infectious, HIV antibody test positive (1-3-6) month), no other pathological blood findings.

B)   Like A but with pathological blood results :
- blood count : lymphocyto / thrombocyto / granulocyto-penie
- decrease of T_H/T_S quotient, with normal T_H but increased T_S count
  This latent period lasts on the average > 10 years, but underweighted patients are below of it. HIV- 1 has got a shorter period than HIV-2

Group III - Lymphadenopathy syndrome (LAS) :

A) - Enlargement of lymph nodes for at least 3 months
  - HIV-antibody test positive
  - Seborrheic dermatosis in $1/3$ or patients

B) A) with pathological blood results (see IIB)

Group IV :

A) - *AIDS Related Complex (ARC)* :
  For the diagnosis ARC 2 clinical and 2 laboratory aspects are needed.

Clinical symptoms :   night sweat > 1 month
  - fever > 1 month
  - diarrhea > 1 month
  - weight loss > 10% without any reason.

Laboratory :   - $T_H < 400/mm^3$
  - T_H/T_S - quotient < 1
  - Increasing -γ globulin (IgG)
  - Granulocyto/Thrombocytopenie or anaemia.
  - Decreasing or vanishing of skin reaction after intracutaneous testing (recall antigen).

! Signs of further progression :
↓Helper -T-cells; ↑β_2 Microglobulin and Neopterine

B) - E) - **AIDS :**

B) *Neurological diseases :*

✪ Subacute HIV-encephalitis with atrophy of the brain
   ✪ motorical slow down
   ✪ psychological changes
   ✪ disorder in concentration and memory
   ✪ dementia complex
   ✪ Myelopathy with degeneration of the spinal cord
   ✪ Weakness and paresthesia of the legs, arms etc.
   ✪ paralysed extremities
   ✪ defecation and uresis disorders
   ✪ peripheral neuropathy
      Neurological disorders are often seen in AIDS
      patients (see-Neuro-chapter for detailed studies)

C) I - *Opportunistic infections* :
   In about 80% AIDS is described through opportunistic infections. The diagnosis is rather complicated
   due to the defect of the immunosystem. Therefore,
   you won't get an evidential serologic result.

Protozoa
   ✪ Pneumocystis carinii → Pneumonia
   ✪ Toxoplasmosis → CNS abscess, pneumonia
   ✪ Cryptosporidiosis → watery diarrhea, tenesmus

Mycetes
   ✪ Candidiasis → esophageal, bronchopulmonal
      spreading
   ✪ Aspergilosis, Histoplasmosis etc.
   ✪ Cryptococosis → Meningitis and Pneumonia

Bacteria
   ✪ Mycobacterium avium/intracellulare (MAI)
   ✪ Salmonella sepsis

Virus
   ✪ Herpes simplex → skin, anorectal oropharyngeal,
      CNS, gastrointestinal
   ✪ Cytomegalovirus → Pneumonia, retinitis, encepha-

litis, gastroenteritis

✪ Papovavirus → progressive multiple leukoencephalopathy

2 - *Other infections* :

✪ Epstein-Barr-Virus (EBV)→Oral leukoplakia

✪ Candidiasis of the mouth

✪ Herpes zoster → from intraocular complications to blindness

✪ Nocardiosis → imitating Tbc, but with early metastases and abscessing infiltrations, which build up fistula. The fibrotic proliferating metastases in the soft tissue are called myocytoma.

✪ Tbc of the lung → in the lower parts of the lung without carvens, but mostly miliary development.

✪ Tbc and AIDS are two potential death bringing allies, combined with drug/alcohol abuse and poverty the prognosis is getting worse.

D) - *Malignoma* :

✪ Karposi's sarcoma (Karposi's Sarcoma Herpes virus):

1. classical KS (elderly men, local)

2. African KS (agressive?)

3. KS in immunosuppressive condition

4. *epidemical KS in AIDS* → generalized with multiple tumours in skin, mucosa of mouth (blureddish nodes), gastrointestines, lymphnodes and other organs; mostly homosexual men

✪ Primary cerebral lymphoma

✪ Non-Hodgkin lymphoma (B-cell type) → CNS ($^1/_3$), extranodular ($^2/_3$)

invasive carcinoma of the cervix

E) - *other diseases in AIDS* :

Wasting syndrome → weight loss > 10%, chronical diarrhoea, weakness, etc.

interstitial pneumonia in children

VII. *HIV infection in children* with own CDC classification:

> P0 class : Infection not sure; infant up to 15 months with HIV antibodies, but in which the infection certainly is not sure.
>
> P1 class : asymptomatical infection
>
> P2 class : symptomatical infection

The latent period (group II) in perinatal infected infants is about 4-5 years.

VIII. *Treatment* : The main columns of a sufficient treatment are a healthy way of living, psychological and social support, prophylaxis/therapy of possible illness and last but not least an antiviral drug therapy.

Drugs which are in use :

Nucleosidanaloga : Ziduvudine (AZT), Stavudin (D4T), Zalcitabin (DDC), Didanosin (DD1), Lamivudin (3TC) : all this drugs suppress the RT_2 and as a result of it the HIV replication. AZT and D4T are liquor passable. AZT decreases the risk of transmission from mother to new-born. Side effects : bone-marrow suppression, neuropathy, acute pancreatitis anaemia, etc.

Protease-inhibitor : Saquinavir, Indinavir, Ritonavir; building up non-infective viruscoates. Side effects: Myositis

Immunmodulator : α-inteferon is used for Karposi's sarcoma therapy

IX. *Prevention* is the most important column to stop this disease, it is even more important as long there is no successful therapy

1. Education and information
2. Safer sex
3. Testing of blood donors and blood products
4. I.v. drug users should take clean equipment.
5. Safe yourself while working with blood, wear gloves, be very careful with syringes, sharp instruments etc. For protection against infected aerosola wear glasses and face mask.
X. *General advice* : HIV and AIDS patients are patients like any other, they should be treated like this. No one has got the right to condem and discriminate them. Imagine, that you could get the infection as well.

Appendix to Chapter II

Bleeding time : This is defined as the time taken for a small skin puncture to stop bleeding. The *normal range is 1 to 9 minutes.* Most commonly it is determined by the Ivy bleeding time technique in which three incisions 1 cm long and I mm deep are made in an avascular area of the forearm and the time for the bleeding to cease is measured. A blood pressure cuff is set at 40 mm Hg over the upper forearm to obstruct venous return. An increase in the bleeding time is due either to inadequate platelet activities or to a failure of vascular contractions though they are usually combined. In thrombocytopenia, it is invariable and usual in thrombocytopathia and Von Willebrand disease. The bleeding time is normal in disorders of the coagulation system while generally clinically significant defects of platelet functions are found only if the bleeding time is prolonged. By Duke method the normal bleeding time is 1 to 4 minutes.

Whole blood clotting time (or simply clotting time): This is the time taken for 1 ml of whole blood to clot at 37° C with control of both temperature and exposure of the blood to the glass surface of the test tubes. The venepuncture should be 'clean' to exclude tissue factors. *The time is normally 5 to 15 minutes if an unsiliconised tube is used and 20 to 60 minutes if the tube is siliconised.* Prolongation of the clotting time occurs if there is a gross deficiency of any of the factors concerned in the intrinsic clotting system or in the common pathway. The test is thus insensitive and in *thrombocytopenia the clotting time is normal* despite a prolonged bleeding time.

Prothrombin time (PT) : This is a measure of the factor VII (concerned in the extrinsic system) and factors X, V, fibrinogen and prothrombin (concerned in the common pathway) and is performed by incubating equal amounts of brain extract, calcium chloride solution and test plasma at 37°C. The time taken for clotting to occur is noted. A control is simultaneously put up and this should clot in 11 to 15 seconds.

Partial thromboplastin time : This and the whole blood clotting time test the intrinsic pathway of coagulation. It is defined as the time required for a ·recalcified citrated plasma to clot. Partial thromboplastin' is nothing but a platelet substitute–*cephalin*,–used to eliminate the variability due to the platelet count. Celite or kaolin is used as a standard surface activator to eliminate variability due to surface factors. The value of PTT with standard technique is 68 to 82 sec; *activated* PTT or APTT is 32 to 46 sec.

Thus the coagulation tests are–

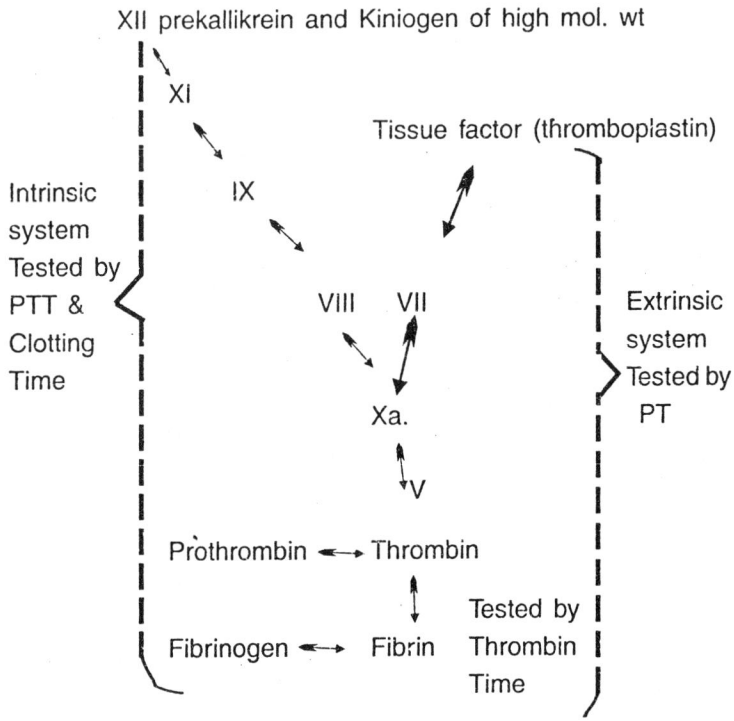

Disseminated Intravascular Coagulation : This is a state of consumption of the coagulation factors resulting from intravascular activation of the coagulative system associated with secondary activation of fibrinolysis. The causes are −

(a) Acute : Sepsis, obstetric emergencies, e.g. abruptio placentae and amniotic fluid embolism burns, shock heat stroke, snake bites, hypergranular promvelocytic leukaemia, haemolysis following transfussion etc.

(b) Chronic : Internal malignancies huge AV malformations (Kassabach-Meritt syndrome), toxaemias, retained dead foetus, malignant hypertension, hepatic cirrhosis with failure etc.

·Laboratory investigations show—(i) low fibrinogen, (ii) thrombocytopenia, (iii) fibrin degradation products i.e. FDP, (iv) prolonged prothrombin time (v) Prolonged PTT, (vi) depressed factor V and (vii) depressed factor VIII.

———————

| CHAPTER 3 | NERVOUS SYSTEM |

It remains an unfortunate fact that most of the students are rather ill at ease while confronting a patient with a neurological problem. Besides being partly due to the inadequacies of training in neurology, this is due mainly to the lack of an adequate grasp on the neuroanatomy, an endless bias towards the rarer disorders leaving the commoner diagnoses aside, and lastly and most importantly, simply due to a lackadaisical approach to history taking.

It is, therefore, urged to maintain always the approach that 'common things are commonly seen'; to ensure a working knowledge at least of the gross anatomy of the nervous system and to develop the habit of insisting on a meticulous history, bordering on obsession. While taking the history the clinician should try to *remain the listener* most of the time. *Cross-check* the facts presented with a relative or a friend. Employ considerable tact in bringing out the problems of sexual activities or alcoholism (that are liable to be concealed for a fear of embarrassment or moral devaluation). *Tailor the interview* to suit the patient but at the same time wait *for the necessary pieces of information* e.g. the momentary lancinating, recurrent jabs of pain of trigeminal neuralgia to emerge. All these and the knowledge of the exact modes of onset and progress of the disease renders the subsequent job of the clinician a very simple task indeed. The history serves to *point out the most important parts of the examination* to be carried out with special care since a confident provisional diagnosis regarding the anatomical site, the extent and the probable nature of the disease process has already been made at the conclusion of the history taking in most, if not all cases. The proper way of conducting the different parts of neurological examination is elaborated in the subsequent pages following a brief outline of neuroanatomy and neurophysiology.

The nervous system is divided into the *central nervous system* consisting of the brain, the spinal cord and meninges, and the *peripheral nervous system* consisting of the peripheral nerves and sympathetic and parasympathetic systems.

The brain is covered by three layer of meninges–(1) two layers of dura matter enclosing the intracranial venous sinuses, (2) the arachnoid matter, and (3) the pia matter, a vascular membrane intimately applied to the surface of the brain and spinal cord. The subarachnoid space between the arachnoid and the piamatter contains the cerebrospinal fluid (CSF) and the blood vessels, A pathological change in the menings produces specific changes in the cerebrospinal fluid.

The brain consists of the forebrain, the midbrain and the hindbrain. The *forebrain* consists of two cerebral hemispheres, each of which consists of an outer covering of *gray matter* composed of nerve cells termed the cortex and an internal mass of *white matter* composed of nerve fibres. The cortex has multiple sulci and gyri of which the *fissure of Rolando* is an important line as it lies between the motor cortex in front and the sensory cortex behind.

The *midbrain* consists of the tectum dorsally the cru of cerebriventrally and the tegmentum centrally. -

The *hindbrain* comprises of the pons, the cerebellum and the medulla oblongata. In continuation of the hindbrain the spinal cord extends from the foramen magnum to the lower border of the first lumbar vertebra. The *midbrain*, pons and medulla together from the brainstem.

Blood supply of the brain

The brain derives its blood supply mainly from the right and the left internal carotid arteries and the two *vertebral* arteries. The *internal carotid* artery has the following principal branches—

(1) the ophthalmic artery which supplies the eyes.

(2) the posterior communicating artery.

(3) the anterior choroidal artery.

(4) the anterior cerebral artery which supplies the paracentral lobule containing the cortical centers for movements of the lower limbs and for micturition as well as defaecation.

(5) the middle cerebral artery which supplies the motor, the sensory and the speech areas.

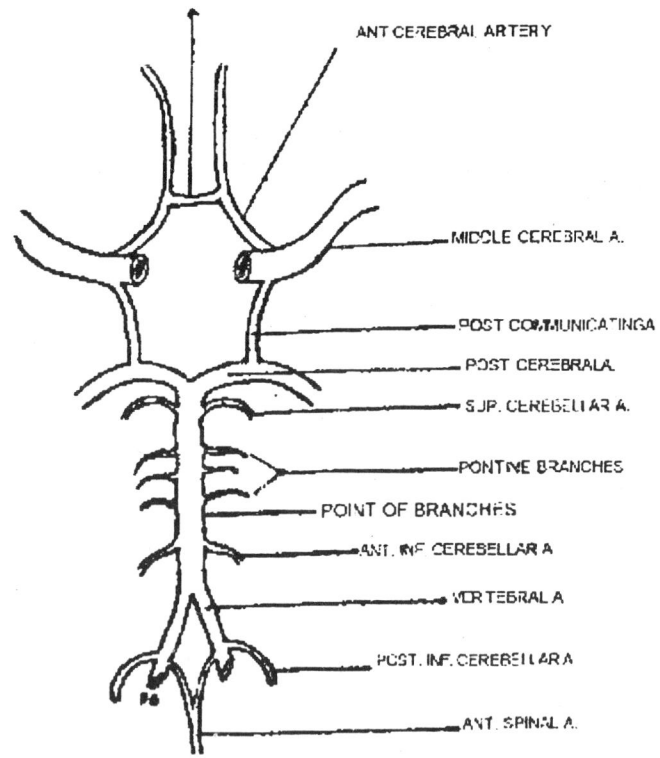

Fig. 3-1 : *The arterial circle of wills*

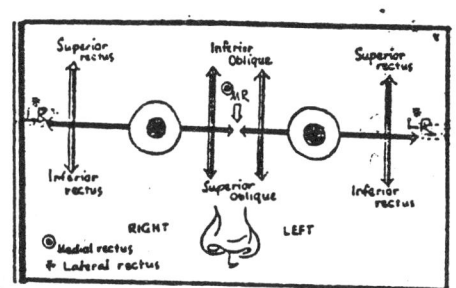

Fig. 3A : Diagrammatic representation of the different eye muscle actions.

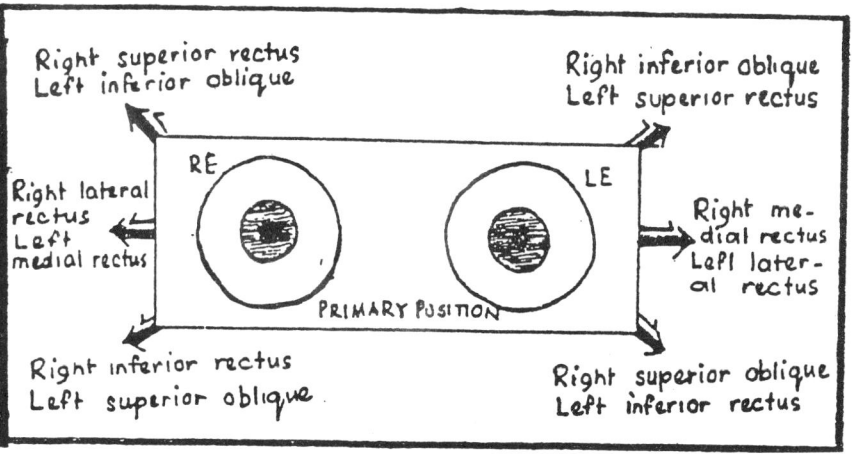

Fig. 3B : Diagram showing the muscles used in the conjugate eye movements in the 6 cardinal direction of gaze.

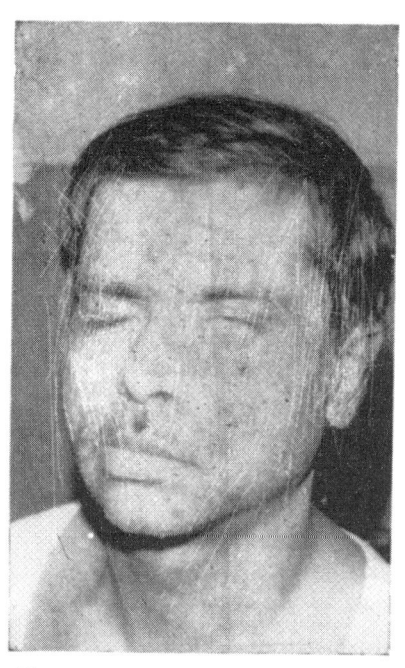

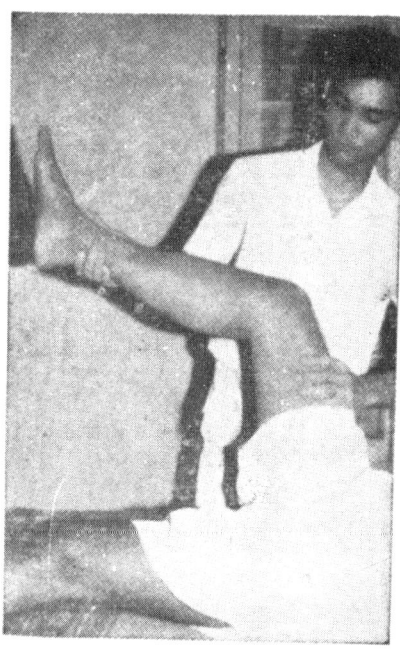

Fig. 3C ; Ramsay Hunt syndrome with left facial paralysic.

Fig. 3D : How to look for Kernig Sign.

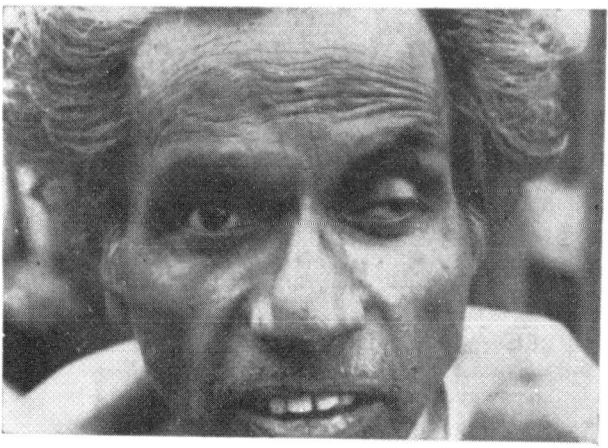

Fig. 3E Left Third nerve Palsay.

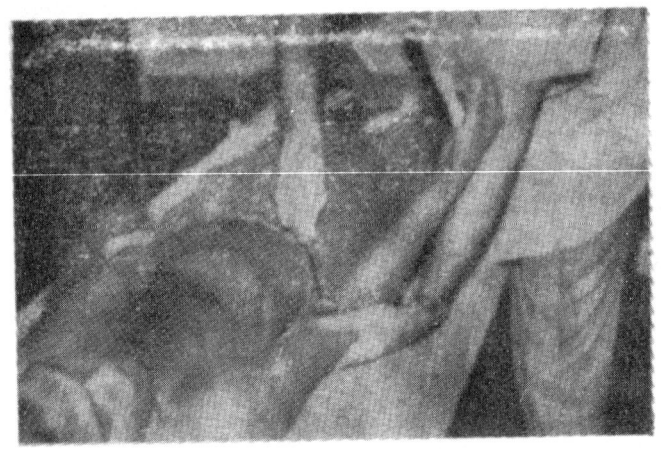

Fig. 3F : Demonstrating how to elicit biceps jerk.

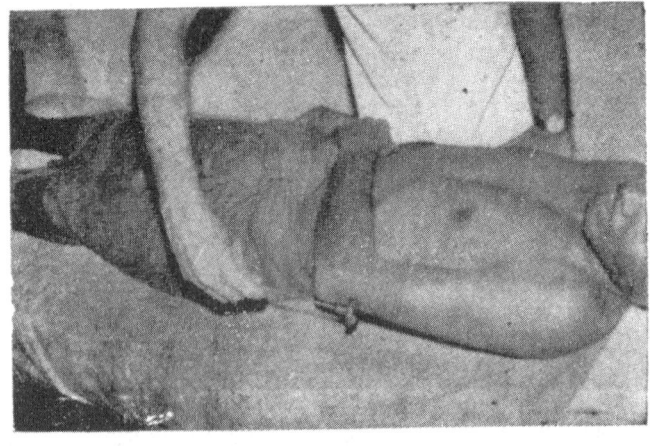

Fig. 3G Elicitation of triceps jerk.

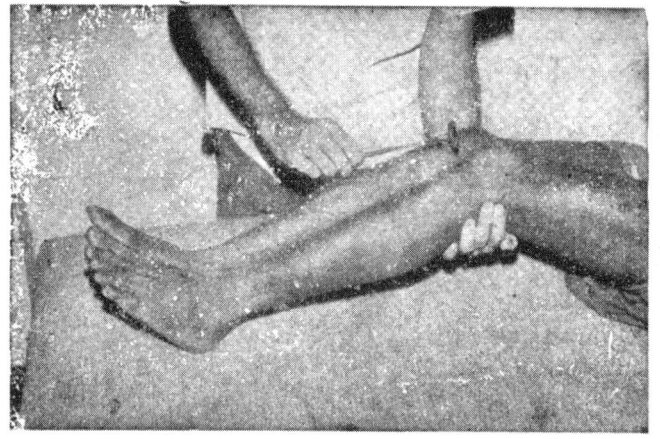

Fig. 3H : Elicitation of knee jerk.

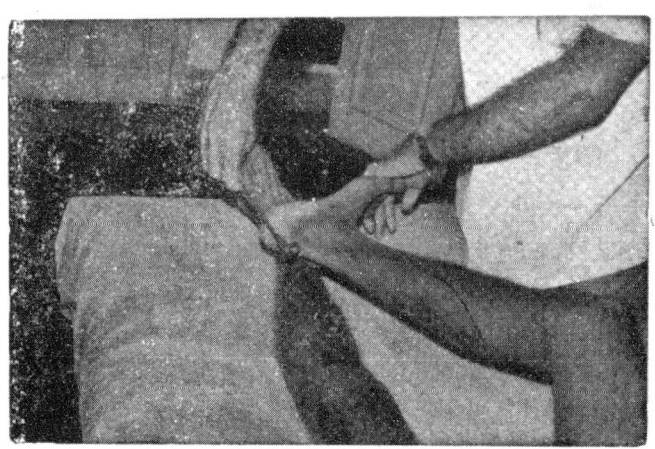

Fig. 3 I : Elicitation of ankle jerk.

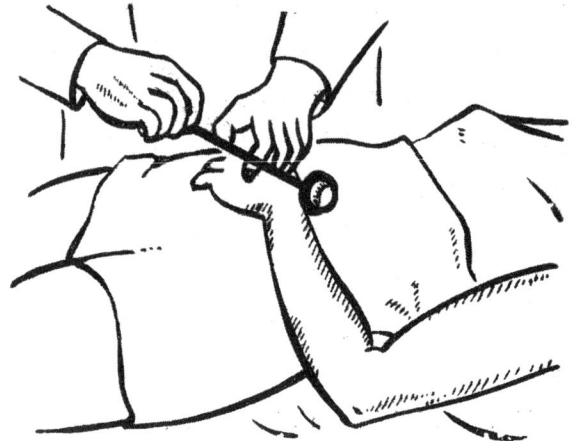

Fig. 3J : Elicitation of Supinator jerk.

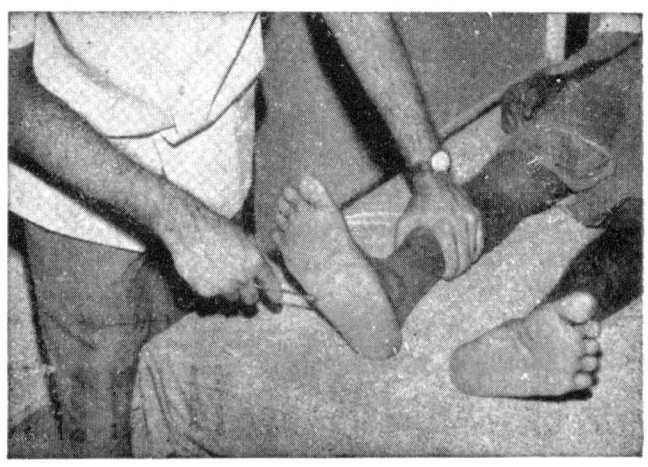

Fig. 3k : Elicitation of the plantar reflex.

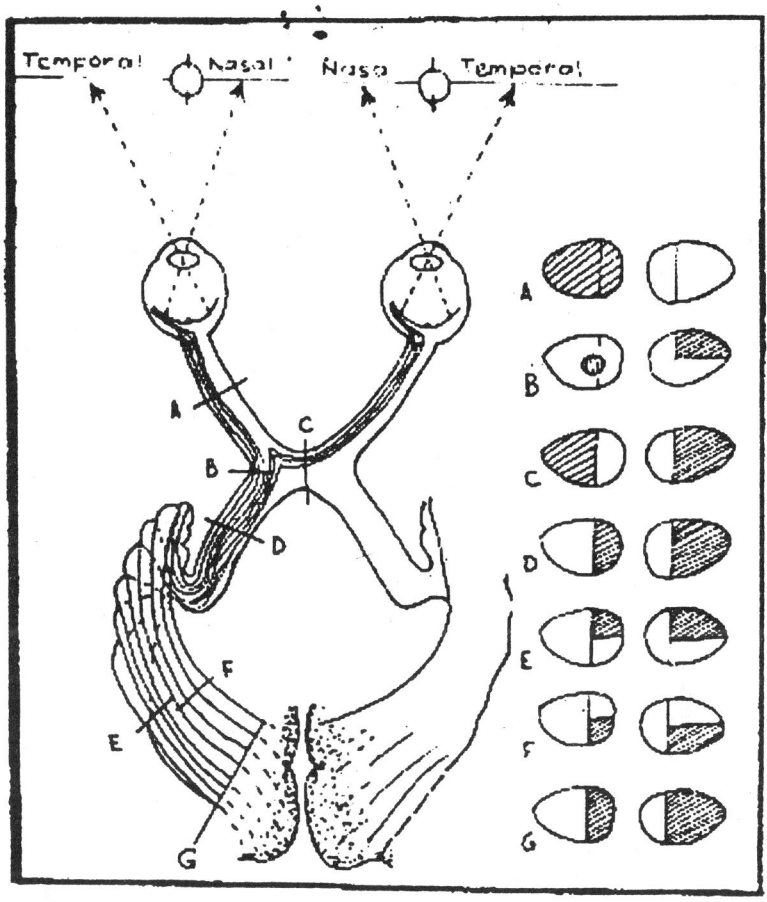

Fig. 3L: Visual field defects produced by lesions at various points along the optic pathway.

A- Complete blindness in left eye. B- Left junction scotoma with right upper quadrantanopia due to lesion of the Wilbrand's Knee. C- Bitemporal hemianopia. D- Right homonymous heminaopia. E, F-Right upper and lower quadrantanopia. G- Right homonymous hemianopia.

The *vertebral* arteries within the skull supply the medulla oblongata and the postero-inferior part of the cerebellum through the posterior inferior cerebellar artery. The vertebral arteries unite at the lower border of the pons to form the *basilar artery* which gives rise to—(1) the anterior inferior cerebellar artery to supply the anterior and inferior parts of the cerebellum. (2) superior cerebellar artery to supply the rest of the cerebellum, and (3) branches which supply the pons.

Ultimately the basilar artery terminates into two posterior cerebral arteries which supply the occipital lobe, including the visual cortex, lower part of the temporal lobe including the crus, and the posterior part of the posterior limb of the internal capsule.

The arterial circle of Willis (Fig 3-1) is formed as follows:

The internal carotid arteries or the middle cerebral arteries are joined to the same sided posterior cerebral arteries by the posterior communicating artery on either side. The anterior cerebral arteries are joined together by the anterior communicating artery. This anastomosis serves to equalise the blood flow to the various parts of the brain and also to furnish collateral circulation in case of occlusion of one or more of the arteries.

Blood supply of the spinal cord

There are two *posterior spinal* arteries arising from the corresponding vertebral or posterior inferior cerebellar arteries. There is *only one anterior spinal artery* formed by the union of a branch from each vertebral artery. Besides these three spinal arteries, there are segmental arteries—cervical, intercostal lumbar and sacral arteries which enter the spinal canal through the intervertebral foramina and course medially along the spinal nerves as *redicular* arteries. The anterior spinal artery is replenished usually by a vessel entering the canal on the C_3 or C_4 root coming from the *thyrocervical trunk*. This upper part of the vessel supplies the spinal cord down to about the T_4 level. The *arteria radicularis magna* or the artery of Adamkiewicz is one of the intercostal arteries which is the main feeder vessel at a variable level of the thoracic spinal cord (arising commonly from the intercostal, artery of the T_{10}, T_{11} or T_{12} segments) and if damaged, usually causes infraction of the whole lumbar enlargement and the spinal cord, up to the midthoracis level.

The anterior spinal artery supplies most of the spinal cord, only the posterior parts of the posterior horns and columns are supplied by the posterior spinal arteries. Venous drainage is basically similar to that of the arterial supply. There are 6 to 11 anterior radicular veins and 5 to 10 posterior radicular veins.

THE MOTOR SYSTEM

Movement of a joints is produced by the contractions of a group of muscles–the *prime movers* along with gradual relaxation of the *antagonists* assisted by the *synergists and the fixators.*

Although many reflex movements act from a spinal level, the *initiation of movement* and the *maintenance of muscle tone* and *posture* depend upon impulses arising from the *higher centres* i.e. the *pyramidal* and the *extrapyramidal* system and the *cerebellum.*

Movements, whether voluntary or involuntary, are the results of contraction or controlled relaxation of one or more groups of muscles and *never* a single muscle only.

A firm base of action is provided by the contraction of the *synergists* which stabilise the joint and by appropriate adjustments of posture. The *postural adjustment* is largely

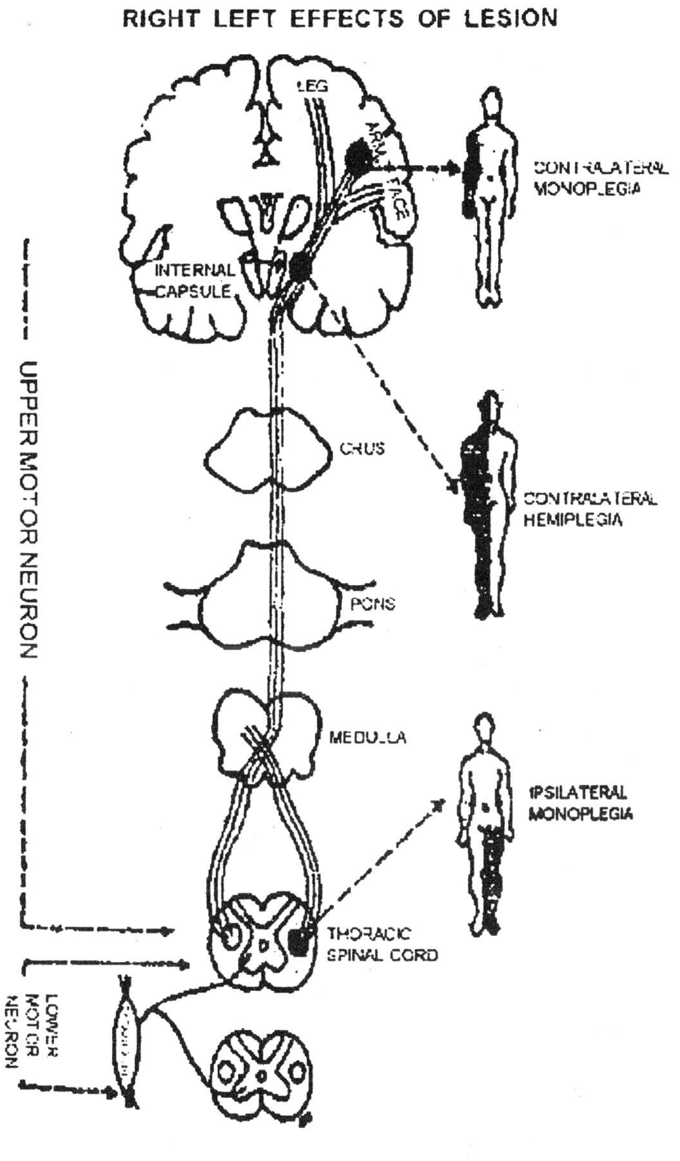

RIGHT LEFT EFFECTS OF LESION

Fig. 3-2 : *The Motor neurones and effects of lesions at different sites*

under the control of the extrapyramidal system and the vestibular and spinal reflexes. Voluntary movements require the participation of the precentral gyrus of the cerebral cortex (motor area) and the timing and degree of a contraction or relaxation of the muscles of synergy are *co-ordinated by the cerebellum*, especially when the movement involves more than one segment of a limb. The excitation of the upper motor neurone from the *motor area of the cortex*, the *extrapyramidal system* and the *cerebellum* are brought directly or indirectly to the *anterior horn cells* of the spinal gray matter or motor cranial nerve nuclei from which the lower motor neurone runs to a group of muscle fibres (motor unit).

Thus the lower motor neurone is *the final common pathway* for all efferent impulses directed at the muscle.

The pyramidal Tract– This tract consists of fibres which connect the cerebral cortex with the lower motor neurones of the brainstem and the spinal cord. The motor fibres arise *mainly* from the motor area (area 4) of the brain which occupies the anterior wall of the central sulcus and the precentral gyrus. *Minor contributions* are made by the fibres which arise from the post central cortex (areas 3 & 2) and subcortical structures.

Localisation of function in the motor cortex is represented in an *inverted* fashion. Areas for the tongue, jaw and facial movements lie in the lowest part of the motor cortex while those for the arm trunk and leg follow successively upwards as the motor area ascends the medial aspect of the cerebral hemisphere. The motor fibres for speech arise from the *Broca's area* in the 3rd frontal convolution on the left side in right handed subjects and usually on the right side in left handed subjects.

From the pyramidal cells the motor fibres pass down the

corona radiata to the *internal capsule*, occupying the anterior two-thirds of its posterior limb bounded medially by the thalamus and the caudate nucleus and laterally by the lenticulate nucleus. The order of representation of the fibres in the internal capsule is face, shoulder, elbow, hand, trunk and lower limb from before backwards. Fibres for the face are in the *anterior limb* those for the tongue and mouth at the *genu* and the rest are in the *anterior two-thirds of the posterior limb* of the internal capsule. The fibres continue downwards to occupy the middle two-fifth of the peduncles of the midbrain in the same order as the internal capsule. The tract becomes broken into scattered bundles as it passes through the pons into the medulla oblongata. The tract is closely related to the emerging motor fibres of the cranial nerves III, IV, VI and XII as it descends through the brainstem.

The corticobulbar fibres conveying impulses to the motor cranial nerve nuclei of the brainstem are closely associated with the corticospinal fibres in the internal capsule and the brainstem.

In the upper end of the medulla oblongata the fibres unite to form a prominent elevation known as the *pyramid* and in the lower end of the medulla the majority of the fibres cross to the opposite side and descend in the spinal cord as *crossed* pyramidal tract in the lateral column. A smaller portion of the pyramidal fibres descend downward in the anterior column as *uncrossed* pyramidal tract and decussate in the anterior commisure. Few uncrossed fibres descend in the crossed pyramidal tract of the same side.

The majority of the pyramidal fibres end in relation with the *internucial cells* and only a relatively small number of fibres synapse *directly* with the motor cells. From the anterior horn cells the fibres pass out through the anterior root of the spinal nerves and are distributed via the peripheral nerves to the end organs in the muscles or glands which they supply. The anterior horn cell and its dendrite up to the motor end plate constitute the *lower motor neurone*. This is the final common pathway for all motor impulses, both voluntary and automatic.

The pyramidal tract conveys impulses to the spinal cord resulting in *volitional movements*, especially the discrete movments of the fingers and hands which form the basis of skillful movements.

The Extrapyramidal System : In voluntary movements, for a perfect functioning of the pyramidal system in the production of skilled voluntary movements the extra-pyramidal system must work side by side since in provides the background on which the pyramidal system operates.

The system includes–(1) caudate nucleus and putamen, (2) globus pallidus, (3) subthalamic nuclei, (4) substantia nigra (5) red nuclei, and (6) reticular formation in the brain stem. The connections of the extrapyramidal centres include fibres from the cerebral cortex and the thalamus. The indirect connections with the lower motor neurones are via the *rubrospinal, reticulospinal, olivospinal* and *vestibulospinal* tracts. Exact function of the extrapyramidal system is yet to be known but it seems to regulate *muscle tone* and *posture, emotional movements automatic movements* and also *associated movments* such as swinging of the arms during walking. Any disturbance of the extrapyramidal system gives rise to–(a) disturbances of the voluntary movements particularly slowness and poverty, (b) disturbances of tone which may be *increased* in Parkinsonism and *decreased* in chorea, and, (c) the appearance of involuntary movements.

The Cerebellum : It is the largest part of the hindbrain and lies behind the pons and the medulla oblongata separated by the floor of the fourth ventricle; in the posterior cranial fossa, covered by the tentorium cerebelli.

The cerebellum receives *afferent fibres* from the spinal cord, vestibular nuclei, cerebral cortex and proprioceptive end organs of the body i.e. the labyrinth and the muscles. The *efferent fibres* act upon the lower motor neurone through its connections via the thalamus, the basal ganglia and the cerebral cortext i.e. the dentato-rubro-thalamo-cortical connexion, The *lateral lobe* of the cerebellum is concerned with the movements of the limbs and the eye of the same side of the body. The *vermis* is concerned with the maintenance of erect posture and equilibrium. Thus the cerebellum has an *ipsilateral control* and regulates the *rate, rhythm, range* and *force* of muscular contraction; maintains *equilibration, muscle tone and coordination* between the voluntary and the automatic movements. Sherrington has, therefore, rightly called the cerebellum as 'the head ganglion of the proprioceptive system.'

THE SENSORY SYSTEM

The functioning of the afferent side of the nervous system is influenced by certain general principles, e.g.–

(a) The environmemt is represented on the opposite side of the cerebral hemisphere.

(b) There are three neurones from the periphery to the cortex to carry the impulse–(i) the first order neurone from the posterior root ganglion, on entering the central nervous system remains on the same side of the environment, (ii) the second order neurone crosses the midline to end in the thalamus and, (iii) the third order neurone begins in the thalamus and reaches the sensory cortex for localisation and discrimination. The thalamus is concerned with crude sensations.

(c) There is no conscious sensation below the level of the thalamus.

The sensory fibres arising from the end organs in the skin and the deeper skeletal tissues ascend in the peripheral nerves, traverse the dorsal root and ultimately enter the posterior column where the fibres undergo grouping into different tracts.

There are mainly two sensory pathways–(1) the spinothalamic tract which carries fibres of pain, warmth and cold and a few fibres of touch, and (2) tracts of Goll and Burdach which carry vibration sense, position sense, pressure sense and the rest of the fibres of touch.

(1) *The spinothalamic Tract*–Consists of 2 columns, the (a) lateral and the (b) ventral spinothalamic tracts.

(a) *The lateral spinothalamic tract*–The fibres carrying the pain and thermal sensations reach the posterior horn cells by the primary neurones. The secondary neurones arising from there cross to the opposite side and reach the lateral column and then run upward. This is the lateral spinothalamic tract. It enters the pons through the medial lemniscus (tractile discrimination and proprioception) and ascends to end in the thalamus.

(b) *The ventral spinothalamic tract*– A few fibres carrying the touch sensation reach the posterior horn cells from where the second order neurones cross to the ventral column of the opposite side at a higher level. The neurones then ascend up the pons and midbrain through the medial lemniscus and end in the thalamus.

(2) *The tracts of Goll and Burdach*–The fibres carrying the position sense, the vibration sense, the pressure sense and the rest of the touch fibres enter the posterior column of the same side and ascend the spinal cord to terminate in the Gracilis and Cuneate nuclei in the medulla from where the second order neurones start and cross to the opposite side to reach the cerebellum. Thus the Gracilis

and Cuneate nuclei and the dorsal grey columns are the sensory relay nuclei for the spinal nerves.

(3) *The fibres from the Trigeminal Nerve* enter the spinal tract, reach the nucleus of that nerve and from there the second order neurone starts and crosses the midline to the opposite side of the medulla and as the quintothalamic and trigeminothalamic tracts it ascends along with the spinothalamic tracts and finally reaches the thalamus.

All these sensory fibres run from the posterior part of the ventral nucleus of the thalamus through the corona radiata to the postcentral gyrus of the cerebral cortex. *The sensory functions of the cortex are, therefore, related to fine touch accurate localisation, tactile discrimination and discrimination of different degrees of thermal sensation and appreciation of size, shape, form, roughness and texture of objects (graphaesthesia and stereognosis).*

Lesions of the sensory nucleus of the thalamus give rise to spontaneous pain of an unpleasant variety in the opposite side of the body and the threshold for pain is frequently raised giving rise to thalamic overreaction and loss of other sensations on the opposite side of the body.

A lesion of the sensory cortex is likely to produce a sensory loss of cortical type over a limited part on the opposite side of the body because of the wide extent of the sensory cortex. Other parietal lobe syndromes are beyond the scope of this book and text-books of medicine and neurology should be consulted for the same.

Scheme of Examination of the Nervous System

Scheme of examination of the nervous system includes (i) examination of the skull; (ii) neck stiffness, Kering's sign. Brudzinski's sign straight leg raising (SLR) test; (iii) higher functions including handedness; (iv) cranial nerves; (v) motor; (vi) sensory functions; (vii) the reflexes;

(viii) the autonomic nervous system; (ix) cerebellar functions; (x) gait and spine.

I. Examination of the skull.

A thorough inspection of the skull for any asymmetry deformity, irregularity, depression or elevation etc. should be done. Look for haematoma or fractures of the skull in a case of head injury. Microcephaly is often associated with congenital idiocy. It is also an important clinical finding in a child with cerebral deplegia (see Sick Children).

The tension of the anterior fontanelle in young children is an important clinical guide to the intracranial pressure. A tense or bulging fontanelle is found in meningitis hydrocephalus etc.

A cracked pot sensation due to springing of the sutures of the skull is highly characteristic of hydrocephalus.

Auscultate the temporal, parietal, and frontal regions and also over the closed eyes for a cranial bruit – this is present in angiomatous malformations and vascular tumours. A bruit over the eyeball is heard in an arteriovenous fistula (carotidocavernous fistula) aneurysms of the internal carotid artery, cavernous sinus thrombosis, angiomas etc.

II. Examination of the neck for neck rigidity head retraction, Kernig's sign, Brudzinski's sign, SLR and carotid artery pulsation.

The neck rigidity and positive Kernig's sign are present in meningitis, meningism, meningoencephalitis, meningomyelitis, subarachnoid haemorrhage, Klippl-Feil syndrome, cervical spondylitis, increased intracranial tension, congenital torticollis, traumatic injuries of cervical spine or soft tissues, multiple myeloma, Still's disease, rheumatoid arthritis and tuberculous diseases of the cervical spine, 'tetanus, strychnine, poisoning, rabies etc.

The *neck rigidity* is tested by lifting the head from the

bed and also turning it from side to side. If the patient is conscious ask him to touch to lower jaw to the sternum with his mouth closed. Passive flexion of the head and neck is prevented by spasms of the cervical extensors. Neck rigidity is sometimes present in cervical spondylosis.

To elicit *Kernig's sign* flex the hip to 90° and then extend the knee to 90°. Now try to straighten the leg while the hip remains flexed. Normally the leg can be easily straightened up to 180°. In meningitis or meningeal irritation particularly involving the posterior roots of the lumbar area, the legs cannot be extended and if extension is attempted forcibly, painful spasms of the hamstring muscles result.

Brudzinski's sign–This is another sign of meningeal irritability. On lifting the head from the bed there will be a flexion of the hip and knee joints or on simply flexing the thigh of one lower limb, the opposite thigh spontaneously gets flexed. This sign is particularly valuable while examining a child. Head retraction occurs in the conditions same as those of neck rigidity. SLR–with the patient supine try to raise one leg first and then the other, keeping the legs absolutely straight without any flexion at knee joints. This passive SLR is possible in normal individuals up to 90° except in those with unusually tight hamstrings. The manouevre puts the sciatic nerve and its root under strain. Also it causes an anterior rotation of the pelvis around a transverse axis thus increasing the stress on the lumbosacral joints and causing pain if the joint is diseased or inflammed. Thus SLR shows a limitation of movement mainly of the affected side, in diseases of the lumbosacral joints and nerve roots. This is also known as *Lasegue's sign* and is a very reliable test for prolapsed intervertebral disc.

The *carotid artery pulsations of the two sides* are compared and any kink, if present, is noted. This is of great clinical significance as carotid artery insufficiency is common in elderly patients leading to cerebral is chaemia.

III. Examination of the nervous system proper.

A. HIGHER FUNCTIONS

(a) Frist of all ascertain whether the patient is *conscious* or not.

Unconsciousness may be due to many different causes for a list of which see Chapter 1 of Part I.

(b) If the patient is conscious, the mental state should be assessed during history taking. *Euphoria* is seen in general paralysis of the insane, multiple sclerosis, opioid addiction, amphetamine intoxication, sometimes in schizophrenia and occasionally in forntal lobe tumours and in association with dementia. The patient may be *confused* or *delirious* in alcohol withdrawal syndrome or in recent vascular episode. Gross *apathy* towards the surrounding is characteristic of Parkinsonism.

(c) The *intellectual capacity* of the patient is noted during history taking. Impairment of the intellectual efficiency is the earliest change in *dementia paralytica.*

(d) *Memory* should be assessed by asking the patient about the past as well as of the recent events. The age, year of passing the school leaving examination, the age of the parents etc. may be asked.

Loss of recent memory, preservation of past memory and confabulation at characteristics of *Wernicke's encephalopathy* with *Korsakoff's psychosis.* This may be due to chronic alcoholism, cerebral arteriosclerosis, postencephalitic psychic disorders and intracranial tumours.

Complete or significant loss of memory occurs in dementia paralytica cerebral arteriosclerosis, bilateral hippocampal lesions, damage of the limbic brain including the hippocampus following encephalitis etc.

Arithmetic ability : After an assessment of the memory, the arithmetic ability is to be determined usually by asking the patient to subtract 7 from 100 with subsequent subtractions of 7 from each remainder.

(e) *Orientation*– This is evaluated by asking the patient about the place where he is being examined, the date and the time etc. to note the orientation regarding time, place and person.

(f) *Delusion*–A delusion means false beliefs that cannot be corrected by an appeal to reason as contrasted to an *illusion* that can be corrected.

(g) *Hallucinations*– These are abnormal sensations arising from the special sense organs in the absence of corresponding external stimuli.

Both delusions and hallucinations are found in vascular, degenerative and neoplastic lesions of the temporal lobe.

(h) *Speech*– Speech is the symbolic expression of thoughts in words and is the mode of communication by meaningful sounds.

Types of speech disorders : (1) Aphasia (2) Dysarthria or anarthria (3) Dysphonia or aphonia.

(I) (a) Motor aphasia–The patient can hear and read but cannot speak due to a lesion in the precentral gyrus and the posterior part of the 3rd frontal convolution of the left side. Loss of power of writing is *agraphia*. Motor aphasia and agraphia constitute *expressive aphasia.*

(b) Sensory or receptive aphasia–The patient cannot understand spoken or written words, vision and hearing remaining normal. The so-called 'word deafness' and 'word blindness' constitute *receptive aphasia.* The site of the lesion is the posterior part of the superior temporal or angular gyrus and a part of the adjacent parietal lobe.

(c) Global aphasia–This is a combination of (a) and (b).

(d) Nominal aphasia (amnesic aphasia)–The patient is unable to name the common objects like watch, pen, knife etc. The lesion usually lies between the angular gyrus and the posterior part of the superior temporal gyrus on the left side and is a common complication of ear infection.

(2) Dysarthria–Dysarthria is a general term indicating defects in articulation and rhythm of speech due to neuromuscular or muscular disorders and not a defect of the higher functions controlling speech. Proper construction and use of words are *not* disturbed. A common example of dysarthric speech is that of an alcoholic, in whom alcohol has affected the centres in the brainstem and cerebellum concerned with the co-ordination of speech musculature. Ask the patient to pronounce the words 'constitution', 'arms and ammunitions' etc. and note whether he can speak with proper articulation. *Spastic dysarthria* is found in pseudobulbar palsy and extrapyramidal lesions such as Parkinsonism. *Flaccid dysarthria* is characteristic of bulbar palsy and recurrent laryngeal nerve palsy. *Ataxic dysarthria* may be found in multiple sclerosis hereditary ataxias, chorea and athetosis.

(3) Dysphonia–Dysphonia is a disorder of vocalization characterised by the production of abnormal sounds from the larynx and is due to a defect of expelling the requisite amount of air across the vocal cords. It may be due to local causes like laryngitis or tumours of the vocal cord. Other important neurological causes include injuries to the recurrent laryngeal nerve from thyroid surgery or infarction of the lateral portion of the medulla (thrombosis of the posterior inferior cerebellar artery) and tumours of the brainstem.

Clinical types of speech disorders are (a) Falling voice (or idioglossia)–Found in defective mental states and cretinism.

(b) Scanning speech of disseminated sclerosis due to lesions in the vermis of the cerebellum.

(c) Slurring speech of dementia paralytica (bilateral lesions of the cortex) and incertain brainstem disorders.

(d) Stammering speech of congenital nature

In this connection it is worthwhile to mention a few special types of higher cortical functions and their derangements, such as agnosia and apraxia.

In visual agnosia the patient fails to recognise common objects which he can clearly see; the path from the retina to the occipital cortex remaining intact. It is the manifestation of a left parieto-occipital lesion in right handed persons.

Apraxia is defined as the inability to carry out a purposive movement in the absence of motor paralysis, sensory loss, or ataxia. This is found in vascular lesions of the parietal lobe, diffuse cerebral inflammatory and degenerative conditions etc.

N. B. – While examining the higher functions note whether the patient is *demented* or not. *Dementia* is the clinical condition characterised by a gradual loss of memory, intelligence, personality and skills, commonly progressive in nature and not associated with unconsciousness. Most commonly it is due to Alzheimer-Senile dementia, but may also be due to multiple infracts, alcoholism, intracranial neoplasms, normal pressure hydrocephalus, chronic drug intoxications, hepatic failure, neurosyphilis, Creutzeld-Jakob disease etc.

B. *EXAMINATION OF THE CRANIAL NERVES*

The cranial nerves are to be examined thoroughly to detect a paralysis or other disorder which may help to localise the site of the lesion.

1. *Olfactory*– To test the smell sensation, the patient is

asked to close his eyes and the test samples soaked in cotton are presented before each nostril separately. Oil of clove, turpentine, oil of lemon, peppermint etc. or other commoner substances may be used. Inability to appreciate the smell of a substance is known as *anosmia*. Anosmia is of three types–unilateral, bilateral and hysterical. *Unilateral* anosmia may be due to a tumour of the olfactory bulb, a tumour of the frontal lobe pressing on the olfactory bulb or tract or by a meningioma. *Bilateral* anosmia may be due to local causes like coryza, atrophic allergic rhinitis hay fever etc. or due to an intracranial cause like head injury or may be due to a congenital disease-Kallman's syndrome. *Hysterical* anosmia can be differentiated from true anosmia using a strong solution of ammonia. One who suffers from true anosmia will not get the smell of ammonia but there will be watering due to trigeminal nerve stimulation; on such phenomenon is noted in the hysterical patient. Perversion of smell, also known as *parosmia* may be found in hysteria, in incomplete olfactory recovery after head injury and occasionally in depressive states. Olfactory hallucinations may be found in temporal lobe epilepsy.

2. *Optic*–Acuity of vision, field of vision, colour vision and ophthalmoscopic examinations are done as a routine while examining this nerve. Students of clinical medicine should know a few basic facts about the visual path and ocular reflexes.

The visual path– The visual path extends from the retina to its termination in the occipital lobe of the cerebral cortex. The two optic nerves converge and meet at the optic chiasma where there is partial decussation of the visual fibres. Nasal fibres cross while the temporal do not. Throughout the entire course from the retina to the occipital cortex, the *visual* fibres are grouped according to the retinal quadrants from which they arise. The optic tract contains uncrossed and crossed fibres from the temporal and nasal halves of the retina respectively. The optic tract terminates in the lateral geniculate body, superior corpora quadrigemina and in the posterior end of the thalamus–the pulvinar. Optic radiation originates from the lateral geniculate body, passes through the posterior limb of the internal capsule and courses backward to the cortex around the calcarine fissure. The superior fibres reach the parietal lobe while the inferior fibres the temporal lobe. The fibres then reach the visual cortex lying above and below the calcarine fissure. Left half of the field of vision is represented in the right hemisphere of the cerebral cortex and vice versa.

In addition to the visual fibres described above the optic nerve and tract contain the fibres that subserve pupillary reflexes. These fibres leave the tract to enter the superior colliculi of the midbrain whence the second order neurone starts and run bilaterally to the Edinger-Westphal nucleus close to the central gray matter, whence the neurones send preganglonic fibres to the ciliary ganglion through the oculomotor nerve and its branch to the inferior oblique muscle. The post ganglionic fibres from the ciliary ganglion traverse the short ciliary nerve to reach the sphincter pupillae. These anatomical facts help to explain the light and accommodation reflexes.

The Light Reflexes are (a) direct and (b) consensual. Light falling on one retina constricts both the pupils. This is because fibres from one optic tract pass to the superior colliculi of both sides. Elicited by shining a bright light on either eye.

Accommodation Reflex : While the patient looks at an infinite distance, ask him to suddenly look at your finger placed near his nosetip. The eyes *converge* and the *pupils constrict*. Explanation–Light falls on the retina→optic nerve

→optic chiasma→optic tract→lateral geniculate body→optic radiation→ visual area in the occipital lobe of the cerebral cotex→(the visual area is connected by the superior longitudinal association tract to the eye field of) the frontal cortex from where the fibres descend through the internal capsule to the nuclei of the oculomotor nerve in the midbrain. From the Edinger-Westphal nucleus the fibres pass to the ciliary and sphincter pupillae muscles and from the central nucleus the fibres supply the medial recti muscles for convergence of the eyes. Accommodation also causes enophthalmos and increased anterior convexity of the lens. Errors of accommodation may be due to problems of refraction, long standing papilloedema with tubular vision, optic neuritis etc.

(a) *Acuity of vision*–This is determined with the Snellen's chart placed six metres from the patient. Alternatively, the patient is asked to count the beams of the ceiling or blades of a fan or the bars of the window. After testing the distant vision by the above procedure, the near vision is tested by Jaeger's chart. Loss of vision in reference to the visual field is known as anopia.

Visual acuity may be defective or even lost in optic neuritis, disseminated sclerosis, Foster-Kennedy syndrome, primary optic atrophy, meningitis pituitary tumour, carotid artery aneurysm, encephalomyelitis, vitamin A deficiency, tobacco smoking and arsenic posioning. Visual defect is generally found from the beginning in papillitis while in papilloedema there is usually not much defect in acuity. Total blindness is due to a lesion in the optic nerve.

(b) *Visual field*–The methods of plotting the *visual field* at the bedside are–(1) In the alert, cooperative patient one of his eyes is covered and the other looks directly into the corresponding eye of the examiner (e.g. patient's right and examiner's left eye) and the object, either a finger or a hatpin is brought from the outside to the centre of the field of vision, holding it equidistant from the patient and the examiner who sit about 18' apart and thus the former's visual field is compared with that of the latter. The patient's blind spot can be aligned with the examiner's one and its size estimated by moving the object outward from the blind spot until it is seen; and also central and paracentral visual field defects can be outlined similarly. (2) Alternatively the examiner holds both hands in the outer part of the visual fields midway, between himself and the patient and moves either or both together instructing the patient to point to the hand moved. This helps in detecting any visual field defect present and also in diagnosing visual inattention seen in parietal disorders when separate testing reveals normal visual fields in each eye. Besides, a homonymous hemianopia can be quickly detected by this method compared to the above. (3) In a patient otherwise uncooperative, field defects can be roughly estimated by quickly moving a hand toward the eyes from different directions when normally there is a blinking response–the *menace reflex*. The different visual field defects and their significance are–

(1) A lesion of the right optic nerve causes *complete blindness* in the right eye with a loss of the direct light reflex e.g., retrobulbar neuritis.

. (2) A partial lesion of the optic chiasma involving only the crossed nasal fibres e.g. in pituitary tumours with suprasellar extension and dilatation of the third ventricle causes *bitemporal hemianopia*. A hemianopia means inability to see object in one-half of the field of vision.

(3) Lesion of the uncrossed temporal fibres of both sides e.g. bilateral aneurysms of the internal carotid artery causes *binasal hemianopia*.

(4) A lesion of the left optic tract by haemorrhage thrombosis tumour or aneurysm causes *right sided homonymous hemianopia* with *Wernicke's hemianopic pupillary reaction,* When light falling on the blind half of the retina evokes a light reflex but there is no accommodation reflex.

(5) Lesions of the left optic radiation cause *right sided homonymous hemianopia* with *normal pupillary reaction to light.* In temporal lobe lesions, the damage of lower fibres lead to *crossed homonymous upper quadrantic hemianopia.* In parietal lobe lesions, the damage of the upper fibres lead to *crossed homonymous lower quadrantic hemianopia.*

(6) Lesions of the upper or the lower lip of the calcarine fissure give rise to *upper quadrantic hemianopia* or *lower quadrantic hemianopia* but the *macular vision persists.* Macular vision may be lost in lesions of the middle cerebral artery.

(7) Bilateral occipital cortical lesions (infraction of the occipital lobe) give rise to *cortical blindness* in which pupillary reactions are normal. Though completely blind, the patient may deny that he is blind. It is most probably due to destruction of visual association areas. This is *Anton's syndrome.*

A lesion of the left occipital cortex causes *right sided homonymous central hemiscotoma.*

N.B.–A *homonymous hemianopia* indicates a lesion of the visual pathway *behind the optic chiasma* and *nothing more* than that if it is *complete.* If it is *identical and congruous,* the lesion is possibly in the *calcarine cortex* and if *incongruous* the lesion is possibly in the *optic tract or radiation in the parietal or temporal lobe.*

(c) *Colour Vision* – Colour vision is tested with bits of cotton wool of different colours or with any object of various colours. Ishihara's chart if available should be used. Inherited colour blindness is X-linked recessive. Compressive lesions of the visual pathways manifest in the *most early stage* as a defect in *visualising red*.

(d) *Examination of the fundus*– The optic disc, the blood vessels, the macular region and the periphery are examined as a routine. Alteration in colour, shape, physiological cupping edge of the disc and its surrounding areas are observed in association with some diseases. Details have been described later in connection with the ophthalmoscopic examination of the fundus.

3. 4 & 6 *Oculomotor, Trochlear and Abducens* [3rd, 4th and 6th cranial nerves]

It is convenient to examine these nerves together as they serve conjointly; innervating the muscles of the eyeball. The 3rd nerve supplies all the muscles of the eyeball except the lateral rectus, supplied by the 6th and the superior oblique, supplied by the 4th. The 3rd nerve carries the pupilloconstrictor fibres whereas the pupillodilator fibres travel via the sympathetic nerve. The 3rd nerve is also responsible for the light and the accommodation reflexes.

First by inspection try to ascertain whether there is any ptosis or not and if there be any, the eyelids will have to be passively elevated for further examination of the ocular movements. Ptosis may be due to (i) 3rd nerve palsy, (ii) Horner's syndrome, (iii) myasthenia, (iv) facioscapular or ocular myopathies, (v) dystrophia myotonica, (vi) congenital causes, (vii) hysteria, (viii) tabes dorsalis, (ix) GPI etc.

N.B.–*Ptosis with miosis signifies Horner's syndrome while ptosis with mydriasis signifies a 3rd nerve lesion.*

Tests–The eye movements are (a) first examined by

asking the patient to look upward, downward, to the right and to the left without introducing any object in his field of vision so as to exclude any *ocular apraxia.*

Next (b) examine with an object (e.g. a pen) about two and a half feet away from the patient. He is asked to follow the object which is moved to either side as well as above and downward, keeping the head fixed. The object is also brought close to the tip of the nose to test the downward and medial movement. If the patient complains of diplopia it will have to be further clarified since there are two images–one internal and the other external. The external one is the false image and if it disappears on closing one eye, there is a paralysis of the muscles of that respective eye. Paralysis of the muscles of one or both eyes causes *strabismus* (or *squint*), i.e. the loss of parallelism of the axes of the eyes. A squint, also may be *paralytic* or *nonparalytic.* The latter is known as *concomitant* or *spasmodic* squint. It is unassociated with diplopia and is equal for all positions of the eyes. On covering the fixing eye, the concomitant squinting eye shows full movements. A paralytic squint is due to paralysis of eye muscles and movement of the eyeball are abnormal, and at least in the early stages there is usually diplopia.

Next examine the (c) *conjugate deviation and (d) ocular fixation.*

Ocular fixation is absent in new-born babies. Some retinal disorder is to be suspected if it is absent in an adult.

Conjugate deviations are of three types–lateral, upward and downward. In *lateral conjugate deviation* the lateral rectus of one eye and the medial rectus of the other contract together. The association of the two eyes in conjugate movements depends upon the integrity of the path which runs from the cerebral cortex to the nucleus of the muscle concerned. The upper motor neurone responsible for the movement starts in the second frontal gyrus and then via the corona radiata through the internal capsule reaches the midbrain and joins the medial longtitudinal bundle. Coursing along the sixth nerve, crosses to the opposite side and goes straight upward to the third nerve nucleus for the medial rectus muscle. Disorders of the *lateral conjugate deviation* may be due to 'spasm' in epilepsy, encephalitis, postencephalitic Parkinsonism, haemorrhage at the pontine level, neoplastic, causes, disseminated sclerosis, encephalomyelitis etc. Disorders of the *upward conjugate deviation* of the eyes is found in midbrain lesions. e.g. pinealoma or in progressive supranuclear palsy (PSP). Disorders of the *downward conjugate deviation* of the eyes may be due to vascular or traumatic causes.

It is also important to remember that whereas a frontal lobe lesion leads to a *contralateral* paralysis of the conjugate gaze, an *ipsilateral* paralysis is caused by brainstem lesions. Hence the *adversive* or *controversive* seizures of frontal area 8 irritation (in which the head and eyes turn to the side opposite the irritative focus).

Just by inspection a 3rd nerve palsy can be detected. *Complete ptosis* due to paralysis of the levator palpabrae superioris, *lateral squint* due to the unopposed action of the lateral rectus and a *dilated pupil* constitute the *triad* of a 3rd nerve palsy.

In a 4th nerve palsy, there are no apparent findings except the inability of the patient of walk downstairs. This is because of paralysis of the superior oblique muscle;–and diplopia on looking downwards and medially. The head may be tilted to the opposite side in a 4th nerve lesion (in an attempt at compensating the disorder).

An internal squint may be found in a 6th nerve palsy due to the unopposed action of the medial rectus.

While examining the (e) pupillary reflexes note initially their size, shape, symmetry margins, colour, presence of a coloboma, if any. Remember that a dilated pupil with minimum or no light reflex may be associated with no paralysis of the eyeball muscles in a 3rd nerve lesion or the reverse may happen. The anatomical basis of this apparently paradoxical phenomenon is simple. The facts are–(i) the pupilloconstrictor fibres of the 3rd nerve lie bundled in a separate group at the superolateral quadrant of the cross-section of the nerve; (ii) this group of fibres have an arterial supply separate from that of the main group which is supplied by a branch from the internal carotid artery. As such, in *medical disorders*, usually, but not always (e.g. diabetes, syphilis, migraine, atherosclerotic etc.) the pupilloconstrictor fibres escape infraction; while in *compressive surgical lesions* the superolateral quadrantic fibres remain most vulnerable to damage, sparing, at least initially the muscles of the eyeball. This, though a broad generalisation, holds good for the common pathological conditions involving the 3rd nerve in clinical practice and the above explanation clarifies the apparent paradox.

Pupillary reflexes are reactions to varying strengths of light stimulus. The pupils generally dilate in dimness and constrict in bright light.

Consensual light reflex– Light falling upon one eye stimulates the centre for pupillary constriction of the same eye as well as that of the other as some of the fibres of the optic nerves decussate at the chiasma; fibres concerned in the reflex also decussate in the midbrain. The reaction in each eye is tested separately by shading the eyes with the edge of the hand placed over the bridge of nose. The consensual reaction of the pupil is tested by focussing light upon one eye and noting the reaction in the other eye, with the patient looking at a distant object to avoid miosis due to accommodation. Lesions of one optic nerve will affect reactions of both the pupils.

Accommodation reflex– Pupils become small on accommodating for a near object. Convergence of the eyes and constriction of the pupils are due to associated muscular contractions. The miosis is also described as the reaction on convergences. Thus the accommodation reflecx is characterised by convergence of the eyeballs, increased convexity of the lens, constriction of the pupils, and also enophthalmos.

In a classical *Argyll Robertson* pupil the pupils are small and irregular, dark or sometimes may be pale due to the presence of neurosyphilitic inflammatory changes, unequal, the light reflex is lost with an intact accommodation reflex, and mydriatics have no effect. This type of pupil is seen in neurosyphilis, rarely in other midbrain lesions, diabetes, amyloidosis. acoustic neuroma, Charcot-Marie tooth disease, brainstem encephalitis etc.

The *reversed* Argyll-Robertson pupil is a rare phenomenon and is seen as a late complication of Von-Economo's encephalitis or post-encephalitic Parkinsonism.

In *myotonic pupil* (Holmes-Adie syndrome) usually there is unilateral involvement and the affected pupil constricts or dilates very slowly. It usually occurs in young women and ankle or knee jerks may be depressed or absent in the fully developed syndrome and thus needs to be differentiated from neurosyphilis.

Effect of scratching the skin of the neck on the ipsilateral pupil (*cilio-spinal reflex*) must be observed when normally the pupil dilates, and any evidence of *Horner's syndrome* like partial ptosis, enophthalmos, constricted pupil, anhydrosis (iodine and starch over the face cause bluish colouration in the normal side but has no effect on the anhydrotic side and impairment of ciliospinal reflexes should be noted. Recent studies indicate that the ciliospinal pupillary reflex is not a reliable sign.

The *Gunn pupil sign or pupillary* escape is the pheno-menon in which the pupil dilates partially following initial constriction despite a bright light shone steadily in one or both eyes and may be found in–(i) optic neuritis or retinitis, classically and (ii) normal individuals, rarely.

The *jaw-winking* or *Marcus Gunn* phenomenon is char-acterised by a momentary retraction of a ptotic eyelid with mouth opening or jaw moving and is a congenital and sometimes hereditary anomaly. This is due to abnormal connections between the central mechanisms involving the levator and the pterygoid muscles and is also known as *trigemino ocular synkinesis.*

Look for (f) *nystagmus* which is defined as a failure of maintenance of posture of the eyes characterised by rhyth-mic, involuntary, and oscillatory movements of the eyes when fixed on an object. It may be due to an *error of refraction, amblyopia, cerebellar diseases, labyrinthine and vestibular* disorders, *affection of the central path concerned in ocular posture*, or a *congenital weakness of the muscles*. Besides these, working for years together in an environment of com-parative darkness may lead to *miner's nystagmus*. Thus it is of localising value in connection with disturbances in brainstem or vestibulocerebellar connections. To test for nystagmus, the patient is asked to look straight and the phy-sician observes whether the eyes remain steady. The pa-tient is then asked to look to his extreme right, to the left and then upwards and downwards. *First degree* nystagmus to the left is seen only on looking to the left. *Second degree* nystagmus to the left is present on looking straight, but increased on looking to the left. *Third degree* nystagmus to the left is present on looking straight in front, increased on looking to the left and also present to some extent on looking to the right. While testing for nystagmus the lateral gaze must not be extended beyond the limit of binocular vision; few irregular nystagmoid (4 or less) jerks of brief duration on full lateral deviation may be confused with nystagmus (5 or more). *Positional nystagmus* : The patient is seated on a couch and his head is rotated about 30^0 to 40^0 towards the observer and then backward in such a way that the inclination becomes 30^0 below horizontal. No nystagmus or vertigo occurs in a normal subject but in *benign paroxysmal positional nystagmus* and in *posterior fossa lesions*, severe vertigo and rotatory nystagmus occur. Sixth nerve may be involved along with the seventh. The former is commonly involved in pontine lesions but at times has a false localising value only.

Nystagmus is broadly classified into *pendular* and *jerk* varieties. The latter is further subdivided into *horizontal, vertical* and *rotatory* types.

An individual congenitally blind or blind since early childhood shows a pendular nystagmus, the mechanism being similar to that of miner's nystagmus.

Normally the visual axes meet at a point at which the eyes are looking since the movements of the two eyes are symmetrical. In *infranuclear* paralysis of the 3rd, 4th or 6th nerve an individual muscle or groups of muscles are affected but in *supranuclear* lesions a paralysis of the conjugate movement occurs.

The medial longitudinal bundle connects the 3rd nerve nucleus to the opposite 6th, is the *first tract* that undergoes *myelinization* in man; and when diseased e.g. in multiple sclerosis causes a disturbance of conjugate eye movements which may be characterised by ataxic or dissociated nystagmus,–the *Harris's sign*.

5. *Trigeminal*–The sensory and motor divisions are tested separately.

(a) *Sensation*–It may be tested by a wisp of cotton wool and a pin over each area of the face supplied by the three divisions of the trigeminal nerve. The *ophthalmic division* supplies the conjunctiva, the lacrymal gland, the medial part of the skin of nose up to the tip, the upper eyelids, the forehead and the scalp as far as the vertex. The *maxillary division* supplies the cheek, the lower eyelid and its conjunctiva, the side of the nose, the upper lip, the upper teeth, the upper part of pharynx, major part of the soft palate and the tonsils. The *mandibular division* supplies the lower part of the face, lower lip, the ear, the tongue and the lower teeth. The sense of taste should be examined in a suspected lesion of the 5th nerve as the taste fibres from the anterior two-thirds of the tongue reach the brain via the lingual branch of the mandibular nerve before joining the chorda tympani nerve.

(b) *Motor function*–The muscles of mastication are examined in the following way :

(i) The patient is asked to clench his teeth and note the contraction of the *masseter* and *temporalis* muscles by inspection and palpation, comparing those of the two sides. These muscles should stand out with equal prominence on each side. If there is paralysis on one side the muscle of that side will be less prominent. The *pterygoids* can be tested by asking the patient to open and close the mouth against resistance.

Alternatively, the patient is asked to open the mouth and

to move the lower jaw from side to side against resistance.

A persistent deviation of the jaw to one side indicates a weakness of the pterygoid (provided it is not due to a dislocated jaw) and the deviation is towards the paralysed side.

(c) *Reflexes*– The cornea is touched lightly with cotton wool while the patient looks to the opposite side and note whether the eyes immediately close or not. Afferent is by the 5th nerve and efferent via the 7th nerve. The *corneal reflex* should be tested for each eye separately. This reflex is absent in herpes zoster, deeply unconscious patients, acoustic neuroma (*earliest manifestation*), and aneurysms or tumours related to the cavernous sinus or orbital fissure. In a 5th nerve lesion there is no response from *either* lid when the diseased side is stimulated, and a normal response from both lids when the normal side is stimulated. In a 7th nerve lesion there is no response from the paralysed side whichever side be stimulated, but if the 5th nerve is normal there will be a response from the normal side even if the abnormal side is stimulated. *Demonstration of jaw jerk :* Ask the patient to partially open his mouth, place your left index finger in the groove under the lower lip and lightly tap by a percussion hammer.

There is normally no reaction or a slight twitching of the elevators of the jaw. It is exaggerated in pseudobulbar palsy, upper motor neurone palsy of the 5th nerve above the level of the pons, and often in disseminated sclerosis. Both afferent and efferent fibres are in the 5th nerve. In paralysis of the mandibular division the jaw moves to the same side of the lesion and there are depressions both above and below the zygoma.

7. *Facial :* The seventh is mainly a motor nerve with a small sensory component, the nervous intermedius of

Wrisberg that conveys taste sensation from the anterior 2/3rds of the tongue and a limited area of the anterior wall of the external auditory canal. It suppiles all the muscles of the face and scalp except the levator palpebare superioris. It also supplies the platysma.

Test : The different facial muscles are tested as follows :

(a) The frontal belly of the occipitofrontalis and the corrugator superciliaries are tested by asking the patient to frown. (b) Next an attempt is made to open the eyelids while the patient attempts to keep them closed. Orbicularis oculi thus tested and if they are acting normally it will be difficult for the observer to open the eyes. (c) The patient is asked to blow up his cheeks and to whistle,—by these the orbicularis oris and the buccinator are tested. (d) the patient is asked to show his upper teeth whereby, the risorius, buccinator, levator anguli oris, and depressor anguli oris are tested. (e) The platysma can be tested by asking the patient to draw down the angles of the mouth while tightening up the neck muscles. (f) The facial expression during emotional states such as during laughing or crying should be observed to detect any 'mimic palsy'.

Taste sensation in the anterior 2/3rd of the tongue is tested by asking the patient to put out his tongue—place some sugar on it, rub and then ask whether it is sweet, salt or sour. Try all the different taste modalities.

Effects of paralysis of the seventh nerve : (i) There is no expression on the affected side of the face. (ii) The nasolabial fold is less prominent. (iii) The eyeball rolls upward to compensate for the failure of the lid to descend when the patient attempts to close the eyes—this is the *Bell's phenomenon.* The eyelashes are not so much rolled in as on the healthy side. The eye is more widely open on the healthy side than on the other. (iv) The mouth is drawn to the healthy side. The patient is unable to whistle; saliva and fluid dribbles from the angle of the mouth of that side and food collects between the teeth and the gum. Air can be made to escape from the inflated mouth more easily on the paralysed side.

Facial paralysis in relation to the site of the lesion : Facial paralysis may be due to (i) a lesion situated above the nucleus involving the pyramidal fibres concerned in the voluntary facial movements (upper motor neurone or *supranuclear* type of paralysis); (ii) a supranuclear lesion involving the fibres responsible for the emotional movements of the face leading to *mimic paralysis*; and (iii) a lesion at the nucleus or below it (*infranuclear paralysis*).

Facial supranuclear paralysis results in the absence of the nasolabial fold, voluntary retraction of the angle of the mouth is weak. blowing and whistling cannot be achieved. Emotional movements of the face are usually not affected. The *lower part of the face is chiefly affected* while the frontalis and orbicularis oculi are usually spared. The *lower motor neurone* type presents with an inability to frown and close the eyes, the nasolabial fold is less pronounced, the angle of mouth is drawn to the side opposite to that of the lesion and the patient can neither blow nor whistle. Thus the *upper* and the *lower* facial muscles are *equally* weakened and the voluntary as well as the emotional movements are affected to an equal extent as the final common path is destroyed. Explanation : The upper facial movements are innervated by *both cerebral hemispheres* and the lower facial movements by the *opposite hemisphere only*. The upper motor neurone concerned with emotional movements have a different course and is separate from the pyramidal fibres. This explains why the emotional movements are *not usually* affected in hemiplegia. A lesion of the opposite frontal lobe damages the fibres for the emotional movements only while the fibres for voluntary movements are spared and, therefore, results in *mimic paralysis*.

The fibres of the facial nerve of its nucleus may be involved in neoplastic lesions of the pons, syringobulbia and disseminated sclerosis. The proximity of the facial and the acoustic nerves in the posterior cranial fossa explains why these nerves are usually affected together; lesions of the cerebellopontine angle (e.g. an acoustic neuroma) gives rise to facial paralysis, loss of taste sensation in the anterior 2/3rd of the tongue and deafness.

Lesions of the geniculate ganglion by herpes zoster will cause loss of taste sensation in the anterior 2/3rd of the tongue with lower motor neurone palsy of the facial nerve and vesicles in the region of the external auditory meatus (*Ramsay-Hunt syndrome*). Hyperacusis occurs because of paralysis of the stapedius.

Causes of facial palsy

It can occur in *supranuclear* lesions i.e. lesions of the cerebral cortex, mid-brain and those just above the pons. *Nuclear* lesions in the pons may be due to vascular causes like haemorrhage, thrombosis or aneurysm; syringobulbia; bulbar polio; tumours at the cerebello-pontine angle and Ramasy Hunt syndrome etc. *Bell's palsy* is the *extracranial* cause, and is a lower motor neurone facial palsy of unknown aetiology. The basic pathology is a nonsuppurative inflammation of the facial nerve in the stylomastoid foramen. *Bilateral facial palsy* is most commonly due to Guillain-Barre syndrome.

8. *Acoustic* : The *cochlear* division is first examined. It is responsible for hearing. Always first exclude the presence of 'wax' in the patient's ear.

(i) Speak loudly at first from a distance of about six feet from the patient and gradually lower the voice while moving closer. Normally the patient should be able to hear the whisper from a distance of 10 to 12 inches.

(ii) Test with the ticking sound of a wristwatch. Stand behind the patient, if possible, ask him to close the eyes and bring the watch gradually close to each ear, in turn, keeping one closed while the other is being examined. Note the distance at which the sound is heard by each ear. Also assess the distance at which an apparently normal ear can hear the same sound under the same conditions. If an impairment is suspected, test with a tuning fork. Normally *air conduction is greater than bone conduction.*

Special tests :

Rinne's test : Air conduction is more than bone conduction in a normal individual. A vibrating tuning fork is applied on the patient's mastoid process with the ear kept closed by the observer's finger. The patient is asked to indicate when he can't hear the sound; the fork is then placed at the external auditory meatus. In middle ear deafness, the sound cannot be heard by air conduction after bone conduction has ceased as the latter is greater than the former. In nerve deafness air conduction is greater than bone conduction though both are less than normal.

Weber's localisation test : A vibrating tuning fork of frequency 256/sec is placed at the centre of the forehead in the midline. A normal individual hears equally on both sides. In nerve deafness localisation is on the *normal* side. In middle ear diseases localisation is on the *affected* side. This is because in nerve deafness both bone and air conduction is reduced whereas in middle ear deafness air conduction is reduced but bone conduction is relatively increased, because ambient noise is excluded.

Another differentiating point between nerve deafness and middle ear deafness is that in the former, the loss of hearing is most marked for high pitched tones while in the latter it is for low pitched tones.

Tests for the vestibular division–History is taken, especially about *vertigo* and *tinnitus*. Look for *positional nystagmus. Caloric test* may be done to investigate the function of each labyrinth separately. The principle of the test is to irrigate each ear with hot or cold water [44⁰C and 30⁰ C. Hyperaesthesia of the auditory nerve or hyperacusis occurs in hysteria and in lesions of the facial nerve due to paralysis of the stapedius muscle.

Tinnitus– A sensation of noises, usually ringing in the ear caused by abnormal excitation of the auditory apparatus or its connections or cortical areas. The commonest cause is a lesion of the internal ear. Iatrogenic causes include administration of drugs like quinine. salicylates and streptomycin. Neoplastic lesions of the auditory nerve (acoustic leuroma) may cause *tinnitus*.

9. 10. *Glossopharyngeal and Vagus*–The nuclei of the ninth, tenth and eleventh cranial nerves are situated in the dorsum of the medulla on the floor of the fourth ventricle and are called the ventral, dorsal and solitarius nuclei. The ventral is the motor and the other two are sensory and autonomic.

Tests–

(a) Taste sensation of the posterior 1/3rd of the tongue (9th) Substances used : Weak solution of citric acid solution of sugar and common salt.

(b) Test for pharyngeal reflex–By tickling the back of the pharynx with a swab stick. This normally initiates coughing and a symmetrical constriction of the pharynx–The afferent via the 9th and the efferent through the 10th nerve.

(c) Test for palatal reflex–Ask the patient to open his mouth and touch the mucous membrane of the soft palate with a cotton swab. The soft palate *normally* elevates, also ask the patient to say 'ah' when the palate should rise symmetrically on both sides. Use a tongue depressor if necessary. Note the normal elevation of the palate during the manoeuvre or for an asymmetry, if there be any. The afferent path is via the maxillary division of the 5th and the 9th; efferent via the 10th. Unilateral response with displacement of the uvula to the normal side may be encountered in a lesion of one 10th nerve and may be absent or diminished in anaesthesia of the palate or lesions of the vagus nuclei in the medulla (e.g. bulbar polio, syringobulbia, lateral medullary or Wallenburg's syndrome), involvement of the vagus in its intracranial course by meningitis, neoplasms, jugular foramen syndrome, carotid body tumour or below that by a cervical lymphadenopathy, thyroid tumours, Hodgkin's disease, oesophageal carcinoma etc.

(d) Ask the patient to speak and to cough and note any hoarseness of the voice, bovine cough, stridor etc. (vide recurrent laryngeal nerve palsy), 'Stridor' may be due to bulbar polio motor neurone disease, syringobulbia, vascular causes, and neoplastic conditions of the cord.

Effects of paralysis of the glossopharyngeal and the vagus nerves.

(a) Loss of taste sensation in the posterior one-third of the tongue means paralysis of the trunk of the glossopharyngeal nerve. Pharyngeal reflex is present only in the normal side.

(b) Movements of the soft palate during phonation gives considerable information. If one side of the palate is paralysed, it will remain, flat and immobile. The median raphe will be pulled to the other side. In bilateral paralysis the palate does not move at all. Regurgitation of the fluid into the nose is a common finding in total paralysis of the soft palate such as due to diphtheritic neuritis.

(c) In unilateral total paralysis of the recurrent laryngeal nerve there is a failure of abduction and adduction of the vocal cord which lies in the cadaveric position. The normal cord crosses the midline to meet the paralysed one and hence phonation is not abolished though there may be hoarseness and difficulty in coughing.

(d) Bilateral total paralysis of the recurrent laryngeal nerve causes paralysis of both vocal cords which lie in the cadaveric position and hence phonation and coughing are lost. Stridor may occur on deep inspiration.

(e) Bilateral abductor paralysis occurs in bilateral lesions of the recurrent laryngeal nerves. Both vocal cords lie close together at or near the midline and fail to abduct on inspiration. This results in serve dyspnoea but voice is little affected and coughing remains normal.

(f) Bilateral adductor paralysis is found in hysterical patients. Aphonia results as the vocal cords are not adducted in phonation.

Causes of 9th and 10th nerve palsy :

(a) Unilateral

   (i)   motor—poliomyelitis, diphtheria, botulism

   (ii) sensory—very rare

   (iii) motor and sensory—lateral medullary syndrome, posterior fossa tumours, syringobulbia, trauma, tumours, bony anomalies.

(b) Bilateral

   (i) Upper motor neurone—bilateral CVA causing pseudobulbar palsy, amyotrophic lateral sclerosis, advanced Parkinsonism.

(ii) Lower motor neurone–progressive bulbar palsy, poliomyelitis toxin.

(iii) Neuromuscular–maysthenia.

Causes of Recurrent Laryngeal Nerve palsy :

(a) Unilateral–Mediastinal neoplasm cervical lymphadenitis, thyroid malignancy, aortic aneurysms, surgical trauma etc.

(b) Bilateral–Enlarged thyroid, cervical lymphadenitis, trauma etc.

In Vocal Cord Palsy the site of lesion can be determined by the following features :

(i) Features of lateral medullary syndrome e.g. ipsilateral cerebellar signs, dissociated sensory loss of same side of face and opposite side of body, ipsilateral Horner syndrome suggest intramedullary lesions.

(ii) Jugular foramen syndrome e.g. 9th and spinal accessory palsy suggest extramedullary intracranial lesion.

(iii) 9th, 10th, 11th, 12th palsies with Horner syndrome suggest a posterior laterocondylar or retroparotid space (extracranial) site of lesion.

(iv) Absences of palatal sensory loss and palsy and absence of pharyngeal sensory loss suggest a lesion below the origin of the pharyngeal branches, usual site possibly is then in the mediastinum.

11. *Spinal Accessory*– It supplies the sternomastoid and the trapezius muscles. It exits from the skull through the jugular foramen and is intimately related with the 9th and the 10th cranial nerves. The cranial part goes with the vagus nerve.

Test – The patient is asked to shrug his shoulders against resistance (by pressing on the shoulder from behind) when the trapezii come into action, and to rotate the head against resistance when the sternomastoid muscle of the opposite side is thrown into prominence. Vertebral border of the scapula becomes prominent in spinal accessory palsy. Paralysis of the sternomastoid causes weakness of rotation of the chin towards the opposite side. In bilateral sternomastoid palsy the head will drop backward. This palsy is usually due to motor neurone disease and dystrophia myotonica.

᾿ N.B.–The UMN fibres controlling the LMN of the sternomastoid muscle is ipsilateral, contrasted to other muscles.

12. *Hypoglossal*– It arises from a nucleus in the lower part of the floor of the fourth ventricle, close to the midline in the preolivary sulcus. It is purely motor and comes out through the hypoglossal canal. It supplies the tongue and the depressors of the hyoid bone.

Test–Ask the patient to protrude his tongue as much as possible. In hypoglossal palsy the tongue will be deviated to one side, in UMN lesions. The tongue is deviated to the *opposite* side ‚of the lesion while in an LMN lesions, it deviates to the same side with weakness and wasting of corresponding half of the tongue; the median raphe becomes· concave on the paralysed side towards which the tip is deviated and the mucous membrane on the dorsum of the paralysed side becomes corrugated with accumulation of food debris between the mucous folds.

This deviation is greater after an LMN lesion than after a UMN lesion. Such a real deviation may be confused with an apparent deviation of the tongue in facial palsy where the mouth is twisted to one side. There may be wasting of the tongue and dysarthria due to paralysis of the muscles; wasting indicates that the lesion is nuclear or infranuclear.

Bilateral LMN lesions cause marked wasting of both sides associated with fasciculation. The *commonest* cause is involvement of the medullary nuclei in motor neurone disease (MND). Nuclear or infranuclear lesion is found in bulbar affection.

Ask the patient to move his tongue and also to bulge out his cheek with the tongue against external resistance. Note any abnormal movements like tremor, fibrillatory twitching or fasciculation and also the power of the tongue muscles.

Affection of the 12th cranial nerve is found in any bulbar lesion–bulbar polio, syringobulbia, MND, vascular lesions, extension of meningitic process into the foramen from which it comes out and in cut-throat injury.

Unilateral paralysis of the tongue does not impair articulation. Bilateral paralysis of the tongue is not usually and isolated finding and in such cases dysrathria and dysphagia are present due to part to paralysis of other muscles.

In *pseudobulbar palsy* (bilateral upper motor neurone affection of the tongue due to involvement of both the corticospinal tracts above the medulla) the tongue becomes spastic, there is difficulty in protrusion, as also dysarthria associated with emotional disturbances. All movements are weak but true wasting does not occur till the late stages and other than bilateral hemiplegia, may occur in MND, Parkinsonism, neoplastic and demyelinative lesions.

(C) MOTOR FUNCTION
Inspection

Inspect the four limbs and trunk to find out their attitudes. In hemiplegia one finds absence of any voluntary movements and the helpless attitude of the affected side of the body.

The *nutrition* or bulk of the muscles, presence or absence of *involuntary movements, muscle tone, power,* and *coordination* of the movements are to be examined systematically with comparison between the two sides.

Look for the evidences of *wasting* of the muscles. If wasting is predominant there will be some amount of flattening of the overlying skin, and in extreme wasting there may be hollowness over the area with prominence of the underlying bony points. It can be confirmed by comparing the measurements e.g. the girth of the part, at fixed points on two sides. The interosseous spaces over the dorsum of the hands should be carefully inspected for depression i.e. guttering, as may be found in MND, spinal tumours, syringomyelia, cervical spondylosis, cervical rib, peripheral neuropathy e.g. due to *Hansen's disease* (commonest) lead poisoning, carcinomatous neuropathy, Pancoast's tumour, brachial neuritis, carpal tunnel syndrome, rheumatoid arthritis syphilitic amyotrophy, old age etc.

The wasting of muscle(s) can be due to LMN lesions, disuse atrophy in UMN lesions, muscular dystrophy, malignancy, thyrotoxicosis, diabetes mellitus, nutritional deficiency etc.

The muscles may be hypertrophied in pseudohypertrophic muscular dystrophy e.g. Duchenne type.

Fasciculations of the muscles should be observed in strong light; these are clonic contractions of bundles of fibres constituting a motor unit and occurs when the neurone of proximal part of the axon of the motor unit is diseased but not totally destroyed, as in *progressive muscular atrophy*. Fibrillation means contraction of individual muscle fibre or a part thereof when the fibre or the corresponding part gets denervated.

A fibrillation is detected by EMG and *not clinically.* Fasciculations may be seen in normal individuals, MND, thyrotoxicosis, early stages of acute anteriorpoliomyelitis, compressive lesions of spinal nerve roots e.g. by prolapsed intervertebral discs, syringobulbia (in the tongue), syringomyelia, rarely during recovery from poliomyelitis, and also in syphilitic amyotrophy, peroneal muscular atrophy, arachnoiditis, myositis and collagen diseases. Note that fasciculations are *best demonstrable* in (i) larger muscles e.g. deltoid, calves etc. by percussing with a hammer, and when gross the muscles may resemble bags of worms, (ii) wasting but not the wasted muscles, and (iii) non-myasthenic subjects by 2.5 mg neostigmine injection and in myasthenic patients by a much smaller dose.

The abnormal movements like tremor, athetosis, chorea, hemiballismus, tics and convulsions should be observed while examining the limbs.

Tremor–This is an alternate rhythmic contraction of the antagonist and protagonist groups of muscles characterised clinically by a more or less regular rhythmic oscillations of a part of the body around a fixed point and usually in one plane. Decide whether the tremor is present at rest–*static tremor*, or movement of the part–*kinetic tremor*. *Intention tremor* appears when the patient is asked to do something such as lifting a glass of water to his mouth. This is found in cerebellar disorders, disseminated sclerosis etc. *Tremor at rest* is characteristically found in Parkinsonism. It is temporarily suppressed when the limb is voluntarily moved. The rate is between 3 and 7 movements per second. *Fine tremor* is characteristic of thyrotoxicosis and chronic alcoholism. *Senile tremor* is found in old age, it may be fine or coarse. *Most common* tremor is that due to nervousness and anxiety.

N.B.–Asterixis or flapping tremors are lapses in maintaining sustained postures; not a true tremor and found in hepatic renal, respiratory failures and other toxic encephalopathies.

Chorea – These are quasipurposive, nonrepetitive jerky

movements of the face, tongue or limbs. They are found in rheumatic affection of the basal ganglia and cerebral cortex (Sydenham's chorea), Huntington's chorea (autosomal domi-nants inheritance); pregnancy (chorea gravidarum); in patients on oral contraceptives; in older age groups (senile or arteriosclerotic); and rarely in haemolytic disease of the newborn,–due to kernicterus and also may be associated with thyrotoxicosis, SLE, polycythaemia vera, hypernatraemia etc.

Athetosis –These are slow, sinuous, writhing move-ments usually of the distant and rarely the proximal parts of the limbs due to degenerative lesions of putamen. These may be congenital or due to difficult labour (leading to cerebral anoxia), Wilson's disease, cerebral arteriosclero-sis, kernicterus, cerebral palsy, overdose of L. -Dopa etc.

Tics –These are nothing but habit spasms which are repetitive and well coordinated. These are found in normal persons as well as in anxiety neurosis.

Hemiballismus – They are involuntary movements of jerky and nonrepetitive nature, limited to one side of the body and are chiefly produced by movements of the proximal group of muscles and there is a great tendency towards rotation of the limbs. Hemiballismus is character-istically found in lesions of the opposite subthalamic nuclei of Luys.

Convulsions–These are widespread and vigorous move-ments produced as a result of clonic contractions of the opposing group of muscles and may be localised to, say, a finger or may become generalised involving the whole body.

These are seen in febrile conditions, grand mal epilepsy, encephalitis, hypertensive encephalopathy, Strokes-Adams syndrome, cerebral anoxia, kernicterus and many other toxic or metabolic encephalopathies.

Spasmodic torticollis is manifested as involuntary movements of the cervical muscles of both sides and may be found in hysteria.

The skin should be inspected for the presence of *trophic changes* and *ulceration*. They are present in lower motor neurone diseases, syringomyelia, tabes dorsalis, diabetic peripheral neuropathy, Hansen's infection, carcinomatous and rheumatoid polyneuropathy and in many other sensory polyneuropathies;—in the form of dryness, roughness and cyanosis of the skin, brittleness of the nails as well as of hairs,. fall of hair, pigmentation, varicosities of veins, ulcers and Raynaud's phenomenon. *Trophic changes* should be looked for on the shin, lateral malleolus, ball of foot, heel, shoulder girdle (over the back) etc. The *trophic ulcers* are usually present over the ball of the foot, lateral malleolus, and back of the sacrum. These ulcers are produced by impairment of sensation from destruction of the vasoconstrictor fibres of the sympathetic system and loss of influence of muscular action upon the circulation

Palpation

First of all confirm the *Wasting* of the muscles by measuring the girth of both limbs at the same particular level above or below the joints. Compare the girths of the two sides.

Now assess the *Tone* of the muscles by noting the posture of the limbs, neck and trunk and by feeling the state of tension of the muscles both at rest and at the time of passive movements of the limb. Tone is defind as the state of sustained and partial contraction of a muscle characterised clinically by a resistance to stretching by passive movements.

The state of tension of a particular muscle is assessed

by passive movement of the limb at the joint. Thus the degree of tone is estimated by handling the limbs and moving them passively at their various joints. *Hypertonia may be spasticity or rigidity and hypotonia* may be due to (i) interruption of the stretch reflex are, (ii) cerebellar disorders, (iii) chorea, (iv) neurological shock etc.

Spasticity means increased resistance to passive movement due to a lesion in the pyramidal tract.

Rigidity means increased resistance to passive movement due to a lesion in the extrapyramidal tract.

Flaccidity means loss of normal muscle tone due to a lesion either in the lower motor neurone or in the posterior column. Hypotonia is, therefore, characteristically found in tabes dorsalis. Hypertonia of the muscles is found in :

(a) Pyramidal tract lesions—This hypertonia is predominantly found in the flexor group of muscles in the upper limbs and extensor group of muscles in the lower limbs i.e. *antigravity* muscles. Hence the characteristic attitude of hemiplegia. This is known as clasp-knife spasticity because it is maximal at the beginning, sustained for a while till it disappears suddenly as the passive movement is continued. [A partial lesion of the higher motor pathway in the spinal cord leads to *paraplegia in extension.* As the disease progresses and involves the extrapyramidal tract, the lesion becomes complete. *Paraplegia in flexion* results from unlimited action of the spinal flexor reflex.]

(b) Extrapyramidal lesion—This type of increased muscle tone is known as rigidity. It may be of two types; *cogwheel* rigidity which is characterised by fluctuant resistance and the other known as *leadpipe* rigidity which is characterised by a steady and continuous resistance to passive movements.

(c) Plastic type of rigidity in midbrain lesion—This is also known as catatonic state. In this type the limb maintains the position in which it is left after a passive movement. There is no resistance during passive movements.

(d) Hysterical rigidity–In hysteria, the muscular resistance increases in proportion to the effort made by the observer to move the limb.

(e) Anxiety neurosis–Muscle tone is increased as the muscles are in a state of tension.

(f) Gegenhalten–This is also known as counterholding and is a peculiar type of variable resistance to passive movement; the patient cannot release the muscle on command and is unable to cooperate since relaxation requires the patient's cooperation Gegenhalten is found in–(i) frontal lobe diseases, (ii) senility, (iii) confusional states etc.

Hypotonia of the muscles is found in :

(a) Diseases of the motor component of reflex arc: poliomyelitis, polyneuritis, peripheral nerve injury etc.

(b) Diseases of the sensory component : tabes dorsalis, herpes zoster, carcinomatous neuropathy etc.

(c) Combined lesions : syringomyelia, compression of cord on root etc.

(d) Diseases of the muscles : myopathies, myasthenia gravis, benign infantile hypotonia etc.

(e) State of neurological shock, chorea and cerebellar lesions.

Clonus–Clonus consists of a series of rhythmical contractions in response to the sudden stretching of a hypertonic muscle. This is associated with hypertonicity and exaggerated deep jerks. Clonus is one of the most important signs of pyramidal tract lesion.

Method of examination of *ankle clonus*–Ask the patient to relax in bed. Raise the knee from the bed by placing your left palm on the posterior aspect of knee joint above the origin of calf muscles. Grasp the distal part of the foot and toes with the help of your right hand and ensure that the heel is not touching the bed. Now suddenly dorsiflex the foot when the calf muscles will be stretched, maintain the stretch, and a series of contractions of the calf are visible. For the demonstration of ankle clonus, a steady pressure on the foot should be maintained in the direction of initial sudden movement.

Ankle clonus is produced by the loss of upper motor control over the first and second sacral segments of the spinal cord (S_1, S_2).

Patellar clonus–Pull the patella with a fold of skin upwards and then suddenly push it down towards the shin and hold it. A series of contractions of the quadriceps will be observed. For the demonstration of the patellar clonus the leg should be in the extended position and a steady pressure on the patella should be maintained. The patellar clonus is also know as *trepidation sign*. The patellar clonus is produced by a lesion involving the upper motor control over the 3rd and 4th lumber segments of the spinal cord (L_3, L_4).

N.B.–Remember that there is nothing diagnostic about an isolated clonus which merely represents an increase in reflex excitability.

There is a condition known as *pseudoclonus* where the number of contractions after stretching of the muscle is usually less than six at a time. This is found in anxiety states, in a strained muscle or in a subject who has had a fright.

Motor power– Test the motor power of the limbs, the shoulder girdle, the rectus abdominis and sacrospinalis, the respiratory muscles, the diaphragm and the muscles of the neck. Individual muscle power should be determined by asking the patient to perform some movements or to work against resistance.

(a) Muscles of the upper limbs–All the muscles of the

upper limb can be roughly tested by asking the patient to hold your hand as firmly as he can. Compare it to that of the normal side. Test for both static and kinetic power by trying to move the patient's limb from a particular position against resistance in the former and by trying to resist the patient's effort of moving the limb in the latter.

(i) Small muscles of the hand—The *opponens pollicis* is tested by asking the patient to touch the tip of the little finger with the tip of the thumb.

The *first dorsal interosseous* is tested by asking the patient to abduct the index finger against resistance.

Dorsal interossei are abductors, hence their power can be assessed by asking the patient to abduct the fingers against resistance. Palmar interossei are the abductors of the fingers and can be tested by placing a card between the fingers and then trying to pull it out.

The *lumbricals* are tested by asking the patient to flex his metacarpophalangeal joints and to extend the distal interphalangeal joints.

The power of the *flexors of the fingers* should be elicited by asking the patient to squeeze your index and middle fingers placed in a crosswise manner.

(ii) Ask the patient to touch the crease on the front of the same wrist joint (*long flexors*).

(iii) Now test the power of the *extensors of the wrist.* Ask the patient to flex the fingers in the form of a first when the hand is held with palm downward. Hold the wrist joint firmly and ask the patient to extend the wrist against the resistance offered by the flat of your hand on the patient's dorsum. Paralysis of the extensors of the wrist (wrist drop) is typically found in peripheral neuropathy with involvement of the radial nerve, classically seen in lead neuropathy.

(iv) Place the hand of the patient midway between

supine and prone positions. Apply resistance by grasping the hand while the patient tries to bend up his forearm. *Brachioradialis* is tested by this technique but it is characteristically exempted in paralysis of the forearm muscles in chronic lead poisoning.

(v) Power of the *biceps* is elicited by asking the patient to bend up the forearm with the elbow firmly placed on the bed. Apply resistance of the flexor aspect of the wrist. The muscle bulk should be inspected for prominence and palpated for texture.

(vi) Ask the patient to straighten out his forearm while trying to keep it flexed by passive resistance and thus the *triceps* is tested. Look for its consistency and bulk.

(vii) The *supraspinatus* and the *deltoid* are tested by asking the patient to lift his arm at a right angle to his side. The first 30^0 of the movement is done by the supraspinatus and the last 60^0 by the deltoid.

(viii) Place the patient's elbow by his side. Ask the patient to rotate the limb outwards with the elbow held in 90^0 flexion. The muscle bulk should be inspected by placing the hand over the *infraspinatus*.

(ix) The *pectoralis* can be put into contraction by asking the patient to clap his hands while attempts are made to keep them apart. Inspect whether both heads of the muscle are thrown into prominence or not.

(x) 'Winging' of the scapula occurs in paralysis of the *serratus anterior.* The deformity can be made obvious by asking the patient to push forward against a wall with his hands. The long thoracic nerve is at fault.

(xi) Grasp the two posterior axillary folds of the patient from behind and ask him to cough repeatedly. Compare the contractions of the *latissimus dorsi* of the two sides.

Lastly raise the two upper limbs in turn straight upwards

and let them go suddenly. The weak or paralysed side falls like a log of wood.

(b) Muscles of the neck–The techniques for assessment of power of the muscles of the neck have been mentioned earlier.

(c) Muscles of the lower limbs :

(i) The *dorsiflexors* and the *plantar flexors* are tested by asking the patient to move the feet up and down respectively against resistance. The observer should keep the ankle fixed by holding it.

(ii) The *evertor* of the foot i.e. the *peroneus tertius* can be tested by asking the patient to turn the foot outwads against resistance. The muscles of the anterior crural compartment i.e. the *invertors* can be tested by asking the patient to turn his foot inwards against resistance. The *tibialis anterior* retains its power while all the others are paralysed in chronic lead poisoning.

(iii) *Extensors of the knee–* Bend up the knee of the patient, place your palm on the sole of his foot and ask him to straighten the limb.

(iv) *Flexors of the knee–* The thigh is flexed and supported with the left hand and the ankle with the right hand. Now ask the patient to pull his leg backwards.

(v) *Extensor of the hip* can be tested by asking the patient to depress the limb against resistance. Knee being kept fully extended, patient's foot should be off the bed.

(vi) *Flexors of the hip–* The knee is fully extended and ask the patient to lift his leg off the bed against resistance.

(vii) *Abductors and adductors of the thigh* can be tested by asking the patient to move the limb away from the midline and towards the midline respectively against resistance.

(viii) *Rotators of the hip* can be tested by asking the patient to rotate the limb outwards and inwards against resistance—the legs being kept fully extended on the bed.

Lastly elevate the two legs in turn and let them suddenly go. The weak or paralysed side falls like a log of wood.

(d) *Rectus abdominis*—Paralysis of the rectus abdominis of one side can be detected by a deviation of the umbilicus to the opposite side when the patient tries to lift his head from the bed. This is known as *Beevor's sign*. Fell for the contraction of the muscles of the two sides. The umbilicus moves upwards if there is a paralysis of the lower segment of the rectus and similarly it goes down if there is a paralysis of the upper segment.

(e) *Sacrospinalis*—The sacrospinalis is tested by inspecting its prominence over the back on extending the head and neck. The patient should lie in prone position.

(f) *Respiratory muscles*—Ask the patient to take a deep breath and count up to 30 at a stretch. Normally one should be able to count up to 30 after taking a deep breath.

(g) *Diaphragm*—Note the movements of the diaphragm by tidal percussion of the chest. The technique of this manoeuvre is discussed in Respiratory System.

The movements of the abdomen should be studied. Normally it bulges during inspiration an retracts during expiration. Inspect the abdomen and see whether there is recession of the epigastrium and hypochondrium during inspiration, as occurs in *diaphragmatic palsy*. This is known as the paradoxical movement of the diaphragm. In this case the lower part of the chest shows an increased horizontal expansion with widening of the subcostal angle during inspiration.

In unilateral paralysis of the diaphragm one side of the abdomen moves better than the other.

N.B.–In an internal capsular lesion, the diaphragm as well as the pharyngeal and laryngeal muscles remain uninvolved.

Quantitative assessment of muscle power : The gradation that is commonly used is as follows :

GRADE 0 – Total paralysis.
GRADE 1 – Just visible or palpable flicker of contraction.
GRADE 2 – Normal movement with gravity eleminated.
GRADE 3 – Normal movement against gravity, not against additional resistance.
GRADE 4 – Full normal movement, but overcomes by resistance.
GRADE 5 – Normal power.

Co-ordination–

It means co-operative action of the prime movers, synergistic, antagonistic and fixator muscles to accomplish a definite act. It is controlled by the sensory system as well as by the neocerebellum.

Co-ordination in the *upper limb* is tested by the *finger nose test.* Explain the whole procedure to the patient and ask him to touch the tip of the nose with the tip of his index finger with the arm drawn out to full abduction while the eyes are open. Next, with the eyes closed ask him to repeat the same. *Intention tremor* occurs at the end of the act and it increases in frequency as the object comes nearer and nearer. Intention tremor is one of the characteristic signs of cerebellar disorders.

Co-ordination of the lower limbs can be elicited by asking the patient to walk on a straight line. It can also be tested by asking the patient to place one heel on the opposite knee and slide the heel downwards, along the shin, first with the eyes open and then with the eyes closed. This is known as the heel-knee test.

Look for *dysdiadokokinesia.* This is the failure of execution of rapidly repeated movements. Ask the patient to flex his elbow to a right angle and then alternately supinate and pronate as quickly as possible. Normally one can continue this at the same rate and rhythm. In cerebellar diseases these movements are clumsy, irregular and jerky. Another method is to ask the patient to clap over the dorsum of one hand with the palm and dorsum alternately of the other hand as quickly as possible. The movements are slow and incomplete if dysdiadokokinesia is present.

Romberg's sign is a special test to **differe**ntiate the ataxia of sensory origin from that of cerebellar origin. The patient is asked to stand with his feet close together. If he can stand with the eyes open, ask him to close them. If the patient sways or falls on closing the eyes the Romberg's test is positive and the ataxia is of sensory origin. If he can -not stand even with the eyes open, the Romberg's test is *then also positive* but the ataxia is of cerebellar origin.

(D) *GAIT*

The gait of a patient suffering from a neurological deficit needs to be observed with keen interest. Gait means posture of the patient during walking. It may be of the following types :

(i) Due to diseases of bones e.g. *limping* gait of talipes equinovarous.

(ii) Due to diseases of joints e.g. *limping* gait of tuberculosis of the knee and hip joints, *waddling* gait of bilateral congenital dislocation of hip.

(iii) Due to diseases of muscles e.g. *waddling* gait of myopathies.

(iv) Due to diseases of the nervous system–

(a) Spastic–e.g. *hemiplagic gait.* This is due to paralysis of the flexor group of muscles of the lower limbs resulting in dragging of the foot. The foot is raised from the ground by tilting the pelvis and the leg is dragged forward in an arc (circumduction).

Another type of spastic gait known as *scissors* gait is found in paraparesis and congenital paraplegia.

In Parkinsonism the gait consist of short shuffling movements, with a posture of flexion and an inability to stop walking suddenly. The patient appears to run to get a hold of his centre of gravity. This is also known as *festinent gait.*

(b) Ataxic–Gait of sensory ataxia is typically found in polyneuritis and tabes dorsalis. In a case of polyneuritis the gait is *high stepping* in type. In case of tabes dorsalis the gait is typically known as *stumping gait*, with a broad base. The feet are lifted too high and brought down to the ground violently.

(c) Reeling–It is typically found in alcoholics and cerebellar diseases. The patient walks on a broad base and the ataxia is present irrespective of whether the eyes are closed or open.

(v) Prosthetic gait–This is due to walking with an artificial limb.

(vi) Functional or hysterical– All types of gait may be present in combination or there may be bizarre movements associated with the gait. These are characteristically absent when there is no observer nearby.

(E) *REFLEXES*

When a muscle with normal innervation is passively stretched by sharp taps, it will actively resist the stretch; and the tension inside the muscle is increased and sustained for a short while. This reflex action is evoked by the stimulation of the stretch receptors i.e. the muscle spindles. The stimulus passes to the anterior horn cells via a monosynaptic arc. The contractions become visible due to potentiation of the sensitivity of the stretch receptor by the contraction of its intrafusal muscle fibres in response to the stretch.

Superficial reflexes are manifested as brisk, short lived contractions of the muscles innervated from the same spinal segment which receives stimulus from the region of the skin supplied by that segment.

Besides the superficial and deep reflexes, the primitive reflexes also should be examined as a routine.

Tendon reflexes :

1. Biceps jerk (C5 & 6)–The fifth and sixth cervical segments of the spinal cord (particularly the fifth segment) are concerned with this deep reflex. Flex the patient's elbow to a right angle with forearm in a semipronated position and let it relax on your hand. Expose the arm fully .up to the shoulder and free the biceps tendon. Place your thumb on the biceps tendon and strike it with the percussion hammer. Use the hammer by moving only the wrist joint. Look at the biceps muscle which will contract in response to the strike, and there will be flexion of the elbow.

2. Supinator jerk (C5 & 6) – The reflex path for this jerk also passes through the fifth and sixth cervical segments of the spinal cord (particularly the sixth segment).

A tap is given upon the radial styloid process. Flexion of the elbow occurs and slight flexion of the fingers often occur also.

If there is a lesion of the fourth or fifth cervical segment of the spinal cord, the reflex will be abolished, but flexion of the fingers occurs. Presence of finger flexion only in absence of elbow flexion or bracioradialis contraction is known as the *inversion* of the radial reflex (Radial reflex is the synonym of supinator jerk). In this condition the biceps jerk is absent and triceps and finger flexion jerks are exaggerated and is caused by cervical disc lesions. syringomyelia cervical trauma, cervical cord neoplasms etc.

3. Triceps jerk (C6 & 7) – Place the hand of the patient over the chest with the elbow flexed. Feel the triceps tendon and tap it just above the olecranon. There is an extension of the elbow. It depends on the sixth and seventh cervical segments of the spinal cord. It is a classical example of the monosynaptic reflex arc.

4. Flexor finger-jerk (C_6 to T_1) – A sharp tap upon the palmar surface of the semiflexed fingers will cause flexion of the fingers and thumb.

5. Knee jerk (L 3 & 4) – The spinal segments concerned are the third and fourth lumbar segments of the spinal cord. Both the knees being passively flexed place your forearm below the knees and ask the patient to relax and divert his attention in some way. Expose the quadriceps muscle and feel the quadriceps tendon below the patella. Now give a sharp tap on the patellar tendon of each side. Extension of the knee occurs. Inspect the contraction of the quadriceps of one side and compare it with that of the other.

Sometimes *reinforcement* (Jendrassik manoeuvre) may be necessary when the reflexes are otherwise unelicitable. For this the patient is asked to clench his teeth with a much pressure as he can or pull out the fingers against one another (the fingers lying together in a hook like fashion). Reinforcement acts by increasing the muscular tone throughout the body by increasing recruitment of the γ (gamma) efferent neurones.

The spinal segments involved in this jerk are L3 and L4;

though according to some they are L2, L3 and L4.

6. Ankle jerk (Sl & 2) – It depends on the first and second sacral segments of the spinal cord. Place the lower limb on the bed so that the leg is flexed at the knee join and it lies everted. Dorsiflex the foot with the help of left hand to partly stretch the tendo-Achilles and strike the tendon on its posterior surface. The calf muscles should be inspected for contractions, and there will be plantar flexion of the ankle. This reflex can also be elicited with the patient kneeling on a chair.

7. Rossolimo reflex–With the patient lying supine, the leg extended and the foot partially dorsiflexed the ball of the foot is struck with the hammer. In UMN lesions and hypertonic states there is a plantar flexion of the great toe at the metatarsophalangeal joint and brisk contractions of other toes. The reflex can be elicited also be flicking one or more of the toes upward. Its counterpart in the upper limb is the *Hoffman reflex*, when, under similar condition, if the terminal phalanx of the patient's middle finger is sharply flicked downwards, the tips of the other fingers flex while the thumb flexes and adducts.

All the tendon reflexes are dependent on particular segment or segments of the spinal cord. A tendon jerk may be affected in the following ways :

(a) Lesions of the corticospinal tract supplying the particular segment of the spinal cord will produce *exaggerated jerks* and this may be found in cerebral thrombosis, cerebral embolism, subarachnoid haemorrhage, disseminated sclerosis, amyotrophic lateral sclerosis cerebral tumours, spinal tumours etc.

Tendon reflexes may be brisker than average in some normal individuals. *Anxiety states* may also cause exaggeration of the tendon reflexes.

(b) Lesions of the anterior horn cells of the segments will produce *loss* of jerk as in acute anterior poliomyelitis, motor neurone disease like progressive muscular atrophy etc.

(c) Lesions of the peripheral nerves (as for example the musculocutaneous nerve in biceps jerk, the radial nerve in triceps jerk and supinator jerk, the femoral nerve in knee jerk and the sciatic nerve in ankle jerk) will cause *diminution or absence* of the jerks.

(d) Jerks are usually lost during the period of neural shock which last for 10 to 14 days and also may be reduced or lost when an excess of spasticity, rigidity or muscle contracture disallow muscle movement.

(e) Jerks may be lost in lesions of the posterior column due to degeneration of the afferent path e.g. in tabes dorsalis.

(f) Jerks may be abnormally prolonged in (i) cerebellar lesions particularly if there is a partial UMN lesions and (ii) myxoedema–the relaxation is especially retarded–the 'hung up' reflex.

Loss of knee jerk is commonly encountered in acute anterior poliomyelitis, acute infective polyneuritis, tabes dorsalis, peripheral neuritis, acute compression myelitis and acute transverse myelitis in the stage of neural shock, Friedreich's ataxia, progressive muscular atrophy and very late stages of muscular dystrophy.

A special importance of elicitation of the ankle jerk lies in the fact that it is often *singly lost without a loss of knee jerk* in subacute combined degeneration of the cord, cauda equina syndrome and rarely in conus medullaris syndrome, taboparesis, Friedreich's ataxia etc. In myxoedema, 'delayed relaxation' of the ankle jerk is a special feature.

In cases of cerebellar syndromes the knee jerks are often *diminished* or *pendular.* The first knee jerk is followed by a series of diminishing oscillations which are 5 or more.

Some other important causes of loss or diminution of deep reflexes include– (i) Diabetes mellitus in which the loss of knee and ankle jerks may be the earliest or even the sole manifestation of polyneuropathy.

(ii) Holmes– Adie syndrome in which the deep reflexes especially the knee and ankle jerks may be affected (see page 88.)

(iii) In sciatica the ankle jerk of the affected side may be lost or diminished.

(iv) In cervical spondylosis the deep reflexes of the upper limbs may be particularly affected.

Superficial reflexes :

Stimulation of an area of the skin by scratching results in a contraction of certain muscles supplied by the same spinal segment. They are dependent upon the *polysynaptic reflex* arcs of which the frontal cortex is a part.

Planter reflex : Ask the patient to relax in bed and grasp the lower portion of the leg above the ankle joint with your left hand. The outer border of the foot is now scratched with a blunt needle or preferably with a key. Start from the heel and draw the needle upwards along the lateral border of the foot and then turn towards but *do not touch* the ball of the great toe in a hockeystick fashion. Look at the great toe for any upward or downward movement at the *metatarsophalangeal* joint as well as the other toes for fanning or plantar flexion. Normally in healthy adults the plantar reflex consists of slight contraction of the adductors of the thigh and the sartorius, and flexion of the outer four toes. With a still stronger stimulus all the toes are flexed on the metatarsus and drawn together; dorsiflexion with inversion of the ankle joint may occur. And with further strong stimulus, violent movements of the limb spreading to the trunk and to the opposite side and sweating along with incontinence of urine may occur. The latter portion is known as the *mass reflex.*

Babinski's sign means extensor plantar response and truely is a physiologic flexion of the big toe. It was described by Babinski in 1896. Physiologically it is a part of the normal flexion withdrawal reflex. Babinski's sign is characteristic of pyramidal tract involvement and is due to disinhibition resulting from UMN lesions. However, the nociceptive spinal flexion reflexes, of which Babinski's sign is a part, do not constitute an essential component of spasticity. The plantar reflex is normally extensor up to the first year of life. It may be absent in coma and lower motor neurone diseases and spinal shock.

Oppenheim's sign–Stroking of the inner border of the tibia results in extension of the great toe associated with some dorsiflexion of the foot in pyramidal tract lesions.

Gordon's reflex–Extension of the great toe associated with dorsiflexion of the foot can be produced by squeezing the calf muscle. Oppenheim's sign and Gordon's reflex are found in progressive diseases involving the pyramidal tract.

Chaddock's reflex–Strike lightly below the lateral malleolus on the outer side of the foot–significance, observation and inferences are same as the plantar reflex. All these three reflexes are seen in extensive or progressive UMN lesions.

Abdominal reflexes : They consist of contractions of the recti abdominis muscles as a result of stimulation of the skin overlying the muscles by scratching with a needle. The strokes must be a gentle one without producing any injury to the skin. They are tested in three regions;–below the costal margin, at the level of the umbilicus and in the iliac fossa. Spinal segments responsible for these reflexes are 7th, 8th, 9th, 10th, 11th and 12th thoracic segments.

The skin should be scratched from outside inwards in the following manner :

(i)   The part of the skin above the level of the umbilicus supplied by the 7th and 8th thoracic segments should be stimulated from outwards parallel to the subcostal arch towards the midline.

(ii)   The umbilical region (9th & 10th segments) should be stimulated horizontally toward the umbilicus.

(iii) The part of the skin below the level of the umbilicus (11th & 12 th thoracic segments) should be scratched from outwards parallel to the inguinal ligament towards the midline, on both sides.

The abdominal reflexes are often absent or undetectable in obese multiparous women. These reflexes are usually diminished or absent in pyramidal tract disorders, herpes zoster or surgical trauma damaging the peripheral nerves or muscles etc. and may be *exaggerated* in psychoneurosis, anxiety, nervousness etc.

In hemiplegia the superficial reflexes are disturbed on the paralysed side.

N.B.–The nociceptive abdominal reflexes are *lost early in multiple sclerosis* while *long retained in cerebral palsy* and MND despite extensive UMN lesions.

Besides the abdominal there are other superficial reflexes which include the following :

(i) Cremasteric reflex (LI)– It is tested by mild scratching of the medial side of the upper thigh from below upwards, where upon the testis is drawn upwards and there is a contraction of the dartos muscle as evidenced by an increase in wrinkling of the scrotal skin. The spinal segment responsible for this reflex is the first lumber segment.

(ii) Bulbocavernosus reflex (S3 & 4)– This consists of contraction of the bulbocavernosus as a result of pinching the dorsum of the glans penis. This depends upon the 3rd and 4th sacral segments.

(iii) The 3rd and 4th sacral segments are also responsible for the *anal reflex* which means contraction of the anal sphincter on scratching the skin near the anus.

(iv) Scapular region–Stroking of the skin of the interscapular region stimulates the cord from the 5th cervical to the 1st thoracic segments, which results in contraction of the scapular muscles.

Primitive reflexes : It has been stated already that the superficial and deep reflexes having been elicited, the student should proceed to the examination of *primitive reflexes* which has been elaborated in Sick Children. Here it is emphasised that these reflexes having disappeared by the 4th to 6th month of life, normally because of and simultaneous with the rapid maturation of the nervous system, may reappear anytime in later life whenever there is a degenerative process involving particularly the cortex. Even these reflexes may continue to persist beyond 4 to 5 months of age in infants with severe neurologic defects. Presence of these reflexes in adult subjects is of more diagnostic value when *they are unilateral*, since their bilateral elicitation does not help in localising the side. Two important such reflexes are–(i) *palmomental reflex* elicited by scratching across the base of the thenar eminence; when a contraction of the ipsilateral mentalis muscle result in a dimpling of the chin and in reflex hyperexcitability or in normal individuals this may be present bilaterally but when present in one side only it indicates a pyramidal tract lesion; (ii) the *blink reflex* or the *glabellar tap sign* in which repeatedly tapping the forehead above the bridge of the nose evokes visible contractions of the palpebral orbicularis oculi that cease after the first few taps in a normal person but continues in many patients with *Parkinsonism* so long as the tapping stimulus is applied but is totally absent in *coma*. Both these are mediated by the 7th nerve. The glabellar tap sign is also known as *Meyerson sign*.

F. SENSORY SYSTEM

A comprehensive knowledge of the paths of different types of sensation and a methodical approach while examining the sensory system will be of great value in the accurate localisation of a lesion. The fibres enter the spinal cord through the posterior nerve root and dissociate to run in the different tracts–some ending in the cord, some in the medulla (Gracile and Cuneate nuclei), while others passing to the thalamus and few directly to the cerebellum to supply the proprioceptive information. Lastly relay from the thalamus goes to the cerebral cortex.

Cutaneous sensations like light touch, pain and temperature and kinaesthetic sensation like joint, vibration, posture, and pressure etc. are the different modes of sensibility.

Light touch is carried by the columns of Goll and Burdach but crude touch or pressure sensation, pain and temperature are carried by the lateral spinothalamic tract and trigeminothalamic tract. Fibres of kinaesthetic sensation pass through the posterior column, cross in the spinal cord and ultimately reach the medial lemniscus where the superior sensory decussation takes palce. Sensory fibres are ultimately destined for the thalamus and a few fibres pass via the internal capsule to the sensory cortex situated behind the central sulcus.

General plan for examination of sensory function : *Spinothalamic sensations* (pain, temperature, and crude

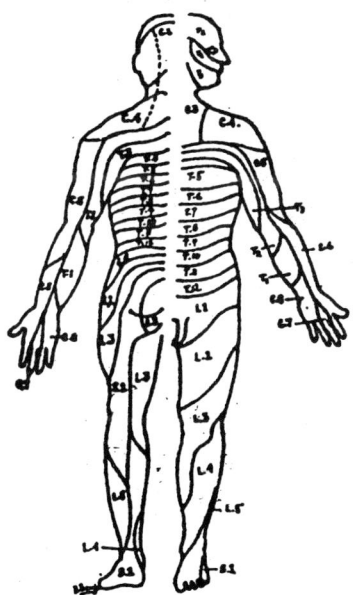

Fig. 44 : *Distribution of Dematomes of the skin.*

touch) are examined first and after that the tests for *posterior column sensations* (like muscles sense, joint sense. vibration sense, appreciation of movement, sense of position and fine touch) are performea as a routine. Lastly the *cortical sensations*–point localisation, two point discrimination, recognition of the size, shape and form (stereognosis), weight discrimination, texture discrimination, graphaesthesia, and sensory and visual inattentions are to be examined gently and cautiously, first explaining the details of the procedure to the patient during every individual test, to get his full cooperation. Zone of hypesthesia or hyperesthesia and abnormal sensations or paresthesia can only be found out after a meticulous search, repeating the tests, and comparing always with the normal side.

N.B.–Instruct the patient to close the eyes while carrying out the actual manoeuvre;–*this is a must.*

Tests : Tactile sensation is examined by touching the skin with wisps of cotton wool, comparing it with the corresponding point on the opposite side of the body. A hairy area must be shaved before testing the area. The different types of responses that are commonly met with in clinical practice are complete loss of sensation (anaesthesia) and pain sensation in the form of pricking or burning;–evoked even on light touch (hyperesthesia) Abnormal spontaneous subjective sensations (paresthesia) may be met within the form of tingling, numbness or pricking. *Spontaneous pain, sensation of heat, walking on cotton wool or pin pricking paresthesia* may be the features of tabes dorsalis, epilepsy, sensory hallucination tetany, hysteria etc.

Perversion of sensation may arise from incomplete interruption of sensory nerve fibres or from a damage to the myelin sheaths as in disseminated sclerosis. *Glove and stocking anaesthesia* is found in peripheral neuritis. Considerable interval between the appreciation of the stimulus and the response of the patient labelled as *delayed conduction* is observed in tabes dorsalis. Superficial pain sensation is tested by pricking with a blunt pin or needle avoiding heavy pressure (otherwise pressure pain may be induced and wrongly interpreted. It must be noted whether the patient can determine the sharpness of the prick. Complete loss of pain sensation (analgesia), partial loss of pain sensation (hypoalgesia) and too much pain on prick (hyperalgesia) are the different variants. *Threshold of pain sensation is raised* in a thalamic and spinothalamic tract lesion and in lesions of posterior ˉoot ganglion or mixed spinal nerves. this is classically known as *hyperpathia* and overreaction is one of its features.

The clinical examination as described above and a history of spontaneous pain may give clues to the diagnosis of neurological disorders. *Spontaneous pain* in the absence of any sensory stimulus may ɔe found in lesions of the thalamus, spinothalamic tract and mixed spinal nerves; and as lightning pain of tabes dorsalis. History of root pain and girdle sensation may indicate the level of spinal compression. *Root pain* refers to irritation of the posterior root ganglion. Radiation of pain along the distribution of the nerve may be helpful in the diagnosis of the level of the lesion or gives an idea of involvement of a spinal nerve, The presence of root pain in paraplegia indicates the possibility of a spinal tumour which is progressively increasing. An *electric shock-like sensation* may be found on flexion or extension of the spine in posterior root lesions and when this radiates down the spine and limbs on sudden flexion of the neck, as may occur in cervical spondylosis, cervical spinal cord tumours, multiple sclerosis etc, it is termed *Barber's chair or Lhermitt's sign.* *Spontaneous pain* may also be found in diabetic neuropathy and in Buerger's disease. *Phantom pain* as expressed by the patient indicates the parietal lobe as the site of the lesion. Constitutional disturbances followed by the appearance of vesicular or bullous rash along the distribution of a spinal nerve and hyperalgesia lead to suspicion of *preherpetic stage* (affection of the posterior root ganglion by the varicella zoster virus).

Temperature sensation is tested by test tubes containing cold and warm water respectively and frequently interchanging them with a view to avoiding error. The thresholds for heat and cold should also be determined. *Dissociated anaesthesia* may be found in syringomyelia. This may occasionally be confused with Hansen's infection. Dissociated sensory loss also occurs in Wallenburg's (lateral medullary) syndrome, conus medullaris syndrome intramedullary intraspinal tumours etc.

Muscle sensation is tested by applying firm pressure on the calf muscle. Deep pain sensation is tested by the above procedure and by squeezing the tendo-Achilles. Muscle sensation is increased in polyneuritis (*Abadie's sign*) myositis, subacute combined degeneration etc. and diminished in tabes dorsalis, syringomyelia, carcinomatous neuropathy etc.

The principle of testing proprioception depends on whether the patient can accurately appreciate passive movements of the joints. When the small peripheral joints of the limbs are severely affected the joint sense is impaired in the terminal interphalangeal joint of the index finger or hallux.

Sense of position and joint sensation are tested by fixing the base of the terminal interphalangeal joint in the index finger and in the great toe with two fingers placed on two sides of the joint. Then the terminal phalanx is moved up and down (within 5⁰ from neutral position) finally leaving it in some definite position and the patient is asked to indicate the direction, whether up or down, first with the eyes open and then with the eyes closed. At least four shots must be missed before concluding that the joint sensation is lost. It is absent in lesions of the posterior column, diabetic neuropathy etc.

Vibration sense is tested by placing the vibrating tuning fork of 128 or 256 cycles per second on the medial malleous, dorsum of the hand and foot, olecranon and wrist joint. If the vibration sense is not appreciated the tuning fork should be applied to more proximal bony prominences of the limb. The test is continued until the level at which vibrations can be appreciated has been determined. The vibration sense in the trunk is tested in the anterior abdominal wall, ribs, clavicles and over the vertebral spine. Absence of vibration sense in old age may be a physiological process. It is lost in lesions of the posterior column, in diabetic neuropathy etc.

Point localisation– The patient is asked to close his eyes and the head of the pin is touched in different areas. He is then asked to open his eyes and point the sites stimulated. Normally there is no difficulty in localising the points stimulated. Two point discriminations are tested by means of a special compass or divider.

Stereognosis– Coins of various size, pen, key etc. are given to the patient and asked to indicate the object only by palpation with the eyes closed. Similarly weight discrimination and texture discrimination are tested with the help of the common objects of identical shape and size. Simultaneous assessment of weight is tested by placing a coin on the outstretched palms. In lesions of the sensory cortex the object in the contralateral and appears lighter than an indentical object in the normal hand. The object on the affected side in a cerebellar lesion appears heavier than it really is.

Graphaesthesia–An alphabet, a number, a simple geometrical figure (e.g. circle or triangle) is inscribed on different parts of the body of the patient who keeps his eyes closed and tries to identify the figure. This is lost on one side in a contralateral parietal cortical lesion.

Tests for perceptual rivalry– Corresponding points on two sides of the body are tested simulatenously by the same stimulus. When the test is done separately, the patient can identify the stimulus but if they are applied simultaneously, the one opposite the site of the lesion in parietal cortex is not understood by the patient.

G. *AUTONOMIC NERVOUS SYSTEM*

The autonomic nervous system may be involved in hypothalamic syndromes, diabetes, spinal lesions particularly of the cervical and thoracic regions etc. The following points should be noted during examination of the autonomic nervous system :

1. Disorders of growth–These are due to associated involvement of the pituitary gland, for example–pituitary infantilism and Frohlich's syndrome (dystrophia adiposogenitalis)

2. Disorders of sleep–Somnolence or insomnia are the characteristic symptoms of the hypothalamic disorder.

3. Disorders of temperature regulation–Hypothermia may be observed in lesions of the hypothalamic region.

4. Genital dysfunctions manifested in the form of impotency and amenorrhoea are commonly encountered in diabetic neuropathy due to involvement of the autonomic nervous system.

5. Postural hypotension–This is also due to involvement of the sympathetic autonomic system as occurs in diabetic

neuropathy progressive autonomic failure with multisystem disease (Shy-Drager syndrome); familial dysautonomia (Riley-Day syndrome) etc.

6. Sweating–Sweating may be excessive or diminished below the level of lesion in the spinal cord, due to involvement of the sympathetic nerves. A lesion of the cervical spinal cord may cause excessive sweating of the whole body. Diabetic neuropathy may present with complaints of sweating only.

7. Diarrhoea–This occurs due to rapid emptying of the intestines as a result of parasympathetic overactivity and is manifested as nocturnal diarrhoea in diabetic neuropathy.

8. Trophic ulcers–These have been described earlier. Raynaud's phenomenon is due to intermittent spasm of the digital arteries.

9. Horner's syndrome–This is characterised by partial dropping of the eyelid, constriction of the pupil, enophthalmos and anhydrosis of one side of the face. This is found in syringobulbia, syringomyelia, thrombosis of posterior inferior cerebellar artery, thoracic outlet syndrome etc.

10. Bladder and bowel functions–Micturition consists of relaxation of the sphinecters and contraction of detrusor muscle allowing expulsion of urine from bladder into the urethra. This is performed by a complex neurogenic mechanism involving the sympathetic and parasympathetic neurones, somatic sensory motor sacral peripheral nerves, S_2, S_3 and S_4 spinal cord segments brainstem 'micturitions' centres, with their spinal an suprasegmental connections.

The detrusor has motor innervation from S_2, S_3, S_4 intermediolateral gray column–the postganglionic fibres arise from parasympathetic ganglia within the bladder wall. In the dome of the bladder sympathetic T_{10}, T_{11} and T_{12}

intermediolateral neuronal fibres stimulate muscle cells via β-adrenoreceptors. The internal sphincter have mostly α-adrenoreceptors innervated by hypogastric sympathetic fibres. External sphincter (striated muscle) innervated by S_2, S_3, S_4 anterior horn cells via pudendal nerves–responding to cholinergic nicotinic effects. Afferent fibres from urethra and external sphincter–S_2, S_3, S_4 segments of spinal cord for reflex activities. Pain sensation from bladder →higher centres via spinothalamic tract and pressure →higher centres via posterior column.

In acute transverse lesion of spinal cord sacral segment function is abolished for several weeks→incomplete detrusor contractions occur.

Micturition centre in the periaquiductal area receives afferent impulses from the sacral segments and sends efferent fibres via reticulospinal tracts to the bladder. If this path remains intact, proper bladder emptying occurs. This centre is controlled from frontal cortex and other higher areas.

Voluntary restraint of micturition is a cerebral affair controlled by frontal lobe paracentral motor regions, i.e. UMN function is inhibitory and variations of this inhibition result in micturition. Thus (i) in complete cord destruction below T_{12} voluntary micturition is impossible; retention with incontinence occurs as the bladder is paralysed with no awareness of fullness; (ii) in sacral gray matter motor neurone diseases or those of anterior roots or peripheral nerves bladder sensation is intact, other features being same as above; (iii) in afferent fibre interruption, as in tabes, primary sensory bladder paralysis occurs resulting again in same disturbances; (iv) in upper spinal cord lesion a reflex neurogenic bladder results, also known as spastic bladder since detrusor becomes overactive as spinal shock subsides, bladder capacity is reduced, precipient micturition and incontinence results; (v) mixed sensory motor and spastic bladder paralysis (mixed neurogenic bladder) results from multiple sclerosis, syphilitic meningomyelitis etc.; (vi) bladder neck obstruction result in stretch injury with atonic or hypotonic bladder wall that undergoes fibrosis; (vii) right or left sided lesions of the posterior part of the superior frontal and anterior cingulate gyrus and intervening association fibres result in loss of control of bladder and bowel functions–this is frontal lobe incontinence and occurs because the patient does not get any warning of fullness of the bladder an imminence of urination; (viii) in nocturnal enuresis there is most likely a delay in acquiring inhibition of micturition.

The anal sphincters as well as the colonic muscles are controlled the same way as bladder and hence bowel disturbances parallel those of the bladder but since the bowel content is solid and less often filled, bowel incontinence is less frequent and less troublesome.

Based on the above anatomical and physiological concepts the following clinical conditions should be noted–

1. A lesion in the afferent side of the arc (tabes dorsalis) causes loss of appreciation of bladder distension. As a result the bladder distends and the urine dribbles away.

2. Interruption of the sacral reflex are (stage of spinal shock in severe damage of the spinal cord) gives rise to retention of urine.

3. Gross lesions of the spinal cord above the sacral segment (transverse myelitis) leads to reflex incontinence i.e. the bladder empties automatically causing repeated involuntary micturition due to damage of the inhibitory fibres. Hesitancy and /or retention of urine may occur due to damage of the facilitatory fibres.

4. Compression of the cauda equina causes retention of urine even though the external sphincter is paralysed.

5. In disseminated sclerosis, incontinence of the urine is the usual manifestation.

6. If the higher control is completely lost, there is a period of retention with overflow from a passively dilated atonic bladder until the sacral reflex begins to function in the way as it does in infancy i.e. automatic bladder emptying.

7. In a frontal lobe lesion, the intellectual disturbance may be associated with failure of inhibition of reflex emptying of the bladder.

Detailed history about difficulty during micturition and percussion of the bladder will be necessary to determine the exact nature of the bladder involvement.

H. CEREBELLAR FUNCTIONS

The cerebellum basically co-ordinates movements by regulating the range, rate, rhythm and force of muscular contraction and maintenance of posture.

The specific functions are − (1) The flocculonodular lobes or archicerebellum (the oldest portion) functions in keeping the individual oriented in space and if damaged, result in truncal ataxia, swaying and staggering, not worsened by eye closing.

(3) The clumen and central lobe or palaeocerebellum (the next oldest portion) controls the antigravity muscles via its effect on cortical stimuli.

(2) The posterior lobe or neocerebellum (the youngest portion acts as a brake on volitional movements particularly those requiring halting activity and fine movements of the hands and when damaged result in dysmetrias, dysdiadokokinesias, intention tremors hypotonia and alteration of gait.

A cerebellar hemispheric lesion will produce ipsilateral signs. The following points should be carefully looked for in a case of cerebellar syndrome :

(i) Hypotonia—The muscles are flaccid both at rest as well as on passive movements of the limbs.

(ii) Pendular or diminished knee jerk—The oscillations are gradually diminishing and are found characteristically in the *knee jerk.*

(iii) Intention tremor—The tremor increases as the target is approached. Termor at rest may also be found as the tension necessary to maintain a posture is affected.

(iv) A movement may be disrupted by incoordination and hypotonia.

(v) Dysdiadokokinesia—Rapidly alternating movements are disturbed and carried out in an irregular, jerky fashion.

(vi) Dyssynergia—The movements covering more than one joint are broken up into their component parts.

(vii) Dysmetria—In this case the fingers overshoot or fall short of the object due to muscular incoordination. There is 'past pointing' of the fingers if the movement is performed with the eyes closed.

(viii) Rebound phenomenon—The limb moves beyond the normal range when resistance is suddenly withdrawn as strong contractions cannot be arrested.

(ix) Disorders of articulation and phonation—In this case, the articulation is irregular, sulrred and explosive.

Scanning speech is found in disseminated sclerosis in which the syllables are separated from each other.

(x) Nystagmus—Horizontal jerky nystagmus is diagnostic of cerebellar diseases. The movements are greater in amplitude but slower in rate when the eyes are deviated to the side of the lesion. (in unilateral cerebellar disease).

(xi) Reeling gait—It is due to cerebellar ataxia and the

head may be tilted towards the side of the lesion when the patient is in an erect posture.

(xii) Romberg's sign–It is positive even when the eyes are kept open (see page 138.)

After examining the motor system, the sensory system and the reflexes, decide whether the lesion is of an upper or lower motor neurone type. Then decide whether there is any involvement of the extrapyramidal system. The principles signs by which a *pyramidal tract lesion is* diagnosed are (1) Loss of a voluntary specific movement and not that of an isolated individual muscle. (2) Muscle groups affected diffusely. (3) Wasting minimal and is due to disuse atrophy. (4) Spasticity. (5) Brisk neep reflexes, (6) absent or diminished superficial reflexes. (7) Presence of clonus. (8) Extensor plantar response. (9) Absence of twitching. (10) No reaction of degeneration in the muscles and a normal EMG.

N.B.–In a UMN lesion the distal muscles performing finer movements are predominantly affected.

A lower motor neurone lesion is characterised by– (1) Paralysis of the individual mucloco and not a specific movement (2) Atrophy and wasting of the muscles are pronounced. (3) Flaccidity and hypotonia. (4) Presence of fasciculation and /or fibrillation (5) Loss of deep reflexes. (6) Planter response flexor or may not be elicitable. (7) Presence of reaction of degeneration in the muscles and EMG shows decreased motor units and reveals fibrillations.

An *extrapyramidal lesion* is detected by–(1) Akinesia, hypokinesia or bradykinesia, i.e. poverty or slowness of associated and voluntary movements with the preservation of power; paralysis of voluntary movements is either absent of slight. (2) Loss of normal postural reflexes. (3) Rigidity, either, (a) *cogwheel rigidity.* when tremor is also present rigidity exhibits an interrupted character, or (b) *lead pipe rigidity*, when tremor is absent, the rigidity is smooth. Rigidity is distributed to flexors of all the four limbs and trunk (except in chorea where there is hypotonia). Hence the flexed attitude of the patient (4) Presence of tremor, chorea, athetosis, dystonia, hemiballismus etc. (5) Monotonous speech. (6) Sialorrhoea because of infrequency of swallowing. (7) Infrequent blinking and masked facies. (8) Absence of sensory changes. (9) Absence of bladder disturbances. (10) Normal tendon reflexes (11) Flexor plantar response. (12) Glabellar tap sign positive.

N.B.–Postencephalitic Parkinsonism is associated with a few features that are peculiar to this condition and these include–

(i) Reversed Argyll Robertson pupil, (ii) oculogyric crises, (iii) seborrhoeic dermatitis of the face and forehead, (iv) severe sialorrhoea, (v) intractable hiccoughs and respiratory tics and (vi) behavioural disturbances.

HEMIPLEGIA

Definition–It is defined as the paralysis of one-half of the body (face, arm and leg of one side) due to a pyramidal lesion.

Causes–There are numerous causes of hemiplegia which can be discussed under two groups, congenital and acquired.

I. *Congenital*–Hemiplegia can occur due to degenerative lesions of the cerebral cortex, lobar atrophy, global sclerosis and cerebral agenesis. Congenital cerebral deformity such as true porencephaly, prematurity and postmaturity may also be the factors.

Hemiplegia being a common condition of infancy and early childhood may be congenital, may be due to birth injuries or may occur as a complication of many acute infective disorders such as whooping cough, encephalitis, meningitis etc.

II. *Acquired*–Hemiplegia can develop due to (a) vascular lesions in the internal capsule, for example, cerebrovascular accidents due to arteriosclerosis; (b) neoplastic lesions for example vascular angioma, cerebral tumours; (c) degenerative lesions of example Schilder's disease, disseminated sclerosis; (d) infective lesions as for example encephalitis, cerebral abscess; (e) traumatic as in head injury : (f) functional as in hysteria.

Spinal (homolateral) hemiplegia–A unilateral lesion of the pyramidal tract in the spinal cord below the medulla and above the fifth cervical segment results in hemiplegia of the same side.

N.B.–It is important to remember that though hemiplegia is almost always spastic, a permanently flaccid hemiplegia rarely results from an associated parietal lobe damage.

Site of lesion of a cerebrovascular accident.

The clinical findings and the anatomical areas of involvement are taken into account when one wants to locate the site of a lesion.

(A) Lesion in the cortex : Here the fibres are widely distributed and hence the lesion does not affect a large area and usually produces monoplegia. Jacksonian convulsion occurs if the lesion is in the precentral cortex. Besides there may be aphasia, astereognosis, anosognosia or homonymous visual field defect.

(B) Lesion at the subcortical level or at corona radiata : The paralysis or paresis predominantly affects one limb. In fact, the whole of the opposite side of the body is affected to some extent as many coverging neurones are damaged. A lesion at the subcortical level can effect the corticospinal tract or it may affect the adjacent thalamocortical sensory fibres resulting in postural insensibility, impairment of tactile discrimination and localisation in the affected limb. A subcortical lesion, therefore, tends to involve more fibres than a cortical lesion of equal size.

(C) Lesion at the internal capsule :

(i) Complete hemiplegia of the opposite 'side as the fibres are closely packed.

(ii) Homonymous hemianopia and hemianaesthesia due to damage of both visual and sensory fibres which lie behind the corticospinal fibres.

A lesion of the brainstem is distinguised from a capsular hemiplegia by–(i) involvement of the cranial nerve nuclei and their motor and sensory pathways at the various levels and also the long ascending sensory tracts in brainstem lesion, and (ii) involvement of the sensory pathways and visual fibres in lesions of the internal capsule.

(D) Lesion at midbrain : Damage to the corticospinal tract at the base of the midbrain by vascular occlusion, tumour or aneurysm may cause a paralysis of the face, arm and leg on the opposite side. The site of the lesion is localised by the presence of a paralysis of the muscles supplied by the oculomotor nerve on the same side of the lesion. This oculomotor palsy with crossed hemiplegia constitutes *Waber's syndrome.*

Damage to the corticospinal tract and red nucleus at tegmentum of the midbrain causes oculomotor palsy on the side of the lesion with contralateral hemiplegia, cerebellar ataxia and tremor. This constitues the *Benedikt's syndrome.*

Damage to superior colliculi at the tectum by a pinealoma causes paralysis of upward gaze, fixed pupil and divergence of the eyes–known as *Parinaud's syndrome.*

(E) Lesion at pons : Damage to the corticospinal tract at the base of the pons by a tumour causes paralysis of the leteral rectus (6th nerve) with or without facial paralysis (7th nerve) of lower motor neurone type on the same side of the lesion and hemiplegia on the opposite side,–classically known as *Millard–Gubler syndrome.*

Foville's syndrome is similar to Millard-Gubler syndrome with the exception that the paralysis of conjugate ocular deviation to the side of the lesion takes the place of the sixth nerve palsy.

A lesion of the tegmentum of pons causes Horner's syndrome (paralysis of ocular sympathetic).

(F) Lesion at medulla :

(i) On the midline above the decussation of the pyramid causes unilateral paralysis of half of the tongue with crossed hemiplegia of the limb due to involvement of the corticospinal fibres to the limb above the decussation together with the fibres of the hypoglossal nerve.

(ii) Infraction of a wedge shaped area of the lateral aspect of the medulla and the inferior surface of the cerebellum due to thrombosis of posterior inferior cerebellar artery or one vertebral artery produces a clinical picture of *(lateral medullary)* Wallenburg's *syndrome.* This is characterised by ipsilateral paralysis of the soft palate, pharynx and vocal cord (from involvement of nucleus, ambigus of vagus, some degree of cerebellar deficiency, hypotonia, incoordination and nystagmus on the side of the lesion. Horner's syndrome, analgesia and thermoanesthesia of the face on the same side of the lesion and on the trunk and limb of the opposite side due to involvement of the spinal tract and nucleus of the trigeminal nerve and spinothalamic tract respectively are the sensory manifestations.

(iii) A vascular lesion at the midline on the decussation

of pyramid damages both corticospinal tracts leading to quadriplegia with unilateral 12th nerve palsy.

(G) Lesion at spinal cord : If the lesion is below the decussation of the pyramid but above the 5th cervical segment, there will be ipsilateral hemiplegia, but the muscles innervated by cranial nerves will be exampted.

Certain special investigations like examination of the cerebrospinal fluid, carotid angiography, pneumoence-phalography, ventriculography, lumber myelography, and electroencephalography etc. are carried out for confirma-tion of the different neurological disorders and also when an operative procedure is to be undertaken.

N.B.–Hysterical hemiplegia can be differenciated from an organic one by *Hoover's sign and Babinski's test*. In the former placing both hands under the heels of the recum-bent patient the examiner asks the patient to press them forcefully when with organic hemiplegia pressure is felt only from the sound leg and to confirm further a hand is placed on top of the nonparalysed foot instructing the patient to raise that leg when in organic hemiplegia no further pressure will be felt by the hand kept under the heel of the paralysed leg which, however, occurs with hysterical hemiplegia. In Babinski's test the recumbent patient is asked to sit up with arms kept in front of the chest;–in a true hemiplegia involuntary flexion of the affected limb occurs while in the hysterical one only the normal limb may be elevated. In this Babinski's trunk-thigh test, in true paraplegia both legs are raised with flexion of the trunk while in hysterical paraplegia neither leg is elevated.

OPHTHALMOSCOPY

The Ophthalmoscopic study of fundus oculi has been in use for more than a century. The fundus examination provides much useful information regarding the diagnosis and prognosis of many ocular and systemic disorders.

The optic disc, the retinal blood vessels, the macular region and the periphery are examined as a routine.

The optic disc–Note the colour, the shape, the physiological cupping, the edge and the surroundings of the disc. The colour of a normal fundus may be described as ranging from orange to vermillion. The disc is paler than the surrounding area. The temporal side of the disc is usually paler than the nasal side. It becomes pale in optic atrophy, severe anemia and disseminated sclerosis. Physiological cupping is a short funnel shaped depression in the centre of the papilla from which the retinal vessels emerge. There may be a good deal of variation in the depth of this cup. In advanced glaucoma the cup becomes deep and steep. The edge of the disc is normally clear and well defind. It may be blurred in papilioedema.

Surroundings of the disc should be inspected for haemorrhages, exudates or chorodial tubercles. A white scleral ring or a dark pigmented ring surrounding the optic disc may be found in normal eyes.

The blood vessels form four groups to supply the four quadrants of the fundus i.e. superior and inferior temporal and superior and inferior nasal. Another branch goes towards the macula known as the macular artery which is thinner, brighter red in colour and is better defined. Light strip is present centrally, light being reflected from the convex wall. Observe the crossing of the vessels and note whether the vessels are narrowed or dilated. Spontaneous venous pulsation is seen in a normal eye but spontaneous retinal artery pulsation is seen only in aortic incompetence and in glaucoma. The arteriovenous ratio, which is normally 2 : 3, is altered due to narrowing of the arteries or dilatation of the veins.

The macular region–It is situated about 2 disc breadth

from the outer edge (temporal border) of the disc. It is darker than the fundus, often surrounded by a halo of reflected light. There is a depression at the centre of the macular region, known as 'fovea' which is lighter in colour and often glitters. A circle of white spots may be found in hypertensive retinopathy. Pathological changes in the macular region produce marked reduction of vision than any other part of the retina.

Periphery–The periphery is usually looked for diabetic retinopathy, retinitis pigmentosa, haemorrhages and exudates.

CHANGES IN THE FUNDUS IN DIFFERENT DISORDERS

Papilloedema–The disc margin is blurred. The physiological cup is filled up, the blood vessels are congested, spontaneous pulsations of the retinal vein is absent and field of vision becomes tubular. The disc becomes swollen as the condition progresses [– 3 dioptres is equivalent to 1 mm of swelling]. This is commonly seen in *malignant hypertension* accompanied by arterial changes, *increased intracranial tension* as in brain tumour, severe anaemia, chronic cor pulmonale (80% of cases) and tuberculous meningitis. An acute form of papilloedema with haemorrhage extending into the vitreous is characteristic of *subarachnoid haemorrhage,*–subhyaloid haemorrhage. *Hydrocephalus* from any cause, *intracranial sinus thrombosis* (by diminishing the absorption of the cerebrospinal fluid) and cerebral abscess may also give rise to papilloedema.Papilloedema may be rarely due to– (i). aqueductal stenosis; (ii) cerebral oedema e.g. in head injury, benign intracranial hypertension, lead poisoning, steroid withdrawal, vitamin A intoxication, post-cerebral anoxia (iii) raised CSF protein e.g. in spinal cord tumours, Guillain-Barre syndrome, hypertrophic polyneuritis;

(iv) metabolic disorders e.g. in hypocalcaemia especially in childhood, malignant thyrotoxic exophthalmos; and (v) circulatory disorders e.g. in superior vena cava syndrome, polycythaemia rubra vera, multiple myeloma, macroglobulinaemia, hyperlipidaemia, temporal arteritis, diabetes mellitus etc.

Optic atrophy–This is commonly characterised by a whitish optic disc which seems prominent; and blood vessels are thin and shiny with complete loss of vision. *Primary, secondary* or *post neuritic* atrophy; and *consecutive atrophy* are the different varieties that are commonly met with. Primary optic atrophy is not preceded by optic neuritis;–the disc is flat and white with clearcut edges. Congenital optic atrophy. Leber's hereditary optic atrophy, hereditary ataxias, tabes dorsalis, retinitis pigmentosa and cerebromacular degenerations are the common examples of primary optic atrophy. *Secondary* optic atrophy is a degeneration of the optic nerve subsequent to optic neuritis. The disc is greyish white and its edges are indistinct. Cerebral tumour, cerebral abscess, meningitis, aneurysm and hydrocephalus are the common causes of secondary optic atrophy.

In *consecutive* optic atrophy, the cause of the atrophy is obvious on retinoscopy. It includes various forms of retinitis and obstruction of the central artery of retina.

Papillitis–This is characterised by an acute onset with pain and gross visual loss but less distension of veins. These features may be seen in retrobulbar neuritis when the disease process affects the part of the optic nerve behind the eye but the disc appears normal in the acute stage of the disease.

Opaque nerve fibres may be detected in normal individuals and is a benign congenital abnormality.

Severity of hypertension is assessed by examination of

the fundus. Narrowing of the arterioles with increased light reflex is found in grade I. Further narrowing of the arterioles and nipping of the veins at the crossing with arterioles is grade II; exudates and /or haemorrhages in addition to above findings is found in grade III. Ultimately papilloedema with or without the above changes develop (grade IV). *Dilatation* of the veins occur in chronic respiratory failure, polycythaemia, papilloedema and diabetes.

Pulsating capillary or retinal vessels may be seen in aortic incompetence.

Flame shaped haemorrhages are seen when bleeding occurs in superficial nerve fibres layers of the retina. e.g. in simple diabetic retinopathy in which haemorrhages may also occur into the inner layers and then appears *dot-shaped.*

Roth spots may be found in infective endocarditis and has the appearance of a 'cotton wool' exudate and consists of aggregation of cytoid bodies. Histologically they are perivascular collections of lymphocytes in the retinal nerve layer with or without oedema and haemorrhage, Roth spots are also known as *Litten's sign.* A very commonly mistaken notion is that Roth spots are boat shaped haemorrhages in the retina.

Cherry red spots may be found in the retina in central retinal artery occlusion. Tay-Sach's disease, carbon monoxide poisoning Gaucher's and Niemann Pick's disease, and Eale's disease.

Fluffy grey exudate close to a retinal vessel may be seen in fat embolism.

Diabetic retinopathy is characterised by microaneurysm, blotchy white cholesterol deposit, dot and /or blot haemorrhages, exudates, features of co-existing hypertension, vitreous haemorrhage, retinitis proliferans, detachment of retina and ultimately' optic atrophy.

Ophthalmoscopic findings of hypertension with *macular star* is diagnostic of hypertension of renal origin.

Choroidal tubercles may be found in miliary tuberculosis and in tuberculous meningitis. These are visible ophthalmoscopically as ill defined rounded or oval yellowish bodies about half the size of the optic disc.

Increased *temporal pallor* of the optic disc may be one of the early positive findings in disseminated sclerosis. Evidence of bilateral retrobulbar neuritis or papillitis may be found in a child suffering from Devic's disease.

The *subhyaloid* haemorrhage is the characteristic of subarachnoid haemorrhage.

Typical *optic atrophy* may be found in subacute combined degeneration of the cord. The *Foster-Kennedy* syndrome due to a tumour of the sphenoidal fissure presents with unilateral optic atrophy due to pressure on the optic nerve, and papilloedema of the opposite side due to increased intracranial tension.

Red globular formation may be the manifestation of retinal angiomatosis.

Cytoid bodies or minute ischaemic infracts are the characteristics of systemic lupus crythematosus. The striking ophthalmoscopic feature of *periarteritis nodosa* is the presence of intraretinal and subretinal exudates and rapid variation in the severity of the fundus lesion.

The outstanding fundal appearance in *leukaemia* is marked tortuosity and fullness of retinal veins and these are nipped by normal arteries. Retinal haemorrhages with pale centres and oedematous disc may be found in later stages of the disease.

Retinal haemorrhage is found in only 2 per cent cases of *purpura.*

Highly coloured fundi with dark engorged and tortuous vessels are seen in *polycythaemia*, whereas haemorrhages, pale disc and vessels may be detected in *anaemia.*

Chorioretinitis and optic atrophy are the ophthalmoscopic findings of *toxoplasmosis.* Disseminated choroiditis indicates previous *syphilis.*

CEREBROSPINAL FLUID AND ITS EXAMINATION

CSF is a modified tissue fluid present in the central nervous system. The central nervous system is devoid of lymphatics and the cerebrospinal fluid replaces them.

FORMATION AND CIRCULATION

It is formed by the choroid plexuses in the lateral ventricles. The vessels lie invaginated in the folds of pia matter. The CSF is probably formed by ultrafiltration and secretion. It passes from the lateral ventricles through the foramina of Monro into the third ventricle→through the aqueductus Sylvii to fourth ventricle and then passes through the foramina of Luschka and Magendie into the subarachnoid space.

It is absorbed again probably by filtration through the arachnoid villi into the venous sinuses of the skull.

Total volume–100 to 150 ml (about 130 ml in normal adults).

Fluid pressure–It depends on a balance between its rate of formation and absorption.

The pressure at the lumbar theca with the patient lying on his side is 50 to 150 mm of cerebrospinal fluid. This must be measured with a properly fitting manometer. An average idea from the rate of escape of fluid from the needle may be obtained (normally 1 drop per second), though this is a very crude method and is not to be recommended.

QUECKENSTEDT'S TEST

The patency of the cerebrospinal fluid pathway is tested by Queckenstedt's test.

Compression of the internal jugular vein gives rise to congestion of cerebral veins, and the consequent rise of venous pressure leads to promptly increased CSF pressure which is reflected in the rise of meniscus in the manometer and is maintained so long as the compression is maintained. Compression of one vein leads to moderate rise of pressure and further rise occurs with compression of the second vein. The CSF pressure promptly returns to normal with release of compression.

So, following compression of the internal jugular vein if there is no rise CSF pressure detected in the spinal manometer (positive result), it suggests complete spinal block either by a tumour or extradural compression, thrombosis of the jugular vein or some interference with the escape of the fluid from the cranial cavity. If, however, there is a small rise it will suggest and incomplete block and in such a case, release of the jugular compression will be followed by a slow return of the meniscus to a former level; or the level may remain unaltered indicating a ball valve type of obstruction. A positive test, therefore, does not occur until the block is almost complete. If no rise occurs either on jugular venous compression or on abdominal compression, the most likely cause in a faulty position of the needle.

Tobey-Ayer test– A failure of CSF pressure to rise with compression of one jugular vein but not the other is indicative of the possibility of a lateral sinus thrombosis.

Method of withdrawal of C S F

1. Lumbar puncture, 2. Cisternal puncture, 3. Ventricular puncture.

It has Indications of lumbar puncture diagnostic values in –

(a) M ingitis of any aetiology.

(b) Cerebrovascular accidents to differentiate cerebral haemorrhage from cerebral thrombosis of embolism.

(c) Differentiating meningitis from meningism by increase in cell count and biochemical studies.

(d) Spinal tumours,–there will be hypotension and xanthochromia and block may be demonstrated.

(e) All cases of neurosyphilis.

The *therapeutic* value of lumber puncture lies in the fact that withdrawal of some amount of fluid leads to a release of increased intracranial tension and hence performd in *benign intracranial hypertension*. Moreover intrathecal administration of drugs may be achieved by injecting through the lumbar puncture needle. Commonly used drugs are streptomycin 5 to 10 mg dissolved in 10 cc distilled water (in tuberculous meningitis) or Penicillin G 10,000 units (6mg) dissolved in 10 cc distilled water or normal saline (in pyogenic meningitis). Also polymyxin (2mg in children and 5 mg in adults), ampicillin (5mg in children and 20 mg in adults); amikacin (3 mg in children 10 mg in adults), erythromycin (10mg in children and 20 mg in adults) and gentamicin (1 mg) all in 10 ml saline or CSF may be administered intrathecally. However, prior to intrathecal injection an equal volume of CSF has to be withdrawn.

Lumbar puncture is carried out at intervals to assess the *prognosis* of the case particularly in pyogenic and Koch's meningitis. But one of the problems that have been encountered in recent years is the development of arachnoiditis following lumbar puncture.

Spinal anaesthesia administration and,

Myelogram and pneumoencephalogram can also be done by lumbar puncture.

Examination of CSF should be done in (i) peripheral neuropathies, (ii) suspected CNS infections, (iii) suspected

intracranial bleeding and (iv) suspected disseminated sclerosis.

Technique of lumbar puncture

Instruments–Sterilised Harri's needle with stellate, a 2
ml syringe and IM needle.

Commonest site–Between the 3rd and 4th lumbar spines
or the 4th and 5th lumbar spines.

Join the highest points of the iliac crests–the line will
pass through the tip of the spine of L4. Puncture the space
above this point.

Procedure–The patient is to be brought to the side of
the bed and is to be kept on his side in an attitude of
hyperflexion by attendants with the knees and chin as
nearly approximated as possible. If the patient appears to
be apprehensive give Inj. Diazepam 5-10 mg IM. Sterilise
the local area by painting with iodine and spirit. If the
patient is conscious, infiltrate the site of puncture with 5 ml
Inj. Novocain (2%).

Next introduce the needle with its bevelled surface
towards the head end. The exact site should be slightly
lateral to the midline and press it forward, upward, and
slightly medially. As soon as the resistance is lost, withdraw
the stellate, let the CSF come out and collect about 5-10
ml of the CSF in several test tubes.

Dry tap– Most commonly it is due to a faulty technique.
Too thick pus, spinal block, lumbar sac filled by a neoplasm
or by a developmental lesion e.g. lipoma or equidermoid
as in spina bifida may be the causes for a genuine dry tap.

Contraindications

Lumbar puncture is *absolutely contraindicated* in
subtentorial or infratentorial tumours particularly in cerebellar tumours as there are chances or herniation of the
medulla into the foramen magnum. It should preferably not

be performed in patients with *papilloedema* and in *cerebral tumours.*

It should be avoided in presence of *local sepsis,* otherwise there is a chance of introducing infection in the CSF.

It is very difficult to do lumbar puncture in presence of bony deformities like kyphosis, scoliosis, ankylosing spondylitis and in cases of osteoarthritis. Decisions to perform lumbar puncture must be tempered with utmost caution in (i) unconsciousness. (ii) headaches, (iii) suspected spinal cord compression which may be suddenly worsened by the alteration of pressure in CSF and (vi) neck stiffness.

EXAMINATION OF CSF

(A) *Ayala Index*–This helps in the diagnosis of *hydrocephalus, subarachnoid block* etc. This index is the product of the volume of CSF removed (say, 10) in ml and final CSF pressure and is normally 5.5 to 6.5. In hydrocephalus or serrous meningitis because of a large reservoir the Ayala index is *greater than* 7.0 and with a small reservoir e.g. in subarachnoid block the index is *less than* 5.

(B) *Physical*

(i) Colour–Normally the CSF is colourless.

It may be *reddish* in *cerebral haemorrhage.* However, sometimes following injury to the blood vessels, while doing lumbar puncture, the CSF may be reddish or even frank blood clot. In cerebral haemorrhage the CSF is deep rosy red in colour and the depth of the colour is constant. On keeping for sometime the supernatant fluid looks yellowish and on microscopic examination, there will be no intact RBC. On the other hand, following trauma, the depth of colour of the CSF should gradually fade, the supernatant fluid is clear and the blood clots. On microscopical examination RBC's will remain intact.

Colour of the CSF may be *yellowish* (xanthochromia) in long standing *spinal block*, *cerebral tumours*, after *subarachnoid haemorrhage*, after an *intracerebral haemor-rhage* or cerebral infraction and in some cases of *Guillain-Barre syndrome* and *subdural haematoma*. In *Froin syndrome* a pronounced yellow colour is associated with a excess or protein (usually more than 500 mg%) and massive coagulation of the fluid and this is found in a *spinal subarachnoid block caused by meningioma, neurofibroma* etc. or in some cases of *Guillain-Barre syndrome*.

(ii) Appearance–Normally the CSF is clear and transparent.

It becomes turbid or frankly purulent in pyogenic meningitis and opalescent and clear in tuberculous meningitis. On standing, in cases of pyogenic meningitis there will be copious deposit at the bottom of the test tube, while in tuberculous meningitis the CSF will clot giving rise to *cobweb coagulum*.

(iii) Tension–The CSF remains clear but under increased tension in tuberculous meningitis, viral encephalitis, cerebral malaria, typhoid meningism, GPI and hypertensive encephalopathy. Normally the CSF should come out at the rate of one drop per second but this is not an index of CSF pressure.

(iv) Fibrin clot–Other than Froin syndrome which is associated with massive coagulation, a 'cobweb' may form in 12 to 24 hrs.–typically in tuberculous meningitis and sometimes in other forms meningitis. neurosyphilis, poliomyelitis etc.

(C) *Chemical*

(i) Protein content : Normal–20-40 mg%.

The protein content is increased in all cases of *meningitis, cerebral abscess, acute poliomyelitis* and in most of the *viral diseases* of the *nervous system*. In *encephalitis lethargica* it is raised slightly. An isolated increased in protein content occurs in many cases of *intracranial tumours* and *spinal block*. It may also be met with *vascular lesions of brain* and in cases of *acute infective polyneuritis*, where dissociated *albumino-cytological* disorder is the characteristic CSF finding. In *mening ovascular syphilis*, the range may be 50 to 200 mg%.

(ii) Glucose content : Normal–50 to 80 mg%.

This becomes *markably reduced in pyogenic meningitis* (0 15 mg), *slightly reduced in tuberculous meningitis* (5-50 mg%). It may also be reduced in *hypoglycaemic* states. A rise in sugar level may be found in *diabetes mellitus* and other *hyperglycaemic* conditions, *encephalitis* and occasionally in *cerebral haemorrhage*.

(iii) Chloride content : Normal 700-750 mg%.

This becomes *markeably reduced* (480 to 650 mg%). in *tuberculous meningitis and slightly reduced* (600–680 mg%) in *pyogenic meningitis*. It may be *increased* in *chronic renal failure*.

(iv) Urea content : Normal 6-20 mg%.

A *high urea* level may be encountered in all conditions which are associated with high blood urea levels.

(v) A phospholipid, *cephalin* is relatively increased in demyelinating disorders.

(vi) Cholesterol and cholesterol ester in CSF is nonspecifically elevated in multiple sclerosis.

(vii) CSF *glutamine* estimation is a valuable and reliable diagnostic test in hepatic encephalopathy.

(viii) High *homovallinic acid* (HVA) content of CSF in Parkinsonism is indicative or poor response to levodopa therapy compared to those with low HVA content.

(D) *Cytological*

Normally the cells are all *lymphocyes* in the range of 0-5 per cmm.

Polymorphonuclear leucocytosis is seen in pyogenic meningitis, while *lymphocytosis* is the characteristic finding in tuberculous and syphilitic meningitis and in viral infections of the nervous system. A *mixed pleocytosis* is seen in some cases of tuberculous meningitis, cerebral and extra-dural abscesses, superior saggital sinus thrombosis and poliomyelitis. A pleocytosis, i.e. excess of cells in spinal fluid indicates meningeal irritation and not necessarily meningeal infection. A *mononuclear pleocytosis* is seen in neurosyphilis, encephalitis, herpes zoster, acute lymphocytic choriomeningitis and after the first few days of the onset of poliomyelitis.

Malignant cells may be found in 10 to 20 per cent cases of *glioma* and 20 to 30 per cent cases of *intracranial metastases*.

(E) *Bacteriological*

Gram-positive cocci like streptococcus, staphylococcus, pneumococcus and gram-negative coccus like meningococcus may be the causative organisms of different meningitis. Acid fast bacilli and rarely gram-negative bacilli like E coli are also seen. Preliminary microscopical examination of a stained smear of centrifused deposits and subsequent culture in the respective media and animal inoculation (M tuberculosis) will finally reveal the nature of the organisms.

(F) *Serological*

VDRL, Wassermann reaction and Kahn test of the CSF are particularly helpful in the diagnosis of tabes *dorsalis* and GPI especially when WR and Kahn test of the blood have been negative. The CSF in neurosyphilis shows– (a) 200–300 cell/cmm, mostly lymphocytes, few plasma cells, (b) total protein 40 to 200 mg%. (c) elevated levels of γ globulins, (d) positive serologic tests of which FTA-ABS is most commonly used while TPI is higly reliable. VDRL slide tests are negative in a good proportion of patient with late syphilis especially in those with neurosyphilis and is then known as *seronegative syphilis*. FTA–ABS and TPI tests are helpful in such cases.

(G) *Special*

Lange's colloidal gold reaction :

The high globulin content of CSF in some diseases will have the power to precipitate gold from a colloidal gold solution. This is tested by adding CSF in gradually increasing dilutions to a fixed amount of colloidal gold taken in test tubes. Precipitation is best observed after 24 hours. The result, thus obtained, if plotted graphically will show a *tabetic* curve in tabes dorsàlis i.e. 1233210000 (when the 3rd and 4th dilutions shows maximum precipitation), a *paretic* curve in GPI and 5% of cases with disseminated sclerosis i.e. 5554320000 (when first 4 or 5 dilutions are precipitated) and *meningitic* curve in meningitis i.e. 0012344310 (where the 6th to 8th dilutions are precipitated).

False positive Wassermann and Lange tests may be found if blood is present in CSF.

(H) *Parasitological*

Rarely in trypanosomiasis, the *trypanosomes* may be found as may be *Toxoplasma gondii* in toxoplasmosis and viable trophozoites of *Naegleria* in amoebic meningoencephalitis etc.

(I) *Microchemical*

Estimation of sphingomyelin, cerebroside, cephalin and lecithin contents of CSF can give an idea of the nature and degree of structural breakdown within the brain.

OTHER SPECIAL INVESTIGATIONS

BIOPSY : (i) *Brain biopsy*–This is done for brain tumours. subacute inclusion-body encephalitis, lipoidosis, leucodystrophy, suspected herpes simplex encephalitis, Alzheimer's disease etc. When other non-invasive investigations have failed or given an uncertain diagnosis.

(ii) *Peripheral nerve biopsy*–A superficial nerve from the dorsum of the foot or the sural nerve is selected. Indications are hypertrophic polyneuropathy, amyloidosis, nerve involvement by Hansen's disease, metachronic leucodystrophy, and diabetic and other toxic neuropathies.

(iii) *Muscle biopsy*–This is done in different varieties of muscular dystrophies, myasthenia gravis, trichiniasis, collagen diseases, and may help in differentiating primary muscle disorders from those *secondary* to primary neural degeneration (e.g. due to Kugelberg-Wellander or Werdnig-Hoffmann syndrome).

Besides these, biopsy of other organs like liver, kidney, lungs, lymph glands, blood vessels (especially arteries) may be required for confirming the suspected aetiological factor.

ROENTGENOGRAPHIC STUDIES : (a) Chest : In each case of suspected intracranial or spinal cord lesion, a P-A view of the chest is taken and this sometimes give an immediate diagnosis.

(b) *Skull* : Either straight X-ray lateral view, postero anterior with 20⁰ downward tilt or Towne's projection are taken. Indicated in traumatic, primary or secondary neoplastic diseases, aneurysms, systemic diseases producing changes in the skull etc. In an X-ray of the skull, look for displacement of normally clacified structures like pineal gland, the flax, choroid plexuses etc. which will demonstrate a change in the size of one part of the brain.

(c) *Computerised axial tomography* : Roentgenographic rays are passed through the skull in a series of horizontal planes. The degree of absorption by different tissues of the rays are then recorded and computerised; finally displayed on a screen. Water, oedema fluid of CSF shows as *dark* areas and bones or calcified structures show as dense *white* areas. Other abnormalities show in differing degree of density. Many different pathological conditions of the brain and skull, spinal cord, vertibral bodies etc., e.g. tumours abscesses, cysts, infracts, haemorrhages, to name a few, can be confirmed by this procedure.

(d) *Carotid angiography* : A radio opaque contrast medium is injected into the carotid artery in the neck and X-ray are taken. The medium can be injected either by introducing a needle directly through the wall of the internal carotid or by introducing a fine cannula into the common carotid through which a catheter may be passed. By the latter method, the bifurcation of the common carotid as well as both internal and external carotids can be studies. *Indications* of carotid angiography include intracranial haemorrhages, epilepsies with focal features, increased intracranial tension particularly caused by a supratentorial tumour, recurrent unilateral paralysis, sudden hemiplegia in young patients without any cardiac disease, unilateral 3rd or 6th nerve paralysis, suspected subdural or extradural haematoma and signs of compression of the optic chiasma. *Digital subtraction angiography* (DSA) is a sophisticated method utilising computer analysis and helps in much better resolution of anatomical defects.

(e) *Vertebral angiography* : It may be performed by direct percutaneous arterial puncture or better by inserting a catheter through the femoral or brachial or axillary artery and guiding the tip fluoroscopically to the entrance of the vertebral arteries. It is *particularly indicated* in subarachnoid haemorrhage with normal carotid circulation, tumours of the occipital regions. stenosis at the origin of the **vertebral** arteries, intrinsic tumours of the brainstem etc. Carotid and vertebral angiography done simultaneously is known as *four vessel angiography.*

(f) *Pneumoencephalography* : A lumber puncture is performed with the patient in sitting posture, and not more than 30 cc air is introduced through the needle with the head positioned suitably so that air enters into the ventricles. It is particularly *indicated* in suspected cases of cerebral atrophy, maldevelopment and low pressure hydrocephalus; post-traumatic and other epilepsies, intracranial neoplasms without raised intracranial tension etc.

(g) *Ventriculography* : Ventriculography is a surgical procedure. The ventricles are punctured through burrholes, and either air or myodil is injected and X-ray taken. In this procedure, there is no danger of tentorial or cerebellar pressure coning. It is *indicated* in cases of raise intracranial tension or suspected cerebral space-occupying lesion where arteriography failed; in posterior fossa tumours acoustic neuromas, and suspected obstruction of the 3rd or 4th ventricles or aqueduct of sylvius.

(h) *Myelography* : It is either *cisternal* or *lumbar* according to the site of puncture. Air or oxygen under positive pressure may be used, but myodil is more commonly employed. It is indicated in any case of suspected spinal cord or root compression, lesions at foramen magmum with Arnold-Chiari malformation, syringomyelia etc. The contrast media *metrizamide* helps in much better resolution, because its penetration is greater than myodil, the viscosity being very low.

RADIOISOTOPE ENCEPHALOGRAPHY :   Principle: Certain radioisotopes, administered orally or intravenously, gets concentrated in abnormal brain tissues after some interval and these areas can be indentified by a scanning apparatus (Geiger-Muller counter) since the abnormal areas emit gamma radiation. Technetium 99m is most commonly employed.

Meningiomas, glioblastomas, metastatic tumours, blood clots and areas of cerebral softening take up the isotope and thus can be detected.

ECHO-ENCEPHALOGRAPHY : By this method the side of a space-occupying lesion can be determined especially where physical signs have failed and in the X-ray *pineal calcification* is absent.

ELECTROENCEPHALOGRAPHY : It is the method by which electrical potential changes from different regions of the brain can be recorded. The electroencephalogram or EEG is the voltage-versus time graph that appears as a number of wavy parallel lines and the abnormal waves are DELTA (<4/sec). THETA (4-7/sec) and rarely high voltage faster waves called SPIKES, while in adults the *normal* waves are ALPHA (8-13/sec) and BETA (faster than 13/sec). Absence of any waves, i.e. a flat EEG is almost always diagnostic of *brain death.* This potentially invaluable investigation, more often than not, is being used as a short-cut way to diagnosis. But it should be emphasised that it only supplements and does not supplant a detailed history taking, cereful neurological and general examination and other radiological biochemical or surgical investigations. The indications are –

(i) Repeated, attacks of disturbances of consciousness.

(ii) Children exhibiting short periods of detachment from surroundings.

(iii) Sudden unexplained episodes behavioural distur-bances.

(iv) Comatose patient with non-localising physical signs.

(v) Suspected cerebral abscess or abscesses.

(vi) Unexplained intellectual deterioration.

(vii) Suspected hypoglycaemia.

(viii) Unexplained dementia.

(ix) Assessment of recovery from encephalitis.

(x) Recording evoked potentials e.g. short-latency somatosensory evoked potentials (SLSEP), brainstem auditory evoked responses (BAER) and pattern shift visual evoked responses (PSVER).

(xi) Monitoring cerebral activity during extensive procedure of modern cardiovascular surgery.

(xii) Indicating the level of anaesthesia.

ELECTROMYOGRAPHY (EMG) : Electrical activity of the muscles can be recorded by an electromyograph. Electrodes used are either surface electrodes attached to the skin or concentric needle electrodes introduced into the muscles EMG is used in investigating peripheral nerve lessions, distinguishing muscular dystrophy from neurogenic atrophy, detecting myositis, localising lower motor neurone lesions, detecting carriers of muscular dystrophy, demonstrating myasthenia and myotonia etc.

N.B.–*Nuclear Magnetic Resonance Imaging (MRI) and Position Emission Tomography (PET) are the latest sophisticated investigative procedures the discussion of which is beyond the. scope of this book.*

Appendix to Chapter III

Paraplegia–types and causes.

The term paraplegia signifies a paralysis of both lower limbs. An acute lesion of spinal cord (during the stage of spinal shock) give rise to a *flaccid paraplegia*. As this stage passes off, *spastic paraplegia* sets in, provided there has been no extensive LMN lesions of the lower limb. The *spastic paraplegia* is predominantly characterised by an increased tone of the extensor muscles of the lower limbs when the spinal cord lesion is incomplete affecting principally the pyramidal tracts only–this is *paraplegia-in-extension*. When the two pyramidal tracts are severely diseased along with other descending pathways, especially the reticulospinal tract, the primitive flexor withdrawal reflexes are released from inhibition and leads to *paraplegia-in-flexion* where the heels remain in proximity with the buttocks.

An *acute paraplegia* is most commonly due to spinal cord trauma associated with fracture dislocation of the spine. It may be due to anterior spinal artery thrombosis, spontaneous haematomyelia due to a vascular malformation, dissecting aortic aneurysm or atheroma causing occlusion of a spinal branch of aorta, rarely in multiple sclerosis.

A *paraplegia of slower onset* is seen in transverse myelitis (postinfectious or postvaccinal), acute demyelinative myelopathy, acute necrotizing myelopathy, an epidural abscess, a tumour with spinal cord compression, paralytic polio, acute idiopathic polyneuritis, epidural or subdural haemorrhage in a bleeding diatheses, sometimes in multiple sclerosis.

A *paraplegia of insidious onset* is seen in infantile diplegia (arms minimally affected), Friedreich's ataxia, hereditary spastic paraplegia, progressive muscular dystrophy, chronic polyneuropathies, lathyrism subacutè combined degeneration, cervical spondylosis, protruded cervical disc, spinal tumours, syphilitic meningomyelitis. tuberculous, arachnoiditis or other chronic epidural infections, motor system diseases, syringomyelia, polyneuropathies and polymyositis. A recently identified cause is the rare *vascular myelopathy*–one of the many different neurological disorders associated with HIV (human immunodeficiency virus) infection. HIV is the agent commonly causing AIDS and formerly known as LAV (lymphadenopathy associated virus) or HTLV (human T-cell lymphotropic virus) III.

Remember the *cauda equina* and *conus medullaris syndromes.* While both cause root pains and sensory loss, the former causes LMN paralysis of sacral roots, *brisk* knee jerks but *absent* ankle jerk and planter response; the latter causes LMN paralysis of lumbar roots with absent knee jerk but brisk ankle jerk and *extensor* plantar response.

———————

CHAPTER 4

SICK CHILDREN

The student of clinical medicine will have to meticulously exercise his knowledge of the art and science of medicine when he ecounters an infant or a child presenting with a morbid process. How to do so is the topic of present discussion. At the outset, it is emphasised that children are very much unlike adult people and the technique of clinical examination discussed in the previous chapters need considerable modification before these are applied to the clinical examination of sick children. Also, more attention need to be paid to the growth and developmemt of the child,–because this builds the basis of the science of paediatrics. Students should always keep in mind that the more constant and narrow spectrum of physiological normals of adults stand out in sharp contrast to the widely variable physical, mental and psychological status of children. A *palpable liver* or an *extensor plantar response* classically illustrates this very point. A one finger palpable liver that would be normal in a child might indicate enlargement of the liver from any morbid process in an adult : and whereas an extensor plantar reflex is a normal finding in at least 70% of all children up to 1 year of age, a similar finding, in an adult carries a very different significance.

Before starting the physical examination the clinical history should be taken very carefully and meticulously. In paediatrics the history is usually obtained from the parents, maternity nurse or midwife. But when the patient is an older child, the history obtained from the mother, should, if necessary, be supplemented by asking him simple questions regarding his symptoms. Beginning with the history of present illness, equire about previous history of the child's development, the family history and finally the social and environmental history.

While taking the history of present illness note the age and sex. Note down the precise order of appearance of symptoms. Note whether the child has been active or lethargic and apathetic to the environment sorrounding him : his appetite and detailed account of feeding, detailed history of vomiting if there has been any : state of bowels and charectar of stools; and changes in weight; cough, breathlessness, mouth breathing, stridor and wheeze. Ask the mother about any history of jaundice, cyanosis, pallor or squatting, involuntary movements and convulsions; dysuria, frequency of micturition, bed wetting, volume and character of urine. Also ask about the behaviour and mood of the child and history of any treatment that he might have received.

In considering the past history, specifically ask for history of birth of the child, the birth weight, the history of immunisation and whether the mother had suffered from any illness during pregnancy or if she have had any abortion or death of a viable child. Note also whether she have had any addiction or have been taking any drug.

Ask the mother about the child's development (see later for milestones of development) and that of bladder and bowel control.

When the history taking has been concluded, proceed to examine the child. Try to gain confidecne of the child with a soft persuasive voice, gently stroking the skin with a finger and giving the child a toy or your pen or if you think it wise, even your stethoscope. However, It might not be possible to follow a strict routine procedure and considerable improvisation may have to be made with persever-ance, depending upon the mood of the child, to have his co-operation.

Physical Examination of the Child
GENERAL EXAMINATION

While taking the history, general inspection of the child will already have given ideas about the child's appearance, demeanour, reactions to environment, sounds uttered by the child and any peculiarity of odour. Any rash present should be examined meticulously to see whether it is rasied or not, erythematous or purpuric, the distribution of the rash and any scratch marks present (see Chapter V)

If the patient is a newborn see whether the vital functions have been established (see page 169 for Apgar score) any gross congenital abnormalities present and presence of any birth trauma.

Weight : Height and weight constitute the most impor-tant measurements of physical development. The child's weight should be noted on the first as well as on all subsequent occations when he is examined. This will help in assessing the nutritional status. At birth the mature child weight about 7lbs; this doubles at 6 months (14 lbs); increases 3 times by 1 year (21 lbs); four times by 2 years (28 lbs) : and becomes 33 lbs at 3rd year. 40lbs at 4 years and about 49 lbs by the 7th year.

Head circumference : An increased or decreased head circomference carries considerable significance in diseases of children. The head circumference is usually measured with the tape placed round the maximal occipito- frontal cir-cumference. At birth, normally it is 13-14 inches. It increased by 1/2 inch per month up to 4 months of age, 1/4th inch per month up to 1 year of age then 1/2 inch per year 5 years of age : finally up to 1/2 inch per 5 years till puberty.

Length : The length or height is an important indicator for growth. The standing height is measured in toddlers and older children. while in infants who are recumbent, the crown to heel length is measured. Sometimes the sitting height or crown rump length may have to be measured. When compared with the crown heel length, the sitting height may be diagnostic of diseases like *achondroplasia*. The relation between the height and weight also should be determined for this will help in detecting *Marfan syndrome, hypothyroidism, wasting* or *obesity.* Stature is said to be significantly short when it is 2 standard deviations below the third centile. The *growth rate* or *height velocity* is high at birth and decreases rapidly during the first 2 years of life; reaching a relatively stable rate of 4-6 cm per year till puberty is attained.

Posture : Note the posture of the child while performing the general examination. Full term babies just after birth normally adopt a posture of partial flexion, and the *preterm infant* when lying supine assumes the so-called 'frog' position. There are wide abduction of the thighs and flexion of the knees and the large head remains turned to one side. Such a peculiar posture is produced by hypotonia and weakness of the muscles. While noting this, also look for spontaneous movements that may be bilateral, rhythmic, fine, or coarse. Remember that only an intermittent clenching of a fist may be the sole manifestation of generalised convulsion in a neonate.

Temperature : This is often forgotten; *it should be routinely recorded.* The thermometer may be placed in the groin in an infant, the thigh being kept flexed on the abdomen; axilla is the site of choice in older children. Occassionally in some cases like neonatal cold injury special low reading thermometers are to be used. Premature infants may show normally a little lower temperature, the normal temperature being about 37⁰C.

Facies and Ear: These should be given special attention since many systemic diseases are reflected in the face and with gradual practice students will find it an interesting clinical exercise to try detecting diseases by looking at the face and ears. The facies can give a clue regarding the emotional state and psychological condition of the child. Facialitics, if present, are readily detected. *Down syndrome* or mongolism is the commonest autosomal abnormality leading to short stature and produces characteristic facial changes including small palpebral fissures sloping laterally upwards, elongated and prominent protruding tongue, a small mouth and prominent epicanthic folds. Mental retardation is invariable. *Gargoylism* (a veriety of mucopolysaccharidosis) can be recognised by presence of a wide nose with depressed bridge and prominent supraorbital ridges and eyebrows. *Cretins* may present with coarse features, a macroglossia, a double chin (due to myxoedematous changes) and bloated cheeks. A *moon face* is caused by adrenocorticosteroid therapy for a prolonged period. *Nephrotic syndrome* causes facial oedema. particularly of the eyelids which may be grossly swollen. Bossing of the forehead is caused by *rickets. Hypertelorism,* that is, increased distance between the eyes may be seen in association with some types of mental retardation and is caused by an abnormal growth of the sphenoid bone. The *sclera* may be *blue* in osteogenesis imperfecta, Ehlers-Danlos syndrome, or Marfan syndrome. *Cataracts* may be present in Laurence-Moon-Biedl-Bardot syndrome, Friedreich's ataxia, Refsum's disease, galactosaemia, aminoaciduria, hereditary nephritis, maternal rubella, or may be secondary in retinitis pigmentosa.

Anaemia can be detected by examining the conjunctival mucous membrane. Also look for abnormal prominence or depression of eyeballs, squint, conjunctivitis, jaundice, haemorrhages, *Brushfield spots* on the iris (a feature of Down syndrome), any other congenital defects of the iris or other abnormalities of the retina.

Examine the external ear : Look for any abnormality of it and of the external meatus. Estimate the position of the ears relative to an imaginary line drawn from the canthi of the eyes. *Low set and malformed ears* are found associated with hypoplastic kidneys, autosomal trisomy, Down syndrome, Noonan syndrome, Turner syndrome and also in Smith-Lemli-Opitz, Klippel-Feil and Pierre Robin syndromes. Auriscope examinations are necessary in cases of infections of the ears.

Head and Scalp : Inspect these carefully, and palpate to detect any swellings; oedema of the scalp at the site of the presenting part is very common just after birth. This is known as *Caput succedaneum*. It should be distinguished from a *cephalhaematoma* which occurs hours to days after birth, remaining localised over individual cranial bones. Examine the fontanelles, assessing their pressures and whether there is a pulsation over the anterior fontanelle which is present normally, synchronous with the apical impulse. The posterior one may be normally close at birth. Measure the head circumference (see page 149). *Hydrocephalus* and *microcephaly* may be respectively associated with *spina bifida and mental retardation*. Examine the hair-line of the neck which may be low in Klippel-Feil syndrome (fusion of multiple cervical vertebare) and Turner syndrome.

A 'mousy' odour of skin, hair and urine with a tendency to hypopigmentation and eczema may be found in *phenylketonuria*–consequences of accumulation of phenylaetate. Press over the parietal bones with the thumb,–it will indent and again spring back in an early stage of rickets. This is known as *craniotabes*. Rerely it may be normally found under 3 months of age. A 'cracked pot' note on percussion over the skull may be found in increased intracranial tension in older children. An important examination is transillumination of the skull. This is done in darkened room with the torch closely applied to the skin. In *hydrocephalus* and *hydrancephaly* the test is positive.

Ausculate for *cranial bruits* over the vertex, occiput, and temporal region, if present, may be due to arteriovenous fistula or gross hypercalcaemia (idiopathic).

Mouth : Examination of the mouth of a child may prove to be a difficult job as even gentle persuation to open it may not be readily obliged by the child. Physical force may then have to be resorted to, but only when all other attempts fail. Inspect the mucous membrane of the mouth, the lips, gums and the tongue to detect signs of dehydration, abnormal colour, vesicles and ulceration, purpuric spots, monilial lesions (which are white, adherent and resembles curd) and Koplik spots. Examine the teeth, particularly for their number and quality; the palate, and also inspect the tonsils for any abnormality of size or for presence of a membranous patch. If the latter is present, *never fail to exclude diphtheria*. If it is possible and neccessary you can also examine the oropharynx with a tongue depressor. If you examine a child with stridor and who cannot swallow anymore, you have to exclude an acute epiglottitis. ATTENTION : But only examine the epiglottis. If you are able to intubate! It may also be caused by a retropharyngeal abscess rarely, which can be felt as a soft fluctuant mass in the posterior pharyngeal wall.

Causes of macroglossia : Hypothyroidism, Down syndrome, Hurler syndrome, amyloidosis and glycogen storage diseases etc.

Causes of high arched palate : Marfan syndrome, trisomy 18 syndrome, Cornelia de Lange syndrome Rubenstein- Taybi syndrome, Turner syndrome and Pierre Robion syndrome.

N.B. *In Marfan syndrome only the cardiovascular and eye changes constitute the major critteria; all other being minor criteria (BMJ, 1988, 296 1347).*

Jaundice : The presence of jaundice should be routinely looked for. To detect jaundice, daylight is better than any artificial light. The skin over the *nose* and *forehead* becomes discoloured yellow. Especially the sclera of the eyes will be found yellowish. Also the skin yellow. Jaundice in a newborn infant may be physiological or pathological. Jaundice of the newborn appearing on the *second or third* day after birth may be due to the familial non-haemolytic jaundice (Crigler-Najjar syndrome). A *protracted course* of physiological jaundice occurs in congenital hypothyroidism. If the jaundice is present at birth or occurs within the first 24 hours after birth, it should be considered pathological and the causes may include; erythroblastosis foetalis, septicaemia, galactosaemia, cytomegalic inclusion disease and rubella. Jaundice appearing between the *third and seventh day* after birth is *most commonly* due to septicaemia but other infections like congenital syphilis, toxoplasmosis or cytomegalic inclusion disease should also be considered. Jaundice after the *first week of life* may be caused by atresia of the biliary tract, septicaemia, rubella toxoplasmosis, cytomegalovirus inclusion disease, alpha-1-antitrypsin deficiency, galactosaemia, idiopathic dilatation of the common bile duct, hereditary spherocytosis, haemolysis due to idiosyncratic reaction to drugs etc.

Jaundice in elder children is very often caused by infection with HA-virus (hepatitis A)–or hepatitis B/ Epstein-Barr-virus.

In all cases you have to take the bilirubin range in the blood.

Cyanosis : Peripheral cyanosis, that may be severe, in the hands and feet of newborn babies, is rarely of any significane by itself. Central cyanosis is *definitely due to pathological causes*, which may be either cardiac respiratory or intracranial. Usally cyanosis is caused by respiratory insufficiency. This may be due either to a primary pulmonary pathology or secondary to damage of the respiratory centre caused by intracranial haemorrhage or anoxia. Cyanosis due to primary pathology in the lungs might be associated with rapid respiration and retraction of the thoracic cage. Irregular, weak and slow respirations might be associated with cyanosis due to damage of the respiratory centres.

If caused by cyanotic congenital heart disease or methaemoglobinaemia, signs of respiratory difficulties are not marked, but in most cases murmur of the heart are recognized. Even hypoglycaemia, bacteraemia and meningitis may present with cyanosis.

Neck : Inspect from the front as well as from the back and try to find out whether there is any shortening, webbing or positional deformity. *Shortening* of the neck is a feature of Klippel-Feil syndrome caused by congenital fusion of the cervical vertebrae and associated with scoliosis; *webbing* is seen in Turner syndrome associated with a broad chest, widely spaced nipples and hypoplasia of breast tissue; *positional* deformity occurs in spasmodic torticollis and head retraction. Look for any limitation of movement.

Neck rigidity : Neck rigidity is in most cases associated

with meningitis and menigeal irritation e.g. by blood in subarachnoid haemorrhage, If there is any sign of neck stiffness. In every clinical examination you have to prove. Inspect carefully for any swellings or dimples. Anomalies present on the posterior midline may sometimes remain connected with the central nervous system. Swellings on the *anterior midline* of the neck may be associated with anomalies of the thyroid gland, whereas those that are more laterally situated may be due to retropharengeal-abscess, cervical adenitis, Lymphadenitis colli (inflammed cervical lymph nodes), cystic hygroma, tumour of the sternocleidomastoid muscles or branchial cyst. Examine the lymph nodes of the neck and at the same sitting look for abnormalities of the lymph nodes at other sites.

Nutrition and Hydration : Assessment of the state of nutrition and hydration is a very important part of general examination. It requires careful inspection and palpation. Redundant skin folds on the medial side of thighs and in the axilla and wasting of the gluteal muscles are evidences for weight loss (undernutrition). Look for the signs of loss of fluid. When fluid loss is 5-10 per cent of the body weight, the eyes are sunken, the fontanelles depressed, skin turgor is lost but there is no *peripheral circulatory* failure. When fluid loss is *more than 10 per cent* of body weight, peripheral circulatory failure sets in. Gently pick up the skin over the chest, abdomen or thighs between the thumb and index finger and compress it to get an idea of the skin turgor. If there is dehydration, the skin will only slowly return to the original position. If dehydration is little distended. The three different types of dehydration, namely, *hypotonic, isotonic* and *hypertonic* dehydrations can be distinguished from one another by a number of signs. These are :

		Hypotonic dehydration	Isotonic dehydration	Hypertonic dehydration
1.	Definition	Loss of Na in excess of water,	Water and Na loss proportionate	Loss of water in excess of Na
2.	Skin Colour	Grayish	Grayish	Grayish
3.	Temperature	Cold	Cold	Hot or cold
4.	Turgor	Severly reduced.	Moderately reduced	Mildly reduced
5.	Feel of skin	Clammy	Dry	Thickened and doughy
6.	Mucous Membrane	Slightly moist	Dry	Parched
7.	Fontanelles	Sunken	Sunken	Sunken
8.	Eyes	Soft and Sunken	Soft and Sunken	Sunken, not soft
9.	Pulse rate	Rapid	Rapid	Moderately rapid
10.	Mental	Comatose	Lethargic	Hyperimitable
11.	Blood Pressure	Very low	Low	Moderately low

Assessment of Development : There are certain well recognised milestones of development which from the basis of assessment of development of a child. A detailed discussion of neurological and physical criteria is obviously beyond the scope of this book. Nevertheless, some of the basic facts given below will help the students in routine clinical assessment of development.

Between 4 and 6 weeks : The child ramains in prone position with the pelvis high and the knees under the abdomen, and smiles at mother. Grasp reflex is positive.

6 weeks : When suspended ventrally, the head is held momentarily in the same plane as the trunk. Tarily in the same plane as the trunk. In abdominal position it is able to turn the head if it is necessary for getting breath. Prone position pelvis high, knees no longer under abdomen and hips are extended. The child follows objects with eyes; grasp reflex negative.

12 weeks : Head is held above the plane of the trunk on ventral suspension, grasps objects momentarily when placed on palm, turns head towards the

source of sound and gurgles responsively **with** smile.

24 weeks : The child sits unsupported by hands, **rolls** from prone to supine position, and also **can** transfer objects from one hand to the **other.**

9 months : The child will pull into sitting position, **crawls** on abdomen, unsupported abdomen and it **may** be able to sit unsupported and can stand **or** biscuits.

10-11 Months : At this age the child should be able **to** stand holding on the furniture.

12-14 months : The child walks with support and **may** speak single words with meaning.

18 months : The child has learnt to walk upstairs with support, scribbles if pencil is given and is able to speak single words with meaning.

BUT YOU HAVE TO KEEP IN MIND THAT EVERY
CHILDS DEVELOPMENT IS DIFFERENT FROM THE OTHER

EXAMINATION OF THE CARDIOVASCULAR SYSTEM

A routine examination of the cardiovascular system should be always done while examining a child;–this will help avoid overlooking an acyanotic congenital heart disease, or for that matter, any lesion of the cardiovascular system. Inspection, palpation, percussion and auscultation are performed in that order.

Inspection : At the onset, look for the signs that could be attributable to a disease of the cardiovascular system, namely, impaired development squatting tachypnoea, central or peripheral cyanosis; clubbing of the fingers and / or the toes; oedema and superficial venous engorgement.

Normally the apical impulse is rarely visible. But ventricular activity will be evident if the child with thin chest wall becomes apprehensive. Abormal precordial pulsation may be visible and there may be bulging of the precordium due to cardiac enlargement. Note whether there are abnormal and excessive precordial pulsation and if there be any, whether it is due to *right* ventricular hypertrophy (occurring in the central and upper parts of the precordium) or due to *left* ventricular hypertrophy (apical impulse is accentuated and precordium is visibly lifted). Also note the position of the apical impulse, it it is visible. Look at the jugular veins, try to assess the jugular venous pressure, and make an idea of the venous pulse wave if the engorged vein is also pulsatile. No doubt this is difficult to assess in young children and also you must keep in mind these are only *hints* and no clinical *diagnosis.*

Palpation : Now start palpation; first try to locate the *apex beat.* It is in left 4th or 5th intercostal space, just outside the midclavicular line in children up to 2 years of age, on or inside the line after that age, and by about 15 years of age the apex beat is usually in the 5th space. There are normal variation to these.

First try to find out if the apex beat is more wide as usual. In this case you get a hint about the enlargement of the heart. Try to ascertain the *character* of the apex beat. It is heaving if the left ventricle has hypertrophied. In case of enlargement of the right ventricle, there will be an abnormal parasternal impulse.

Carefully note if there is any *thrill*, distinguishing it from the palpable vibrations arising from respiratory tract secretions. Find out whether it is systolic or diastolic and also the area of maximum intensity. A systolic thrill at the lower left parasternal area may be due to a *VSD*, and another at the left base may be due to either *pulmonic stenosis* or *PDA*. A systolic thrill at the base of the heart that is also palpable in the suprasternal notch may be due to *aortic stenosis.*

Examine the *radial pulse* for rate, rhythm and volume and try to detect any collapsing character. Normally the pulse rate in infants lies between 100 and 130/min; in children up to 6 years it is 100-120/min, and about 90-100 /min between 6 and 10 years of age. *Sinus arrhythmia* is a normal feature in children;–the heart rate increases on inspiration and diminishes on expiration. Compare the radial pulse of the two sides and also the femoral with the radial pulse. If the femoral pulse is delayed or weak or absent, palpate the interscapular region to detect pulsation of collateral vessels that may be present in coarctation of the aorta.

Percussion : Since the advent of radiological investigation facilities percussion of the heat has lost its value in the detection of enlargement of the heart of pericardial effusion. Still, it is more suitable in children than in adults because of thinner chest walls in children. Determine the site and extent of cardiac dullness which may be increased in cardiomegaly or pericardial effusion and diminished in emphysema of the lungs.

Auscultation : In clinical examination auscultation gives one of the best hints of heart diseases. Auscultatory signs or cardiovascular diseases in children are essentially the same as that in the adults. The heat sounds in infancy are more sharp in quality that in the adults. The second sound may be normally split in any area. A third heart sound is a *normal* phenomenon in children. Soft, ejection systolic murmurs–the 'functional' 'Velocity', or innocent' murmurs– may be normally heard in children. Such a murmur varies with posture, may disappear in the erect position, decreases on inspiration and is not associated with cardiomegaly. It disappears as the child grows. The *venous hum*–resembling a continuous or machinery murmur–may be audible at the base of the heart in the normal child. It disappears with compression of the vein and has *no pathological significance.*

Congenital heart diseases are more frequent in children than acquired ones. Of the acquired heart diseases the *commonest* after 5 years of age is rheumatic carditis. It may be associated with the *Cary Coomb murmur (soft and middiastolic)* at the apex, pericardial rub and systolic murmurs. The *commonest congenital cyanotic* heart disease in children is *Follot's tetralogy* (others being total anomalous pulmonary veinous drainage, tricuspid atresia, truncus arteriosus, transposition of the great vessels and pulmonary atresia or aortic atresia). Fallots tetralogy is pulmonary stenosis, ventricular septal defect, dextropositioned aorta with the aortic root overriding the defect and a right ventricular hypertrophy. It is characterised by central cyanosis, clubbing, systolic thrill and murmurs in the pulmonary area, single second sound Congenital *acyanotic* heart disease that may be found in children in order of decreasing frequency are VSD, ASD, PDA, coarctation of the aorta, aortic stenosis and fibroelastosis. In VSD there is a large systolic murmur at the left sternal edge. If it is a small whole the systolic murmur, is loud. A large defect effects a calm systolic murmur, in *pulmonic stenosis* and ASD there is a systolic murmur in the pulmonary area; in PDA there is a continuous machinery (Gibson's murmur) on the left sternoclavicular joint or below the left clavicle. In *aortic stenosis*, there is an ejection systolic murmur radiating to the neck and in *coarctation* of the aorta there are easily audible murmurs over the back. Murmurs due to rheumatic valvular heart diseases are less frequently encountered than the above murmurs.

Blood pressure : Blood pressure recording is an important part of examination of the cardiovascular system, but it is often neglected because of difficulties to determine it in infants and young children. While the pressure is recorded, the child should be in supine or sitting position. The width of the blood pressure cuff should be about two-thirds that of the upper arm. The pressure may be measured by the auscultatory, palpatory or flush method. In the auscultatory method, the first Korotkow sound is indicative of systolic pressure. The diastolic pressure is recorded both at muffling as well as at disappearance of the sounds as usually the former is higher and the latter lower than the true diastolic pressure. The mean of the two is taken. Sometimes the pressure in the thigh may have to be recorded, as for instance, when coarctation of the aorta is suspected. The cuff should be suitably wide, covering two-thirds of the surface area. Normally the pressure recorded from the thigh is about 20 mm Hg higher than that of the arm. In the child the arterial pressure varies with the age, height and weight and straining, excitement, coughing etc may elevate the systolic pressure by 40 to 50 mm Hg. The average blood pressure in the arm in a newborn is about 80/50 mm Hg. 85/60 mm Hg at 4 years 95/65 mm Hg at 8 years, 100/70 mm Hg at 10 years and about 110/75 mm Hg at 13 years. Many temporary variations of blood pressure occur during adolescence before the stable level of an adult is attained.

Criteria for detecting heart disease in children

Certain guidelines put forward by Nadas have proved useful to detect heart diseases in children. Nadas' criteria, as these are known, include 4 major and 5 minor criteria. At least one major or two minor criteria need to be present for the diagnosis of an organic cardiac lesion. The criteria are : –

(a) Major :
> (i) A grade 3/6 (or more) systolic murmur.
> (ii) A diastolic murmur.
> (iii) Central cyanosis.
> (iv) Congestive cardiac failure.

(b) Minor :
> (i) A systolic murmur less than grade 3/6 in intensity.
> (ii) An abnormal second heart sound.
> (iii) An abnormal electrocardiogram.
> (iv) An abnormal chest roentgenogram.
> (v) An abnormal blood pressure.

EXAMINATION OF THE RESPIRATORY SYSTEM

A complete examination of the respiratory system includes inspection, palpation, percussion and auscultation of both the anterior and posterior aspects of the chest.

Inspection : Look at the *movements* of the chest and count the respiratory rate. In a newborn the respiratory rhythm is irregular and the rate is about 40/min. *Tachypnoea* is said to be present if the rate is 60/min or more and present for at least 1 hour. *Tachypnoea* may be caused by congenital heart diseases, respiratory diseases, cerebral haemorrhage or hyperventilation caused by metabolic acidosis. In acute respiratory tract infection in children and infants very little signs are present so that respiration rate assumes the greatest value in such cases. The respiration rate should not be counted while the child is crying of feeding. The respiratory *rhythm* may be abnormal in a premature newborn infant, asphyxia just after birth, pneumonia etc. The *rhythm* normally is inspiration→expiration→ pause. In respiratory or cardiac failure, Cheyne-Stokes breathing may be seen.

Look for any obvious *deformity* of the chest. It may be pigeon shaped, funnel shaped or alar chest and rickety rosary or Harrison sulcus may be present. With the child's head placed exactly in the midline look for symmetry of the chest.

Note if there is any *intercostal* suction, which, if present, may be due to diphtheria, a foreign body impacted somewhere in the upper respiratory tract, acute laryngotracheobronchitis, asthma pneumonic etc.

Normally the *lateral* diameter of the chest is greater than the *anteroposterior* diameter in older children. If it is reversed, a long standing disease like asthma should be suspected.

Inspiratory stridor may be present with milder degrees of upper respiratory tract obstruction e.g. epiglottitis, laryngotracheitis. If the obstruction increases, the stridor becomes both inspiratory and expiratory. Respiratory distress, as occurs with severe respiratory infection produces grunting respiration. Presence of *wheeze* is indicative of smalll airways obstruction, such as asthma asthmatic bronchitis, acute bronchiolitis; mycoplasma pneumoni or foreign body etc.

Palpation : By palpating the chest only palpable rhonchi, local tenderness or subcutaneous emphysema may be detected. It is not of much value in the examination of the respiratory system in children.

Percussion : Percussion of the chest in preterm infants is of no value and *should not be done*. Gentle percussion of more mature neonates, however, may be helpful to detect pneumothorax and displacement of cardiac dullness. It should be remembered that because of thinner chest walls percussion note in infants or children is usually more resonant than that in adults. By detecting an alteration of percussion note, pleural effusion and extensive pneumothorax can be diagnosed.

Auscultation : During ausculation, breath sounds should be examined all over the chest, comparing the sounds of one side with those of the other, Normally the breath sounds are either harsh vesicular or puerile. *Crepitations*, which are usually fine may be present at lung bases signifying pneumonia, heart failure etc. *Coarse rhonchi* may be caused by upper respiratory tract infections that are conducted down the bronchial tree to the chest surface. Vocal resonance and vocal fremitus can be perceived only if the child cries. Among the added sounds a *friction rub* is liable to be easily missed during auscultation unless it is searched for all over the chest.

EXAMINATION OF THE ABDOMEN

Inspection : First inspect the stump of the *umbilical cord* and if possible examine the cut surface of the umbilical cord. One umbilical artery in place of two normally present may indicate visceral malformation. *Umbilical hernia* or infection of the umbilical stump should be looked for. Note the condition of the skin of the abdomen. The skin is shiny and tense in a distended abdomen and looks lax and wrinkled if the child has recently lost weight. Respiration in a child is mainly abdominal and loss of respiratory movement of the abdominal wall may be due to peritonitis or other intra-abdominal diseases. Look for a *visible peristalsis*. It may be present in alimentary tract obstruction, the commonest cause of which in neonates, especially males, is *congenital hypertrophic pyloric stenosis.* If the bladder is distended, if will be seen in the hypogastrium as a central round swelling. Look for engorgement of abdominal veins which may be present if there is portal hypertension.

Palpation : Palpation of the abdomen is best carried out with the patient lying supine and the examiner sitting by the side of the patient. If the child cannot be laid down palpation of the abdomen has to be done with the child sitting on the lap of the mother. First examine the *skin* by trying to pick it up between the thumb and the forefinger. Loose folds of skin indicates recent weight loss. The severity and type of dehydration, if present, can also be ascertained (see page 151). By gentle palpation look for *tenderness* and *rigidity.* Tenderness will be reflected in the facies of the child. Also find out if there is an area of rebound tenderness. Next palpate for a *pyloric swelling* that may be present in congenital hypertrophic pyloric stenosis.

Palpate the *liver*–its edge sometimes may be normally felt up to 2 cm below the costal margin. The normal liver is soft in consistency. The kidney and in about 10% cases. the *spleen* may be palpable in a *normal* infant. The spleen also becomes palpable in nutritional anaemia, congenital haemolytic anaemia, and also quite commonly in infections of all types. Palpation of the suprapubic region may reveal a *distended bladder* and if the child has not passed urine in the past 24 hours, it may be due to obstruction of the lower urinary tract. While palpating the abdomen, do not miss enlarged *mesenteric lymph nodes.* Other lumps that may be felt are–faecal masses in the descending colon, nephroblastoma (Wilm's tumour), neuroblastoma, a sausage-shaped intussusception etc. A hernia may be palpable as a soft swelling in the inguinal region and if it becomes strangulated, it will feel hard, tender and irreducible.

Percussion : Free fluid in the abdomen can be detected by percussion and shifting dullness and fluid thrill will be positive. If distension of the abdomen is present, whether it is due to gas, fluid or a solid mass can be made out by percussion.

Auscultation : Auscultation of the abdomen is done as a routine procedure for any evidence of *increased* peristalitic sounds due to *intestinal obstruction* from any cause or *diminished* peristaltic sounds due to post-diarrhoeal abdominal distension which is common in children, or due to *peritonitis.*

Finally inspect the *perineum* and see whether the anus is patent and normally positioned. If a newborn has not passed meconium within 36 hours after birth in the presence of a patent anus, intestinal obstruction might be the cause. Perform the rectal examination with the little finger. In Hirschsprung's disease, (*congenital aganglionic megacolon*) the finger is gripped all around by a norrow segment of the rectum. The genitalia should be inspected for congenital anomalies.

EXAMINATION OF THE NERVOUS SYSTEM

The conventional method of neurological examination as has been described in the chapter on Nervous System, will be readily applicable to the older child. However, it is not so in the younger children and especially the neurological examination of an infant requires a much more objective approach and as the infant or the young child is not sufficiently developed to co-operate with the examiner, assessment of intellect and behaviour is rather difficult. But with practice one can improve upon one's art of clinical examination.

First make an assessment of the *level of consciousness.* The child may be unconscious, semiconscious, drowsy, unresponsive or hyperexcitable and this may be caused by cerebral injury at birth or after that by meningitis, encephalitis, or post-epileptic states etc. Next look for disorders of *posture and movement.* In meningitis neck stiffness may be present, in poliomyelitis and nerve injury (e.g. of the brachial plexus) there will be obvious limitations of movements. Chorea, athetosis or choreo-athetotic movements, if present– may have resulted from *kernicterus* or *acute rheumatic fever.* Intention tremor may be detected when the child tries to get at an object. Also look for convulsive movements and as has been stated earlier, intermittent clenching of a fist may indicate this. Rarely *myoclonic* spasms will produce what is known as Salaam attacks– the sitting child suddenly and transiently falling forward or bowing his head.

Look for *incoordination* as the child makes some movement, and for *abnormality of gait* as he walks. It may be scissors, ataxic hemiplegic, spastic, staggering or waddling gait.

Observe the *general attitude* of the child. Letharge, irritability, tremor and exaggerated reflexes,–all may be caused by the birth injury, infections hypoglycaemia or hypoxia. When the child cries or tries to talk look for any abnormality.

If there is any *strabismus*, find out whether it is paralytic or concomitant. In concomitant strabismus the eyes maintain the same relative position in any direction of gaze. Find out which one is dominant and which is the squinting eye by alternately covering the eyes.

Test hearing by making a sound about half a metre away from the child. Normally the child will turn its head towards the source of sound.

Look af the face of the child to detect *facial palsy*. This can be easily detected when the child cries.

Next assess the muscle tone of the infant by ventral suspension, i.e. suspended by the examiner's hand under the abdomen, and note the position adopted by the infant. Tone can also be assessed by passive movements of the limbs. Persistent abnormalities of tone signify neuromuscular dysfunction.

Deep reflexes may be elicited by briskly tapping the appropriate tendon with the flexed middle finger or a small hammer. Certain *primitive reflexes* that are normally present in the infant up to 4 to 6 months of life should be routinely tested as a part of neurological examination. While testing these, the head of the infant must be kept in midline.

(i) *The Moro reflex*–It can be elicited by two methods. Ideally hold the infant supine on your right hand and support the back of the head with your left hand. Now allow the head to fall by a few centimeters. The infant responds with abduction of upper arms, and extension of the elbows and fingers followed by flexion and abduction. The reflex can also be elicited by making a sudden noise e.g. by clapping the hands. The Moro reflex, present at birth disappears by 4th or 5th month of life. It is considered abnormal if present after the 6th month. Absent or decreased Moro reflex signifies central nervous system depression; and if exaggerated, indicates cerebral irritation by any local or general metabolic cause.

(ii) *Sucking reflex*–It can be elicited by introducing a clean finger into the infant's mouth. Its absence indicates either CNS depression or a cerebral birth injury. It is normally present at birth and persists till voluntary control is achieved.

(iii) *Rooting reflex*–It can be elicited by gently caressing the cheek near the angle of the mouth,–the infant responds by turning the head towards the stimulated side and also opens the mouth and protrudes the tongue. Its absence signifies depression of the CNS. It is normally present up to 2 to 4 months of life.

(iv) *Grasp reflex*–Place a finger across the palm of the infant when the infant's fingers will flex around that finger. It is present from birth to 3rd or 4th month of life.

(v) *Asymmetrical Tonic Neck reflex*– To elicit this, rotate the head of the infant to one side with the body in supine position. Extension of the arm of the same side and flexion of the knee of the opposite side is the normal response. It disappears normally by the 4th month of life, and persistence even after the 6th month is found in spastic cerebral palsy.

(vi) *Glabella tap*–Gently tap the glabella, both the eyelids of the neonate will blink.

The plantar reflex is normally extensor in most children up to 1 year of age and the change into adult type occurs after that. In suspected cases of meningeal or nerve irritation, try to elicit the Kernig's and Brudzinski's signs. The former is a late sign of meningitis in children and neck rigidity is more reliable.

Appendix to Chapter IV

(A) *Causes of Convulsion in Children*

It has been estimated that during the first five years of life, about 5% of all children suffer from convulsions. Convulsions that are characteristic of major epilepsy are rare in the new born because of low electrical activity of the cerebral cortex. The commoner causes of convulsions include :

(a) Newborn period

1. Cerebral defects of malformation. 2. Birth asphyxia. 3. Intracranial haemorrhage e.g. because of difficult forceps delivery. 4. Hypoglycaemia. 5. Hypocalcaemia, tetany. 6. Other electrolyts are not in normal range e.g. hyponatraemia. 7. Infections due to group B-Streptococcus, Staphylococcus, Gram-negative bacteria and pyogenic

meningitis. 8. Neonatal tetanus. 9. Kernicterus 10. Rare metabolix syndromes e.g. pytidoxine dependency, Phenylketonuria.

(b) After newborn period

1. Pyrexia, Benign febrile convulsions. 2. Breath-holding convulsions. 3. Epilepsy, infantile spasms. 4. Syncope. 5. Cerebral trauma. 6. Acute infantile hemiplegia. 7. Hypertension, haemolytio-uraemic syndrome (HUS), Disseminated intravascular coagulation 8. Sickle cell crisis. 9. Infections, toxic shock, Kawasaki disease. 10. Metabolic condition-hypoglycaemia, dehydration, head stroke Di-George-syndrome Reye-syndrome, Phenylketonurie etc. 11. Migraine 13. Drugs poisons.

B. Causes of Diarrhoea in Children

Frequent pasage of loose watery stools is known as diarrhoea and diarrhoea associated with vomiting with or without pyrexia is due to gastroenteritis. Peak incidence of diarrhoea in children occur between 6 and 9 months, the common causes include—

(a) *Infective*

1. Viral : Rotavirus infection is the commonest cause of diarrhoea and Astrovirus, Norwalk, Calcivirus etc may. also cause it.

2. Bacterial :

(i) Enteropathogenic and enteroinvasive E coli. (ii) Enterotoxigenic E coli (iii) Vibrio cholerae. (iv) Klebsiella. (v) Shigella. (vi) Campylobacter. (vii) Yersinia. (viii) Salmonella. (ix) Clostridium difficile.

3. Parasitic :

(i) Giardia Lambila, (ii) Entamoeba histolytica, (iii) Balantidium coli, (iv) Trichuris trichiura, (v) Strongyloides, (vi) Ankylostoma etc.

4. Mycotic : (i) Candida albicans.

(b) *Non-infective*

1. Allergy to cow's milk protein. 2. Irritable bowel

syndrome. 3. Congenital megacolon (in neonates). 4. Congenital lactase deficiency. 5. Cystic fibrosis. 6. Short bowel syndrome. 7. Sprue (tropical and non-tropical). 8. Intestinal lymphangiectasia. 9. Congenital chloridorrhoea. 10. Acrodermatitis enteropathica.

(C) *The APGAR Scoring System*

The Apgar scoring system was devised by Virginia Apgar for the assessment of vital functions of the newborn. The newborn infant is examined at 1 and 5 minutes after birth. Based on the scoring system of the five signs the ideal score is 10. If it is less than 7, the vital functions are significantly depressed and immediate resuscitative measures are to be instituted. The Apgar score is also indicative of prognosis for survival, particularly of preterm infants. The scoring system is based on the table given below :–

Score → Vital Functions ↓	0	1	2
Skin colour :	Pale or bule	Body pink but hands and feet blue.	Completely pink.
Heart rate :	Nil	< 100	> 100
Respiration :	Absent	Slow and irregular	Strong cry
Muscle tone :	Limp	Some flexion of the limbs	Active movement
Reflex irritability :	No response	Grimace only	Cry, cough or sneeze

(d) *Normal Electrocardiogram in Children*

Interpretation of the electrocardiogram of children reuires a basic knowledge of the normal patterns. These vary so much from normal patterns of adults that a normal electrocardiogram is liable to be misdiagnosed as abnormal and vice versa. Before trying to learn the normal electrocardiographic pattern of children, students should recapitulate their knowledge of foetal circulation and of the changes in foetal circulation that occur after birth.

In the foetal life, the lungs remain in collapsed state and the resistance of the pulmonary circulation is of the same magnitude as that of the systemic circulation. As a result of this, the right ventricle of the foetus is of the same size as that of the left ventricle. After birth, as the neonate starts respiring, the lungs expand with air–new vessels open up and vessels that are already patent becomes enlarged–the *pulmonary resistance falls*. Simultaneously, since the low resistance placental circulation is cut off, the *systemic resistance increases*. The sum total effect of this is that with increased load on it, the left ventricle gradually increases in size and because of decreased load, the right ventricle becomes relatively small. These haemodynamic changes occur over a period of *hours to days* and are reflected in the electrocardiogram. The essential features of the normal electrocardiogram in infants are :–

(1)   In the normal full term infant the precordial lead QRS complexes exhibit right ventricular predominance. In leads VI, V3 and V4 the R waves are tall and S waves are shallow, hence the R/S ratio is more than unity. In V6 there is an rS complex (the r wave is small and S wave is deep).

(2)   The QRS axis lies between 120^0 and 140^0 (which is abnormal right axis deviation in an adult).

(3)   T waves that are upright in leads VI, aVL and V6 just after birth, become negative in matters of hours to days.

(4)   After few days, the T waves again become upright in leads VI, V2, aVF and V6 and inverted in VI and aVR.

(5)   The electrocardiogram of premature bebies is usually the same as of full term infants, but some may show generalised low voltage complexes.

(6)   As the infant matures, the picture of right ventricular predominance is gradually replaced by the normal adult pattern of left ventricular predominance (rS in lead VI and q RS in V6).

(7)   T waves are normally inverted in leads VI to V3 and may remain so in leads VI, V3 and V4 till adolescence.

————

THE SKIN AND ITS APPENDAGES

CHAPTER 5

A careful examination of the skin and its appendages enables the clinician to detect the different varieties of cutaneous diseases and not infrequently provides valuable clues to the diagnosis of internal maladies.

To arrive at a correct dermatological diagnosis, the usual sequence of history taking and clinical examination are to be followed up by a proper utilisation of laboratory and instrumental aids.

HISTORY

Although it is true that some skin lesions can be diagnosed on sight with a high degree of confidence, a detailed history is indispensable for evaluation of the aetiological factors and effective planning of management. In addition to a general history, the following special points should be investigated.

Cutaneous symptoms : The subjective symtoms consist of pruritus, burning, tingling pain and numbness.

Pruritus : Itching or pruritus is defind as an unpleasant cutaneous sensation which provokes the desire to rub of scaratch the skin. It is by far the most common cutaneous symptom. It may be more prickling or tingling or its severity may be of intolerable intensity. It may be spasmodic or contineous. Pruritus may be a symptom of a cutaneous disorder of it may be a manifestation of some underlying systemic diseases.

Pruritus may be a prominent feature of some *dermatological* disorders, especially :

E.C.D (II)–34

Scabies. Dermatitis herpetiformis.

Atopic dermatitis. Lichen simplex.

Milaria Pediculosis.

Insect bites. Urticaria

Lichen planus Dematophytosis (ringworm).

Failure to detect an overt or covert cutaneous cause necessitates consideration of, and evaluation for a possible underlying systemic illness. The *systemic causes* or generalized pruritus include :

(a) Matabolic and endocrine : Hyperthyroidism. Diabetes mellitus Carcinoid syndrome.

(b) Renal : Chronic renal failure.

(c) Hepatic : Obstructive biliary disease.

(d) Malignancy : Lymphoma. Leukaemia Multiple myeloma, Abdominal cancers.

(e) Haematologic : Polycythaemia vera.

(f) Drugs : Opiates.

(g) Psychic : Delusion of parasitosis.

Other symtoms :

Pain–It may be deep boring or burning as in herpes zoster, throbbing, as in furuncles, carbuncles or cellulitis,

Numbness–Loss of sensation in skin lesions (together with thickening of superficial nerves) is pathognomonic or leprosy.

Dryness–It is frequent complaint of elderly people.

Seborrhoea–Excessive greasiness of the skin may be physiological. It is said to be one of the features of Parkinsonism, especially the postencephalitic type.

About the skin lesions, the following points should be investigated.

Onset of the skin lesions

Site of onset

Character of the lesions: the patient should be asked to

describe the original lesions and any subsequent change in their appearance or character.

Extension : Rate of enlargement and pattern of extension should be noted.

Topical therapy : Self-treatment is universal. If often changes the appearance of the lesions.

Possible role of psychological factors should be thoroughly explored as they are of importance in initiating, aggrovating or perpetuating a wide variety of dermatoses.

EXAMINATION OF THE SKIN

The patient should always be examined in a good light, preferably daylight. Ideally, the entire skin should be examined routinely and the following points should be noted.

I. The form of the individual lesions.

II. The pattern of the lesions and their spatial relationship to each other.

III. The distribution of the lesion over the body.

1. *The Individual Lesions*

Macules. A macule is a circumscribed area of change in normal skin colour without elevation or depression of the surface. Macules may very widely in shape and size. They result from hyperpigmentation or hypopigmentation or permanent vascular abnormalities of the skin (e.g. capillary haemangioma) and transient capillary dilatation (*erythema*).

Telangiectases are permanent dilatations of blood capillaries that may or may not disappear with the pressure of a glass slide *(Diascopy)*. They are non-pulsatile, fine, bright red lines or netlike patterns on the skin. They are usually macular. Telangiectases may be found in (i) hereditary haemorrhagic telangiectasia (ii) SLE, (iii) DLE, (iv) dermatomyositis, (v) scleroderma, (vi) radiodermatitis, (vii) xeroderma pigmentosum and (viii) rosacea.

Haemorrhages into the skin occur in various conditions. Extravasated RBCs and pigments of haemoglobin breakdown result in macular lesions. If *less than 1 mm* in diameter, they are referred to as *petechiae; from 2 mm to 5 mm in diameter, as purpuric spots*; and if larger as *ecchymoses*. Petechiae and purpuric spots do not disappear when they are pressed on by a glass slide (diascopy). Disappearance of the redness in diascopy suggests erythema due to *vascular dilatation*. Some important examples of macular lesions :

(i)   Disseminated small, erythematous : Drug rash, syphilis

(ii) Confluent, large, erythematous : Capillary haemangioma.

(iii) Brown, small : Junctional naevus. Freckles.

(iv) Cafe-au-lait : Neurofibromatosis. Albright syndrome.

(v)   Hypomelanotic : Vitiligo, Leprosy, Tuberous sclerosis, Post-inflammatory leukoderma.

(vi) Scaly : Pityriasis versicolor. Pityriasis rosea.

Papules : A papule is a circumscribed, solid elevated lesion, by convention under 1 cm in diameter. Papules may result from localised hyperplasia of cellular components of the dermis or the epidermis; from localised cellular infiltrates in the dermis, or from metabolic deposits. A careful observation of the colour and other morphologic characteristics of the papules is important Examples—

(i)   Red, scaly   : Psoriasis

(ii) Disseminated,
      coppery red   : Syphilis

(iii) Itchy, shiny,
      violaceous   : Lichen planus

(iv) Yellow, soft   : Xanthoma

(v) Brownish or
    black   : Melanoma, pigmented
                           basal cell carcinoma.

(iv) Dome shaped,
     pearly white and
     umbilicated   : Molluscum contagiosum.

All erythematous papules should be examined by *diascopy* (firmly pressing a glass slide over the skin lesion) as a yellow brown colour or appears in the papules found in lupus vulgaris, sarcoidosis and lymphoma (*apple jelly nodule*).

Nodules– A nodule is a palpable, circumscribed, solid, round or ellipsoidal lesion. A nodule can be located in the epidermis or extend into the dermis or subcutaneous tissue. A nodule may result from benign or malignant proliferations of the epidermal squamous cells or melanocytes as in basal cell carcinoma, viral wart, melanocytic naevi and malignant melanoma.

Nodules in the dermis or subcuits result from inflammation, neoplasm or metabolic deposits.

Example : Tuberculosis, late syphilis, deep mycosis, xanthomatosis, lymphoma, metastatic lesions, erythema and foreign body reactions.

A *gumma* is a granulomatous, subcutaneous lesion of tertiary syphilis.

Plaques– A plaque is an elevation above the skin surface that occupies a relatively large surface area. It may result from confluence of papules as in psoriasis and *lichen planus*. Plaques of *discoid lupus erythematosus* show atrophy and erythema. Yellowish plaques are found in *necrobiosis lipoidica diabeticorum* (NLD) and *xanthomatosis*.

Wheals– A wheal is an evanescent flat-topped elevation of the skin. There is a rapid shifting of lesions from the involved to the uninvolved skin of the adjacent area. These lesions are pale red in colour and varies widely in size: Wheals are the *characteristic lesions of urticarical reactions*. Production of wheals in response to stroking of the skin : (*Darier's sign*) is pathognomonic of *urticaria pigmentosa* also known as *systemic mastocytosis*).

Vesicles and Bullae– A vesicle is a circumscribed elevated lesion containing fluid. A vesicle with a diameter greater than 5 mm is a *bulla*. Vesicles and bullae result from a cleavage at various levels of skin. The cleavage may be within the epidermis (i.e. untraepidermal) or at the dermo-epidermal interface (i.e. subepidermal). Vesiculobullous lesions result from a wide variety of causes including physical and chemical trauma, allergy, infection and genetic factors. Some example of vesiculobullous diseases :

(i)   Trauma   :   Friction blisters,
                         Bullae due to irritant chemicals.
(ii)   Infections   :   Impetigo, herpes simplex, herpes
                         zoster, Pariola, varicella.
(iii) Allergy   :   Eczema, Contact dermatitis
(iv)   Immunological (damage mediated by autoanti-
                         bodies) :
                         Pemphigus, Pemphigoid
                         Herpes gestations
                         Dematitis herpetiformis.
(v)   Genetic   :   Epidermolysis bullosa.

Pustules : A pustule is a circumscribed elevation of the skin containing purulent exudates. They may be follicular in location or may be unrelated to hair follicles. Pustules are found in sycosis barbae, acne vulgaris and impetigo. A *furuncle* is a deep, necrotising form of folliculitis. Furuncles may coalesce to form a *carbuncle*.

Atrophy– Atrophy of the epidermis result in a thin

semitransparent skin. It may be a manifestation of (i) the normal aging process or may occur in diseases like (ii) discoid lupus erythematosus. Dermal atrophy results in a depression of the skin which may be found in (iii) striae of pregnancy or (iv) Cushing syndrome, (v) scleroderma, (vi) dermatomyositis and (vii) chronic rediodermatitis.

Sclerosis– It is a circumscribed or diffuse hardening or induration of the skin. This may be found in *scleroderma* or *chronic lymphoedema*. These may prevent the pinching of a fold of skin over the dorsal aspect of the toes or fingers;–this is *Stemmer's sign*.

Scaling– Visible desquamation of the skin is evident as scaling. Fine, greasy scaling is found in *pityriasis capitis* (dandruff). Silvery, mica like, lamellated scales, which on removal leaves multiple bleeding points (*Auspitz's sign*) is characteristic of *psoriasis*. Scaling is also a feature of *pityriasis rosea* or *secondary syphilitic lesions* of skin. *Exfoliative dermatitis* is characterised by a generalised inflammatory erythema with scaling. It may occur as a sequela to various cutaneous diseases, as a cutaneous manifestation of internal diseases, particularly lymphomas, or it may be caused by various drugs.

Comedones (blackheads). These are horny keratotic lesions filling the orifices of pilosebaceous follicles. These lesions are characteristic of acne vulgaris.

In addition to the above, skin lesions may be in the form of excoriations, ulcers, fissures, crusts, scars etc.

II. *Shape and Arrangement of Lesions*

The shape of individual lesions and their arrangement in relation to each other is often of diagnostic importance. Three distinctive patterns are :

(A) Linear, (B) Annular, and (c) Grouped.

(A) *Linear lesions*–Many dermatoses occur in linear forms. The linearity of the lesions may be determined by:

   (a)   Liner contact with exogenous agents; as in contact allergic dermatitis.

   (b)   *Koebner's phenomenon* : Appearance of new lesions by non-specific trauma, over previously uninvolved skin Linear lesions by this mechanism occur in psoriasis, lichen planus, vitiligo and plane warts.

   (c)   Development anomaly; as in epidermal naevi.

   (d)   Course of vessels; sporotrichosis, thrombophlebitis.

   (B)   *Annular lesions*–Annular or arciform appearance of lesions may result from coalescence of individual lesions or by central clearing of a circular lesion. This type of lesion may be observed in– Dermatophytosis, urticaria, erythema multiforme, psoriasis, leprosy, sarcoidosis and lupus erythematosus.

   (C)   *Grouped lesions*–Papules, wheals, nodules or vesicles may be arranged in groups. This type of arrangement may be encountered in : Herpes simplex and herpes zoster, Urticaria, Dermatitis, herpetiformis, Insect bites, Plane or common warts.

III. *Distribution of lesions*

Distribution of cutaneous lesions over the body may be local, regional or generalized. Distribution pattern of lesions in some dermatoses are so characteristic as to help in diagnosis. For example, *psoriasis* affects the extensor surfaces, particularly the knees, elbows, sacral areas, and also the scalp; atopic dermatitis mainly involves the flexural regions. The factors influencing the distribution of dermatoses include :

(a) Exposure to exogenous agents–*contact dermatitis.*

(b) Exposure to ultraviolet light–lesions occurring over the areas exposed normally to sunlight, e.g. *SLE, DLE, porphyria.*

(c) Regional variation in distribution of appendages–*acne vulgaris*, a disease of the pilosebaceous follicles occur over areas where these are more abundant i.e. face, chest or back. *Hydradenitis suppurativa*, an inflammatory disease of the apocrine glands, occurs on apocrine gland bearing areas like axillae or groins.

(d) Regional variation of surface environment of skin : candidiasis occurs over areas of warm moist skin like genital and submammary regions.

(e) Dermatomal pattern : Herpes zoster is a classical example.

INSTRUMENTAL AND LABORATORY AIDS IN DERMATOLOGIC DIAGNOSIS

1. *Wood's light*–A source of ultraviolet light from which all visible light has been excluded by Wood's filter (made of nickel oxide) is an useful tool in the diagnosis of certain skin diseases. Some of its important uses are :

(i) Detection of scalp ringworm by demonstration of fluorescence of hairs.

(ii) Demonstration of prophyrins in prophyria.

(iii) Confirmation of pigmentary disorders (e.g. in epiloia).

2. *Patch testing*–With the help of standard preparations of different allergens accurate assessment of contact sensitivity is done.

3. *Microscopic examination of scales, serum crusts, hairs and nails.* Gram's staining and cultures of serum and

exudates should be done if the lesions are suspected to be of bacterial or yeast origin.

Scales, hairs and nails are examined for *mycelia* of fungi if dermatophytosis is suspected. The material is first cleared with 10% potassium hydroxide and warmed gently. Fungal cultures are done in Sabouraud's medium.

Scrapings from the base of vesicles or bullae are stained with Giemsa's stain and examined microscopically. Presence of *acantholytic cells* indicates *pemphigus* group of disorders. Giant multinucleated cells are found in *herpes simplex, herpes zoster* and *varicella*. When cells from the base of the vesicles are microscopically examined; this is known as *Tzanck test*.

4. *Laboratory diagnosis of scabies*—Clinically diagnosed by pruritus and presence of burrows (linear or serpiginous elevations of skin in the form of a ridge, 0.5-1 cm in length) and papulovesicles in characteristic distribution over the flexural aspects of wrists, interdigital areas, buttocks, and umbilical region. Scrapings are done from burrows of papulovesicles and examined microscopically for demonstrating mites, ova or faeces of the parasites.

5. *Dark ground illumination test*–Serum from ulcers over the genitalia are examined for demonstration of treponems.

6. *Serologic test for syphilis*–The reagin tests like WR or VDRL are done. Specific tests like TPI, TPHA or FTA-ABS are confirmatory.

7. *Skin biopsy*– It is an easy and safe procedure. May be done by punch or excision. H & E and special stains are done as required.

8. *Immunofluorescence tests*–Most valuable in the diagnosis of connective tissue diseases and bullous dermatoses. Classical example is the *lupus band test* that confirms the diagnosis of SLE.

THE HAIR

Normal human hairs can be classified according to cyclical phases of growth. *Anagen hairs* are growing hairs, *catagen hairs* are those undergoing transition from growing to the resting phase and *telogen hairs* are resting hairs that fall off after some three months.

Human hair is also typed as *lanugo, vellus, or terminal hair. Lanugo hair* is the fine hair present on the body of the foetus. It is replaced by vellus and terminal hair. Vellus hairs are fine, soft, usually light coloured, and characteristically seen in children's faces. *Terminal hairs* are coarse, thick and dark.

Hair performs no vital functions in man, yet it has immense psychological importance, Any deviation from the culturally acceptable amount of hair may be a cause of great distress for the affected individual. The principal disorders related to hair are *hypertrichosis, hirsutism* and *alopecia.*

Hypertrichosis– It is defined as the growth of hair which in any given site is coarser, longer of more profuse that is normal for the age, sex and race of the individual. While dealing with such a case, the following causes should be kept in mind :

1. Congenital : Congenital hypertrichosis lanuginosa, a rare disorder characterised by persistence and extensive growth of lanugo hair since birth. An acquired, excessive growth of lanugo hairs in the later ages is said to be reliable cutaneous marker of internal malignancy.

2. Circumscribed developmental defect : Hypertrichosis with melanocytic naevi.

3. Inherited metabolic disorders : Porphyria
                                    Hurler's syndrome.

4.   Endocrine causes   :   Hypothyroidism

			Hyperthyroidism Head injuries (possible pi tuitary and diencephalic mechanism).
5.	Drug induced	:	Diphenyl hydantoin Corticosteriods Streptomycin Diazoxide Penicillamine Psoralens.
6.	Other conditions	:	Severe malnutrition Anorexia nervosa Dermatomyositis.

Hirsutism–It is the growth in the female of coarse terminal hairs in partially or wholly adult male sexual pattern. The most common type is found on the upper lip only, with some noticeable hairs in the preauricular area. Hirsutism is an androgen dependent syndrome and it may be a sign of virilism.

Causes :

Adrenal

Congenital adrenal hyperplasia.
Cushing's syndrome
Virilizing adrenal tumours.

Ovarian

Polycystic ovary (possible the commonest cause of idiopathic hirsutism, 92% in one recent study) Virilizing tumours.

Pituitary

Acromegaly.

Drugs

Androgens
Phenytoin

Minoxidil

Glucocoticosteroils

Diazoxide.

Idiopathic

No clear cut endocrinological factors can be implicated.

Others :   May be associated with obesity, anorexia nervosa or rarely genetic disorders.

Alopecia–Loss of scalp hair is a frequently encountered complaint. It may occur as a circumscribed patchy area of hair loss, or the process of hair loss may be more diffuse, uniform and continuous.

Alopecia may be

Chronic diffuse alopecia– In which the following possible factors should be assessed :

1. *Androgenic alopecia* (also known as male type alopecia or common baldness) – It is a genetically determined androgen dependent condition showing itself during the late twenties or early thirties by gradual loss of hair, chiefly from the vertex and frontotemporal regions. The anterior hair line recedes so that the forehead becomes high. In women, this type of alopecia occurs mostly at the vertex or diffusely.

2. *Telogen effluvium*— It is characterised by loss of telogen (resting) hairs following some stresses, e.g. (i) prolonged pyrexia, (ii) prolonged and difficult child birth (iii) surgical shock and severe blood loss, (iv) stopping contraceptive pills, (v) myocardial infarction, (vi) CVA, (vii) bereavement or other psychological stress etc. While normally some 50 to 100 hairs fall off daily, in telogen effuvium about 300–400 are lost per day.

Anagen effluvium is the fall of growing hairs leading to diffuse alopecia and may occur following exporsure to cytotoxics or in thallium poisoning (vide 4 below).

3. *Nutritional and metabolic*–Kwashiorkor marasums and iron deficiency anaemia may result in diffuse hair loss.

4. *Drugs*–Anticoagulants, antimitotics and antithyroid drugs (thiouracil) carbimazole) are important causes of diffuse alopecia. Hypervitaminosis A is also associated with diffuse hair loss.

5. *Severe chronic illnesses*– Carcinomas, lymphomas and impaired hepatic function as in cirrhosis may result in this type of alopecia.

6. *Idiopathic*–Some individuals, particularly women of 30 to 50 years of age may present with diffuse alopecia without any apparent cause. The possibility of androgenic alopecia should be kept in mind.

(B) *Circumscribed alopecia*– Circumscribed loss of hair may be (i) scarring (non-cicatricial) or (ii) scarring (cicatricial, associated with destruction of hair follicles). (i) *Alopecia areata* is the commonest cause of non-scarring circumscribed alopecia. It is characterised by rapid, circumscribed loss of hair in patches, chiefly affecting the scalp, the beard area, the eyebrows and the eyelashes. There is no subjective symptom and the condition is frequently self limiting and heals spontaneously. *Trauma*, in the form of traction, friction of hair pulling may result in localized area of non-scarring alopecia. A common example is the *neonatal occipital alopecia* occurring due to friction of pillow. *Trichotillomania* or hair pulling tics may occur in emotionally unstable children and result in patches of non-scarring alopecia.

(ii) Cicatricial or scarring alopecia is the end result of a variety of pathological processes which cause destruction of hair follicles. Some important causes of scarring alopecia are :

1. Developmental   Aplasia cutis
                               Epidermal naevi
2. Traumatic   Burns
                               Radiodermatitis
                               Mechanical injuries.
3. Infections   Dermatophytosis, Lupus
                               vulgaris, Leprosy Syphilis,
                               Folliculitis, Curbuncles etc.
4. Neoplastic   Basal cell carcinoma
                               Metastatic carcinoma.
5. Dermatoses of miscellaneous pathogenesis :
                               Lichen planus
                               DLE
                               Scleroderma.

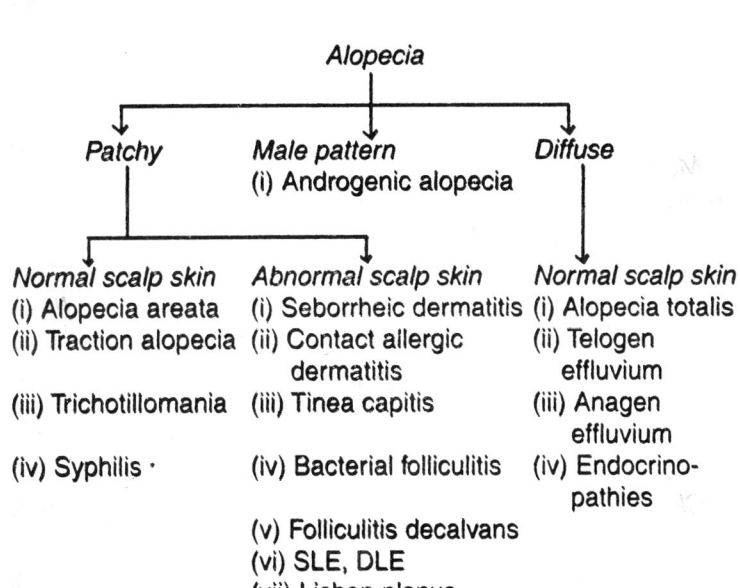

Alopecia

Patchy   *Male pattern*   *Diffuse*
                  (i) Androgenic alopecia

Normal scalp skin	*Abnormal scalp skin*	*Normal scalp skin*
(i) Alopecia areata	(i) Seborrheic dermatitis	(i) Alopecia totalis
(ii) Traction alopecia	(ii) Contact allergic dermatitis	(ii) Telogen effluvium
(iii) Trichotillomania	(iii) Tinea capitis	(iii) Anagen effluvium
(iv) Syphilis ·	(iv) Bacterial folliculitis	(iv) Endocrino-pathies
	(v) Folliculitis decalvans	
	(vi) SLE, DLE	
	(vii) Lichen planus	
	(viii) Morphoea	
	(ix) Lupus vulgaris	
	(x) Radiotherapy.	

The Nails

Various dermatoses and systemic diseases are associated with nail changes. Some of the important nail disorders are described here.

Pitted nails–Small pinpoint depressions in an otherwise normal nail are found in psoriasis, alopecia areata, eczema, and ringworm involving the hand. Though onycholysis is the most characteristic nail lesion of psoriasis, it is usually belived that the presence of 20 or more nail pits in an individual is suggestive of psoriasis. Besides, nail pits may be the earliest of all manifestations of psoriasis.

Beaus' Lines– These are transverse furrows on the nail plate that progress distally as the nail grows. They result from temporary arrest of function of the nail matrix and may be caused by measles, acute febrile illnesses, local trauma etc.

Half and Half nails–These show the proximal half of the nail white and the distal half red or pink. These are said to be associated with renal failure.

Mee's lines–Single or multiple white transverse bands on the nail, described as a sign of inorganic arsenic poisoing

Muehrcke's lines–These show narrow, white transverse bands occurring in pairs. They are associated with hypoalbuminaemia. They may disappear when serum albumin level is normalized.

Terry's nail–The distal 1 to 2 mm of the nail is of normal pink colour; the rest of the nail is white. These changes have been noted in patients with cirrhosis.

Clubbing and koilonychia have been dealt with elsewhere.

Onycholysis–It is the spontaneous, painless separation of the nail from its bed, usuallly beginning at the free margin and progressing proximally. It may occur without any apparent cause, or it may be due to psoriasis, fungal infection, eczema or local trauma. Impaired peripheral circulation may also be responsible. Rarely photo-onycholysis may occur after therapy with photosensitizing drugs like demethyl chlortetracycline any exposure to sunlight.

Azure half moons are found in Wilson's disease. *Red half moons* are associated with chronic renal failure.

The yellow nail syndrome is characterised by slowly growing pale or greenish yellow nails that are thin, overcurved in their long axis, easily shed and slowly replaced. Often associated with lymphoedema and different thoracic disorders e.g. chronic bronchitis, bronchiectasis and pleural effusion.

Splinter haemorrhage in the nail bed is caused by local trauma, infective endocarditis trichinosis (60-70% of cases) and rheumatoid arthritis. These may also be found in psoriasis or fungal infections. These are also rarely associated with uninfected mitral stenosis, peptic ulcer, systemic hypertension and malignant neoplasms.

N. B.–*Onychia* means inflammation of the nails and is usually septic in origin but may be due to trauma, tuberculosis or syphilis etc; leuconychia totalis is a rare congenital abnormality where the whole nail plate is white; *pachyonychia congenita* is a condition of thick and hard nails that are firmly attached to the nail beds; and very rarely nails may be *absent in congenital ectodermal dysplasias,*

Erythema Nodosum

This is a nodular erythematous eruption affecting the extensor aspects of the legs, less commonly the thighs and forearms. Females in their third and fourth decades of life are predominantly affected. The erythematous nodules are tender and warm. run an acute course and regresses in about 3 to 6 weeks showing bruise-like colour changes without scarring or atrophy. Causes of erythema nodosum include : Streptococcal infection, tuberculosis, and drugs like sulphonamides and bromide. Less common causes are lymphogranuloma venereum. Yersinia infections, ulcerative colitis, Crohn's disase, leukaemia, Hodgkin's disease and administration of oral contraceptives.

Erythema nodosum leprosum is an acute, widespread eruptiori occurring in patients with leprosy at or near the lepromatous end of the spectrum. It is clinically and histologically distinct from the erythema nodosum described above.

APPENDIX TO CHAPTER V

(A) Patients presenting with a rash in the butterfly distribution is a common diagnostic problem. The possible causes are—(i) *Light hypersensitivity* e.g. due to *albinism, porphyria, pellagra* or *drug induced* e.g. barbiturates, phenothiazines, sulfa drugs etc. (ii) *SLE*, (iii) *Acne rosacea,* (iv) *Tuberous sclerosis–adenoma sebaceum, (v) Scleroderma. (vi) Chronic discoid lupus erythematosus* etc.

(B) A periorbital bluish red oedema,–heliotrope' erythema is the dermatological hall mark of *Dermatomyositis* and may be associated with scaling erythema of sun exposed areas in the butterfly distribution.

(C) Inflammatory scaling of the whole skin surface (exfoliative erythrodema) may be caused by (i) psoriasis, (ii) allergy to drugs e.g. golds antimalarials, sulphonamides, phenylbutazone etc. (iii) severe contact dermatitis, (iv) atopic dermatitis, (v) seborrheic dermatitis, (vi) underlying lymphomas, (vii) Sezary syndrome (viii) mycosis fungoides etc. The last two belong to the group of T cell malignancies.

(D) Palmar and solar hyperkertosis is quite common and may be due to (i) barefooted walking, (ii) secondary syphilis, (iii) Rieter's disease–keratoderma, "blenorrhagica, (iv) hypovitaminosis A, (v) chronic inorganic arsenic poisoning, (vi) underlying visceral malignancy, genetic etc.

INDEX

NB–I and II respectively indicate Part I and Part II of the book.